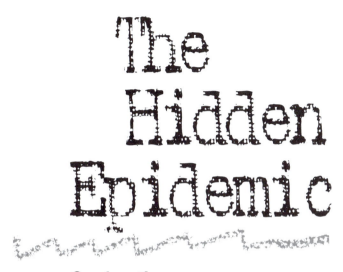

The Hidden Epidemic

Confronting
Sexually Transmitted Diseases

Thomas R. Eng and William T. Butler, *Editors*

Committee on Prevention and Control of
Sexually Transmitted Diseases

INSTITUTE OF MEDICINE

Division of Health Promotion and Disease Prevention

NATIONAL ACADEMY PRESS
Washington, D.C.   1997

National Academy Press • 2101 Constitution Avenue, N.W. • Washington, D.C. 20418

NOTICE: The project that is the subject of this report was approved by the Governing Board of the National Research Council, whose members are drawn from the councils of the National Academy of Sciences, the National Academy of Engineering, and the Institute of Medicine. The members of the committee responsible for this report were chosen for their special competencies and with regard for appropriate balance.

This report has been reviewed by a group other than the authors according to procedures approved by a Report Review Committee consisting of members of the National Academy of Sciences, the National Academy of Engineering, and the Institute of Medicine.

The Institute of Medicine was chartered in 1970 by the National Academy of Sciences to enlist distinguished members of the appropriate professions in the examination of policy matters pertaining to the health of the public. In this, the Institute acts under both the Academy's 1863 congressional charter responsibility to be an adviser to the federal government and its own initiative in identifying issues of medical care, research, and education. Dr. Kenneth I. Shine is president of the Institute of Medicine.

Funding for this project was provided by Centers for Disease Control and Prevention, Glaxo Wellcome, Inc., The Henry J. Kaiser Family Foundation, National Institute of Allergy and Infectious Diseases, NIH Office of Research on Women's Health, Ortho-McNeil Pharmaceutical, and SmithKline Beecham Pharmaceuticals. Any opinions, findings, conclusions, or recommendations expressed in this publication are those of the author(s) and do not necessarily reflect the view of the organization or agencies that provide support for the project.

Additional copies of this report are available from the National Academy Press, 2101 Constitution Avenue, N.W., Box 285, Washington, D.C. 20055. Call 800-624-6242 (or 202-334-3313 in the Washington metropolitan area), or visit the NAP on-line bookstore at **http://www.nap.edu.**

Library of Congress Cataloging-in-Publication Data

Institute of Medicine (U.S.). Committee on Prevention and Control of
    Sexually Transmitted Diseases.
        The hidden epidemic : confronting sexually transmitted diseases /
    Thomas R. Eng and William T. Butler, editors ; Committee on
    Prevention and Control of Sexually Transmitted Diseases, Institute
    of Medicine, Division of Health Promotion and Disease Prevention.
            p.   cm.
        Includes bibliographical references and index.
        ISBN 0-309-05495-8
        1. Sexually transmitted diseases—United States. I. Eng, Thomas
    R. II. Butler, William T. III. Title.
        [DMLM: 1. Sexually Transmitted Diseases—prevention & control—
    United States. 2. Sexually Transmitted Diseases—epidemiology—
    United States. 3. Health Policy—United States WC 144 I59 1997]
    RA644.V4I495   1997
    614.5'47'0973—dc21
    DNLM/DLC
    for Library of Congress   97-4218
                                                                         CIP

RA644
.V4
I495
1997

Printed in the United States of America.

The serpent has been a symbol of long life, healing, and knowledge among almost all cultures and religions since the beginning of recorded history. The image adopted as a logotype by the Institute of Medicine is based on a relief carving from ancient Greece, now held by the Staalichemuseen in Berlin.

COMMITTEE ON PREVENTION AND CONTROL OF SEXUALLY TRANSMITTED DISEASES

Catherine M. Wilfert, Professor of Pediatrics and Microbiology, Department of Pediatrics, Division of Infectious Diseases, Duke University Medical Center, Durham, North Carolina

Jonathan M. Zenilman,[†] Associate Professor of Medicine, Division of Infectious Diseases, Johns Hopkins University School of Medicine, Baltimore, Maryland

Staff

Thomas R. Eng, Senior Program Officer
Leslie M. Hardy, Senior Program Officer (through July 1995)
Jennifer K. Holliday, Project Assistant
Marissa Weinberger Fuller, Research Associate
Michael A. Stoto, Director, Division of Health Promotion and Disease Prevention

---

[†]Served through September 1995.

Preface

This report focuses on the hidden epidemic of sexually transmitted diseases (STDs) in the United States: the reasons why it has not been controlled, and what we, as a nation, need to do differently to confront this problem. The main objective of this report is to educate health professionals, policymakers, and the public regarding the truths and consequences of STDs in the United States. This report is also a call for a bold national effort to prevent these diseases.

Through this report, we hope to improve awareness and knowledge regarding the scope and impact of STDs and demonstrate why all Americans should be concerned about these diseases. At a minimum, we hope to ignite open discussion in both private and public arenas regarding STDs and their prevention. We believe that encouraging open discussion around STD prevention will eventually lead to greater understanding, closer cooperation, improved STD-related services, and lower rates of STDs in the United States.

In the course of this study, the committee was impressed with the fact that STDs are extremely complex health problems without easy solutions. Discussions regarding effective prevention of STDs can easily become emotionally and politically charged because many people have strongly held views about sexuality. Some readers will not agree with all the committee's findings or recommendations. Undoubtedly, there are excellent ideas and solutions that the committee has not addressed. The important thing, however, is that ideas are shared, discussed openly, and lead to positive action. We strongly encourage all readers to view potential solutions to the STD epidemic with an open mind and to consider all the possibilities for confronting these diseases and their burden on individuals and our country. Not to do so would be a tragedy of enormous consequences.

Thomas R. Eng, *Study Director*
William T. Butler, *Committee Chair*
Washington, D.C. 1997

Acknowledgments

This report represents the collaborative efforts of many organizations and individuals, without whom this study would not have been possible. The committee extends its warm thanks to the organizations and individuals mentioned below.

The staff of the following organizations and agencies provided critical advice and data in preparing this report: Advocates for Youth (Kent Klindera), the Agency for Health Care Policy and Research (David Atkins and Carolyn DiGuiseppi), Alan Guttmacher Institute (Pat Donovan, Jackie Forrest, Lisa Kaeser, and Dave Landry), the American Academy of Pediatrics (Victor Strasburger), the American Cancer Society, the American Medical Association, the American Social Health Association (Peggy Clarke, Joan Cates, and Nikki Vagnes), Association of Reproductive Health Professionals, Association of State and Territorial Health Officers, Center for Media and Public Affairs (Dan Amundson), the Centers for Disease Control and Prevention (Susan DeLisle, Shahul Ebrahim, Alan Friedlob, Joel Greenspan, Robert Johnson, William Kassler, William Levine, Judy Lipshutz, Frank Mahoney, Eric Mast, John Miles, John Moran, Craig Shapiro, Jack Spencer, Mike St. Louis, Cathleen Walsh, Judy Wasserheit, and Gary West), East Coast Migrant Health Project (Oscar Gomez), The Henry J. Kaiser Family Foundation (Suzanne Delbanco), National Association of Nurse Practitioners in Reproductive Health (Susan Wysocki), the National Cancer Institute, the National Center for Farm Worker Health (Bobbi Ryder), the National Commission on Correctional Health Care (Ed Harrison), the National Institutes of Health, Ogilvy Adams & Rinehart, Planned Parenthood Federation of America, Sexuality Information and Education Council of the U.S. (SIECUS)

(Carolyn Patierno), State Family Planning Administrators (Lynn Peterson), and the World Health Organization (Antonio Gerbase and Kevin O'Reilly). The following colleagues also provided valuable assistance to the committee: Jane Brown, Margaret Chesney, Jim Kahn, Laura Koutsky, and Richard Rothenberg.

The following persons generously shared their knowledge with the committee through their active participation in the committee workshops: Sevgi Aral, Cornelius Baker, Bobbi Baron, Marie-Claude Boily, Stanley Borg, Robert Bragonier, Allan Brandt, Ward Cates Jr., William Darrow, Gray Davis, Frank Beadle de Palomo, Caswell Evans, Jonathan Freedman, Mindy Thompson Fullilove, Carol Glaser, James Goedert, James Haughton, William Kassler, Paul Kimsey, Janet Kirkpartick, Edward Laumann, William Levine, Steve Morin, Kevin O'Reilly, Frank Plummer, John Potterat, Gary Richwald, Tracy Rodriguez, Philip Rosenberg, Alfred Saah, Marilyn Keane Schuyler, Stanley Shapiro, Sten Vermund, and Maria Wawer.

The directors and staff of the following facilities and programs graciously hosted the committee during its site visits to Atlanta and Chicago. In Atlanta: The Center for Black Women's Wellness; DeKalb County Board of Health (Stuart Brown); Emory/Grady Teen Services Program; Fulton County Health Department STD Clinic (Ruby Lewis-Hardy and Pradnya Tambe); Georgia Department of Human Resources, Epidemiology and Prevention Branch (Jack Kirby and Mark Schrader); Grady Memorial Hospital Family Planning Program; Kaiser Permanente, Prevention and Practice Analysis Department; SisterLove, Inc., West Central Health District (Dee Cantrell); West End Medical Centers, Inc.; and Women's AIDS Project. In Chicago: Austin Community Academy Teen Health Clinic; Blue Cross Blue Shield of Illinois; Chicago Department of Public Health (John Wilhelm); Chicago STD/HIV Prevention Program (Romina Kee and Lisa Krull); Cook County Hospital HIV Primary Care Center, Smart Start Program, Women and Children HIV Program; Erie Family Health Center; Illinois Department of Public Health (John Lumpkin and Charlie Rabins); Night Ministry; Ounce of Prevention Fund, Toward Teen Health Program, Orr Adolescent Health Center; Planned Parenthood of Chicago; Stop AIDS Chicago; Vida Sida; and West Town Neighborhood Health Center, Young Adult Clinic.

The following individuals participated in the planning meeting for the study: Charles Carpenter (chair), Peggy Clarke, Jim Curran, Mary Faye Dark, Gray Davis, Patsy Fleming, Helene Gayle, H. Hunter Handsfield, Maurice Hilleman, Penny Hitchcock, Mark Hounshell, James Kahn, Lawrence Lewin, Heather Miller, Constance Nathanson, Geoff Nichol, Michael Osterholm, Nancy Padian, Thomas Quinn, Mark Smith, P. Frederick Sparling, Beth Unger, Judy Wasserheit, Roy Widdus, and Zeda Rosenberg.

Of particular note, the following individuals directly contributed to the report by drafting commissioned papers in their areas of expertise. A review paper on the relationship between substance use and STDs by John Beltrami, Linda Wright-DeAguero, Mindy Thompson Fullilove, and Brian Edlin was critical to the report, and sections of their paper were replicated in the discussion of substance use and STDs. A paper by Jeffrey Kelly provided important background for the drafting of sections regarding behavioral interventions in STD prevention. Marie-Claude Boily's important work on modeling the impact of STDs on HIV transmission is included as an appendix. In addition, Joanna Siegel's major review of the economic costs of STDs was the primary basis for the committee's cost estimates and is also included in the appendix of the report.

Numerous staff at IOM, the National Research Council, and the National Academy Press (NAP) contributed to the development, production, and dissemination of this report. Leslie Hardy served as study director during its first year; Marissa Fuller organized the committee's site visits and provided research assistance; Jennifer Holliday provided comprehensive administrative support; Mike Stoto, Karen Hein, and Ken Shine provided valuable advice and direction; Mona Brinegar handled the financial accounting of the study; Mike Edington provided editorial assistance; Claudia Carl and Janice Mehler coordinated the report review process; and Dan Quinn and Molly Galvin coordinated press activities. NAP staff included Dawn Eichenlaub (book production); Barbara Kline Pope and Brooke O'Donnell (marketing); Estelle Miller (page layout); Francesca Moghari (cover design); Terrence Randell (Internet listing); and Sally Stanfield (editor). In addition to IOM staff, we are grateful to Andrea Posner for her numerous valuable editorial contributions, to Caroline McEuen for copy-editing, to Kim Greene for assistance with the survey of managed care organizations, to Linnea Eng for proofreading, and to Mary Fielder and Ron Nelson for their research assistance.

The following agencies and organizations and key staff generously provided funding and generated support within their institutions for this study: the Centers for Disease Control and Prevention (Jim Curran [now with Emory University], Helene Gayle, Jack Spencer, and Judy Wasserheit), Glaxo Wellcome, Inc. (Gray Davis), the Henry J. Kaiser Family Foundation (Suzanne Delbanco and Mark Smith), the National Institute of Allergy and Infectious Diseases of the National Institutes of Health (NIH) (Penny Hitchcock), the Office of Research on Women's Health of NIH (Vivian Pinn and Anne Bavier), Ortho-McNeil Pharmaceutical (James Kahn), and SmithKline Beecham Pharmaceuticals (Vincent Ahonkai, Paul Blake, and Geoff Nichol). Their willingness to sponsor a study on the prevention and control of sexually transmitted diseases is no small commitment, given the sensitive and controversial nature of this public health issue. Their encouragement and support are gratefully acknowledged.

Contents

APPENDIXES

The
Hidden
Epidemic

Executive Summary

Sexually transmitted diseases (STDs) are hidden epidemics of tremendous health and economic consequence in the United States. They are hidden from public view because many Americans are reluctant to address sexual health issues in an open way and because of the biological and social factors associated with these diseases. In addition, the scope, impact, and consequences of STDs are underrecognized by the public and health care professionals.

Of the top ten most frequently reported diseases in 1995 in the United States, five are STDs. Rates of curable STDs in the United States are the highest in the developed world and are higher than in some developing regions. Approximately 12 million new cases of STDs, 3 million of them among teenagers, occur annually. The committee estimates that the annual direct and indirect costs of selected major STDs are approximately $10 billion or, if sexually transmitted HIV infections are included, $17 billion. Along with the human suffering associated with STDs, this cost is shared by all Americans through higher health care costs and taxes. STDs represent a growing threat to the nation's health and national action is urgently needed.

The term "STD" denotes the more than 25 infectious organisms that are transmitted through sexual activity, along with the dozens of clinical syndromes that they cause. The spectrum of health consequences ranges from mild acute illness to serious long-term complications such as cervical, liver, and other cancers and reproductive health problems. Women and infants bear a disproportionate burden of STD-associated complications. A variety of women's health problems, including infertility, ectopic pregnancy, and chronic pelvic pain, result from unrecognized or untreated STDs. From 1973 through 1992, more than 150,000 U.S. women died of causes associated with STDs (including HIV infec-

1

tion) and their complications. Women are particularly vulnerable to STDs because they are more biologically susceptible to certain sexually transmitted infections than men and are more likely to have asymptomatic infections that commonly result in delayed diagnosis and treatment. Active infection with STDs during pregnancy may result in a range of serious health problems among infected infants, including severe central nervous system damage and death. Adolescents are at greatest risk of STDs because they frequently have unprotected sexual intercourse, are biologically more susceptible to infection, and are likely to have social problems that significantly increase their risk.

STDs are difficult public health problems because of the "hidden" nature of these diseases. The sociocultural taboos related to sexuality are a barrier to STD prevention efforts on a number of levels. Effective STD prevention efforts also are hampered by biological characteristics of STDs, societal problems, unbalanced mass media messages, lack of awareness, fragmentation of STD-related services, inadequate training of health care professionals, inadequate health insurance coverage and access to services, and insufficient investment in STD prevention.

Although the barriers to STD prevention are formidable, STDs can be prevented by intervening at multiple points with behavioral, biomedical, and structural interventions on both individual and community levels. These and other effective interventions, however, are not being fully implemented or utilized. Because STDs are complex diseases that are associated with a variety of social issues and involve a wide spectrum of stakeholders in the community, a collaborative, multifaceted approach to STD prevention is essential.

Conclusions and Recommendations

The committee concludes that an effective national system for STD prevention currently does not exist and, as a result, STDs are a severe health burden in the United States. Many components of the system need to be redesigned and improved through innovative approaches and closer collaborations. In addition, programs that address important gaps in the current fragmented system of services have not yet been designed and implemented. The committee's recommendations are outlined below and presented in complete detail in Chapter 6.

In formulating a strategy to prevent STDs, the committee developed the following vision statement to guide its deliberations.

Vision

An effective system of services and information that supports individuals, families, and communities in preventing STDs, including HIV infection, and ensures comprehensive, high-quality STD-related health services for all persons.

This vision and the committee's proposed model for improving STD prevention are founded on a multifaceted approach to prevention, shared responsibility and active participation by individuals and the community, coordination of related programs, and adequate resources and support for implementation.

To realize this vision, the committee recommends that:

- **An effective national system for STD prevention be established in the United States.**

The committee envisions a system based on national policy, coordinated at all levels, and composed of local, state, and national prevention programs. A national system is essential because STDs are a threat to the nation's health, because many interventions are most effectively or efficiently developed and implemented at the national level, and because STDs do not recognize geographic borders.

To establish a national system for STD prevention, the committee recommends four major strategies for public and private sector policymakers at the local, state, and national levels:

1. Overcome barriers to adoption of healthy sexual behaviors.
2. Develop strong leadership, strengthen investment, and improve information systems for STD prevention.
3. Design and implement essential STD-related services in innovative ways for adolescents and underserved populations.
4. Ensure access to and quality of essential clinical services for STDs.

Before describing the recommended tactics for these four strategies, the committee makes the following recommendations regarding two important concepts that need to be incorporated into a national strategy to prevent STDs: the impact of STDs on HIV transmission and the impact of STDs on cancer.

- **Improved prevention of STDs should be an essential component of a national strategy for preventing sexually transmitted HIV infection.**
- **Government agencies and private organizations concerned with cancer prevention should support STD prevention activities as an important strategy for prevention of STD-related cancers.**

Strategy 1: Overcome barriers to adoption of healthy sexual behaviors.

Barriers to effective STD prevention efforts include biological, social, and structural factors. One of the primary obstacles is this country's reluctance to openly confront issues regarding sexuality and STDs. Failure to acknowledge and discuss sexuality impedes STD education programs, open communication between parents and their children and between sex partners, balanced messages from mass media, education and counseling activities of clinicians, community activism for STDs, and behavioral research.

Catalyzing Change Through Open Discussion and Promoting Awareness and Balanced Mass Media Messages

A new social norm of healthy sexual behavior should be the basis for long-term prevention of STDs. This is because in one way or another all interventions to prevent STDs are partly dependent on, and must be integrated with, healthy behaviors. In order for societal norms regarding sexual behavior to change, open discussion of and access to information regarding sexual behaviors, their health consequences, and methods for protecting against STDs must occur. Therefore, the committee believes that a significant national campaign to foster social change toward a new norm of healthy sexual behavior in the United States is necessary. An independent entity is needed to promote a social norm of healthy sexual behavior because, based on experience with past initiatives, limitations on government agencies regarding public education programs related to sexuality are particularly problematic.

Lack of awareness regarding STDs and misperception of individual risk and consequences are major barriers to healthy sexual behavior, especially among adolescents and young adults. Lack of open communication and information regarding sexuality and STDs fosters misperceptions and may actually encourage high-risk sexual behaviors. Increased awareness regarding STDs should result in increased individual motivation to prevent STDs and should improve the detection and management of STDs by clinicians. A national campaign to increase public and health care provider awareness of STDs requires active participation of both private and public agencies and organizations to succeed.

Despite their current lack of involvement in promoting healthy sexual behaviors, the mass media can be extremely powerful allies in efforts to prevent STDs by increasing knowledge and changing behavior. Mass media messages that promote healthy sexual behaviors will facilitate needed changes in social norms regarding sexual behaviors because mass media help define these norms. Children and adolescents are particularly exposed and susceptible to explicit and implicit messages in such media. Many adolescents are not receiving appropriate information regarding STDs and sexual behavior from their parents or other sources. Therefore, mass media companies should disseminate information regarding STDs and healthy sexual behaviors, including delaying sexual intercourse and using condoms, with a special focus on reaching adolescents and young adults. Comprehensive public health messages regarding STDs, including HIV infection; sexual abuse; and unintended pregnancy are essential.

With respect to the above issues, the committee makes the following recommendations:

• **An independent, long-term, national Campaign should be established to (a) serve as a catalyst for social change toward a new norm of healthy sexual behavior in the United States; (b) support and implement a long-term national initiative to increase knowledge and awareness of STDs and promote ways to prevent them; and (c) develop a standing committee to function as an expert resource and to develop guidelines and resources for incorporating messages regarding STDs and healthy sexual behaviors into all forms of mass media.[1]**

• **Television, radio, print, music, and other mass media companies should accept advertisements and sponsor public service messages that promote condom use and other means of protecting against STDs and unintended pregnancy, including delaying sexual intercourse.**

Improving Professional Skills in Sexual Health Issues

It is important that clinicians and other professionals develop knowledge and awareness of sexual health issues and become comfortable discussing them. This will enable clinicians to utilize clinical opportunities to effectively counsel patients regarding healthy sexual behaviors, and therefore improve clinical care for STDs. Communicating effectively with patients regarding sexual health is a particularly critical skill for clinicians and other professionals, but most are not adequately trained in communication and counseling skills.

With respect to the above issues, the committee makes the following recommendation:

• **The Health Resources and Services Administration, health professional schools and associations, and schools and associations for training educators should support comprehensive sexuality training for health care professionals, educators, and researchers in order to increase their comfort working with sexual health issues and to increase their effectiveness in sexual behavior counseling.**

Supporting Sexual Health Behavior Research

Population-based surveys and studies of STD-related health behaviors are

---

[1]This recommendation condenses three recommendations presented in Chapter 6.

critical for monitoring population trends in health behaviors, developing effective interventions, and evaluating program effectiveness. Such research, however, has been severely criticized by some policymakers and interest groups. This committee, while recognizing the sincere concerns expressed, strongly believes that research regarding STD-related health behaviors, especially among adolescents, is critical to STD prevention. Federal funding and support for sexual health behavior research is essential. The committee found no evidence that asking questions regarding sexual activity increases sexual activity among survey respondents. Restrictions on collecting behavioral information from adolescents would seriously jeopardize behavioral research and the ability to prevent high-risk behaviors among adolescents. The committee also believes that the objectivity and integrity of the peer-review process for scientific research should be protected.

With respect to the above issues, the committee makes the following recommendation:

• **The National Institutes of Health and other federal agencies should continue to support research on health behaviors, including sexual behaviors, and their relationship to STDs.**

Strategy 2: Develop strong leadership, strengthen investment, and improve information systems for STD prevention.

Developing Leadership and Catalyzing Partnerships

To build an effective national system, highly visible and strong leadership and support are needed from both the public and private sectors, and especially from elected officials. Among public agencies, the Department of Health and Human Services, especially the Centers for Disease Control and Prevention (CDC), and state and local health departments have critical leadership roles. The public sector must continue to play a major role in preventing STDs, but does not have the resources or the organizational reach to fully implement a national system of STD-related services. The private sector must therefore take more responsibility.

The barriers to an effective national system for STD prevention are found in government, private sector organizations, and political factors and social norms. Overcoming these barriers is a challenge that requires the active participation of all levels of government, the private health care sector, businesses, labor leaders, the mass media, schools, and many community-based organizations. In developing and implementing a national system for STD prevention, it is important that stakeholders be involved in all steps of the process; however, a formal mechanism for collaboration among agencies and organizations does not exist. Therefore, a neutral forum is needed to maximize the range of participants and to catalyze the collaborative process.

With respect to the above issues, the committee makes the following recommendations:

• **Private sector organizations and clinicians should assume more leadership and responsibility for STD prevention.**
• **Federal, state, and local governments, through the leadership of their respective health agencies, should ensure that all persons have access to comprehensive, high-quality STD-related services.[2]**
• **An independent, long-term national Roundtable should be established as a neutral forum for public and private sector agencies and organizations to collaboratively develop and implement a comprehensive system of STD-related services in the United States.**

Strengthening Investment

To establish an effective system of STD prevention, a substantially greater investment from both the public and private sectors is needed. The current national public investment in STD prevention is not commensurate with the health and economic costs of STDs. The committee estimates that only $1 is invested in STD prevention for every $43 spent on the STD-associated costs every year. Similarly, only $1 is invested in biomedical and clinical research for every $94 in STD-related costs. For every $1 spent on early detection and treatment of chlamydial infection and gonorrhea, $12 in associated costs could be saved. Investing in preventive services and research will avert substantial human suffering and save billions of dollars in treatment costs and lost productivity. Additional funding for STD prevention should come from local, state, and federal governments and from the private sector. Private health plans, in particular, need to increase support for STD-related services that benefit their enrolled population, and ultimately benefit the health plan's financial status. In addition, because STDs are emerging infections and a global public health problem, the United States has a national interest in preventing STDs worldwide. Despite the problems in the current system of categorical funding for STDs, moving to a system of block grants for STDs would have a devastating impact on STD prevention because STDs will fare poorly in competing with other more visible and "acceptable" health conditions for funding.

With respect to the above issues, the committee makes the following recommendations:

---

[2]This recommendation condenses three recommendations presented in Chapter 6.

- Federal, state, and local elected officials should provide additional funding for STD prevention.
- The CDC should retain and immediately redesign categorical funding for STD programs.
- The federal government, through the Department of Health and Human Services and the U.S. Agency for International Development, and international organizations, such as the World Health Organization and the World Bank, should provide resources and technical assistance to global efforts to prevent STDs.

Improving Surveillance and Other Information Systems

National surveillance and other information systems for STDs are important in monitoring and evaluating a national system for prevention. Data from these information systems are critical to long-term program planning as well as to day-to-day management of programs. The current surveillance system needs enhancement because it does not give accurate estimates of disease incidence. This is because not all persons with STDs seek medical care and because many clinical encounters with health care professionals, especially in private sector settings, are not reported. It is critical that a systematic, comprehensive evaluation of the national surveillance system be conducted to describe the attributes of the system and to provide guidance for future improvements. STD surveillance systems should include and link information from public sector, community-based, and private health care professionals. Special emphasis should be placed on educating clinicians about reporting and on collaborating with and collecting data from private sector providers, including health plans.

With respect to the above issues, the committee makes the following recommendations:

- The CDC should lead a coordinated national effort to improve the surveillance of STDs and their associated complications and to improve the monitoring of STD prevention program effectiveness.
- Federal, state, and local STD programs should encourage and provide technical assistance to employers and other purchasers of health care (including Medicaid programs), managed care organizations and other health plans, and other health care professionals to develop and utilize information systems that effectively integrate preventive services performance data with community health status indicators and STD program data.
- STD-related performance measures should be included in the Health Plan Employer Data Information Set (HEDIS) and other health services performance measures to improve quality-assurance monitoring of STDs.

Strategy 3: Design and implement essential STD-related services in innovative ways for adolescents and under-served populations.

Adolescents and underserved populations require special emphasis in an effective national system for STD prevention because they are at high risk for STDs and they do not have adequate access to STD-related services. Innovative methods for delivering STD-related services to such populations should immediately be designed and implemented because these groups are difficult to reach through traditional clinical settings and approaches.

Focusing on Prevention

A national strategy for STDs should emphasize prevention because averting illness is desirable, many STDs are incurable, and STD-related complications may be irreversible. Effective prevention programs are usually the result of extensive research and evaluation and continuous quality improvement. They should be regularly modified based on the epidemiology of STDs and continuous evaluation of programs. Prevention-related research allows program managers and policymakers to maximize the effectiveness of interventions and available resources. Areas of prevention-related research that should be emphasized include determinants of sexual behavior and sustained behavior change; determinants of initiation of sexual intercourse among adolescents; influence of social and other community-related factors on risk of STDs; interventions to improve condom use and reduce high-risk behaviors; effectiveness of sexual risk behavior assessment and counseling; biomedical interventions that do not rely primarily on individual behavior, such as vaccines; female-controlled prevention methods; cost-effectiveness of interventions; methods for preventing STDs among disenfranchised populations; interventions for preventing STDs among persons of all sexual orientations; and methods to assess prevention program effectiveness.

With respect to the above issues, the committee makes the following recommendations:

• **The National Institutes of Health and the CDC should continue to support and expand both basic and applied research in STD prevention.**
• **The National Institutes of Health, the Food and Drug Administration, and pharmaceutical, biotechnology, and medical device companies should collaboratively develop effective female-controlled methods for preventing STDs.**

Focusing on Adolescents

Although many of the severe health consequences of STDs manifest themselves among adults, these complications usually result from infections acquired or health behaviors initiated during adolescence. By the twelfth grade, nearly 70 percent of adolescents have had sexual intercourse, and approximately one-quarter of all students have had sex with four or more partners. Therefore, a national strategy to prevent STDs needs to focus on adolescents. The committee believes that adolescents should be strongly encouraged to delay sexual intercourse until they are emotionally mature enough to take responsibility for this activity. However, most individuals will initiate sexual intercourse during adolescence, and they should have access to information and instruction regarding STDs (including HIV infection) and unintended pregnancy and methods for preventing them.

Many school-based programs and mass media campaigns are effective in improving knowledge regarding STDs and in promoting healthy sexual behaviors, and these two interventions should be major components of an STD prevention strategy. The committee believes that there is strong scientific evidence in support of school-based programs for STD prevention, that adolescence is the critical period for adopting healthy behaviors, and that schools are one of the few venues available to reach adolescents. Given the high rates of sexual intercourse among adolescents and the significant barriers that hinder the ability of adolescents to purchase and use condoms, condoms should be available in schools as part of a comprehensive STD prevention program. There is no evidence that condom availability or school-based programs for sexuality or STD education promote sexual activity.

STD-related clinical services for adolescents, including hepatitis B immunization, should be expanded through school and student health clinics, because adolescents are less likely than adults to have health insurance and they infrequently use regular health care facilities. Adolescents who are not enrolled in school also need access to clinical services. Because confidentiality is a major concern for adolescents, they should be able to consent to STD-related services without parental knowledge.

With respect to the above issues, the committee makes the following recommendations:

- **A major part of a national strategy to prevent STDs should focus on adolescents, and interventions should begin** *before* **sexual activity is initiated, which may be before adolescence is reached. Interventions should focus on preventing the establishment of high-risk sexual behaviors.**
- **All health plans and health care providers should implement policies in compliance with state laws to ensure confidentiality of STD- and family-planning-related services provided to adolescents and other individuals.**
- **All school districts in the United States should ensure that schools**

provide essential, age-appropriate STD-related services, including health education, access to condoms, and readily accessible and available clinical services, such as school-based clinical services, to prevent STDs.

• All health plans, clinicians, and publicly sponsored health clinics should provide or arrange for hepatitis B immunizations for their infant, adolescent, and adult patients according to the Advisory Committee on Immunization Practices (ACIP) guidelines. Given the difficulty in reaching adolescents in health care settings, public health officials should ensure that adolescents who are not immunized in health care settings are immunized through school-based or other community programs.

Establishing New Venues for Interventions

Although services for disenfranchised groups, including substance users, sex workers, the homeless, prisoners, and migrant workers, do not have popular support, these populations represent reservoirs of infection for the entire community. Innovative methods and alternate venues for intervention are needed because these groups are difficult to reach through traditional health care settings. Nontraditional venues for delivering STD-related services, such as prisons, drug treatment clinics, the streets, and other sites where high-risk persons gather, are appropriate sites for preventive services. Health departments should establish linkages with programs that serve populations at high risk for STDs, and government agencies should coordinate their various STD-related programs, because the lack of coordination and unevenness of services have resulted in critical gaps in service coverage. To contain persisting epidemics of STDs among disenfranchised persons, new biomedical, epidemiological, and behavioral tools should be developed collaboratively by the public and private sector.

With respect to the above issues, the committee makes the following recommendations:

• Federal, state, and local agencies should focus on reducing STDs among disenfranchised populations (e.g., substance users, persons in detention facilities, sex workers, the homeless, migrant workers).

• Prisons and other detention facilities should provide comprehensive STD-related services, including STD prevention counseling and education, screening, diagnosis and treatment, partner notification and treatment, and methods for reducing unprotected sexual intercourse and drug use among prisoners.

• The National Institutes of Health, the Food and Drug Administration, and the CDC should work with pharmaceutical and biotechnology companies to develop improved STD diagnostic tools (e.g., rapid saliva and urine tests) that are suitable for use in nontraditional health care settings (e.g., prisons, mobile clinics, the streets).

Strategy 4: Ensure access to and quality of essential clinical services for STDs.

Both public and private sector clinical services for STDs are currently fragmented, inadequate, and, sometimes of poor quality. This situation leads to coverage gaps, inadequate access to services, and ineffective clinical care.

Ensuring Access to Services in the Community

Access to services is facilitated by expanding the availability of STD-related services through primary care and by coordinating services at the local level. Universal and timely access to curative and preventive services are supported by eliminating financial barriers to obtaining health services, minimizing other barriers, ensuring that patients are not stigmatized, and ensuring that services are culturally appropriate. Given the broad spectrum of risk groups, access to STD-related services in multiple settings—including private sector clinics, family planning clinics, prenatal clinics, adolescent and school-based clinics, HIV clinics, community health centers, and other settings not traditionally targeted by STD programs—is important. STD-related services need to be incorporated into primary care because primary care fosters ongoing relationships between the clinician and the individual, increasing the likelihood of effective preventive interventions and early detection of STDs. In addition, incorporating STD-related services into primary care may increase access to and improve quality of STD-related care.

Each community has responsibility for ensuring universal access to comprehensive STD-related services. However, because communities differ widely in their health needs and capacity to support a system of STD-related services, the organization of community STD-related services should be tailored to local needs and conditions. Depending on local situations, health departments should incorporate STD-related services into public and private primary health care services. Depending on epidemiologic patterns, health insurance coverage, population density, and other community characteristics, they may continue to support dedicated public STD clinics, or may shift such services to community-based clinics or the private sector.

With respect to the above issues, the committee makes the following recommendations:

• **Comprehensive STD-related services should be incorporated into primary care, including reproductive health services.**
• **Local health departments, with the assistance of the state health department and in consultation with the community, should determine how to provide high-quality, comprehensive STD-related clinical services that meet federal and state quality standards most effectively in their communities.**

Improving Dedicated Public STD Clinics

There is wide variation in the quality, scope, accessibility, and availability of services provided by dedicated public STD clinics, and these clinics need significant improvement. Many local health departments operate dedicated public STD clinics that are isolated from other public health and clinical services and for which quality monitoring and assessment have not been priorities. The committee supports incorporating STD-related services in primary care settings, but it also believes that dedicated public STD clinics should continue to be an important component of STD prevention. In some situations these clinics are the primary providers of STD-related services for the uninsured and provide an important focus for STD prevention in the community. In all cases, health departments operating dedicated public STD clinics should ensure that these clinics collaborate with community-based health clinics (including family planning clinics and school-based programs), university and hospital medical centers, and private sector health care professionals to improve access and quality of care. Standards to maintain access to confidential services and to monitor quality should be developed for STD-related services provided by public STD clinics, health plans, and public-private sector arrangements.

With respect to the above issues, the committee makes the following recommendations:

• **Based upon local conditions and health department determination, dedicated public STD clinics should continue to function as a "safety net" provider of STD-related services for uninsured and disenfranchised persons and for those who prefer to obtain care from such clinics.**
• **The CDC, in collaboration with state and local health departments, should ensure that services provided by dedicated public STD clinics are of high quality.**
• **Health professional schools, including schools of medicine, nursing, and physician assistants, should partner with a local health department for purposes of STD clinic staffing, management, and professional training.**

Involving Health Plans and Purchasers of Health Care

The committee believes that if certain concerns are adequately addressed, there is substantial potential for managed care to improve the quality of and access to STD-related services. Compared with other health plans, the structure and resources of most managed care organizations allow for improved coordination and integration of care, accountability of services, incentives to provide preventive services, and monitoring of service quality. However, the current performance of managed care in STD prevention has not yet lived up to its potential. With very few exceptions, STDs are not high priorities among health plans, and few are involved in activities to prevent STDs in the larger community beyond plan members. Managed care organizations and other health plans should take more responsibility for providing STD prevention services, both among plan members and in the community in which they operate. By supporting such activities among plan members and in the community, significant health care costs associated with serious complications of STDs will be averted; health plan members will be less likely to be exposed to infected partners or to acquire reinfections; and long-term complications of STDs will be prevented among current and future plan members in the community. Employers, government agencies, and other purchasers of health care services are vital to ensuring that health plans provide comprehensive, high-quality STD-related services. Most local health departments have not developed billing arrangements with health plans; since most public sector providers are not in managed care networks, their services are considered to be "out of plan" and not reimbursable.

With respect to the above issues, the committee makes the following recommendations:

• **Health plans should provide for or cover comprehensive STD-related services, including screening, diagnosis and treatment, and counseling regarding high-risk behavior for plan members *and their sex partners*, regardless of the partners' insurance status.**
• **Federal, state, and local health agencies should educate employers, Medicaid programs, and other purchasers of health care regarding the broad scope and impact of STDs and the effectiveness of preventive services for STDs.**
• **Health plans, including managed care organizations, should develop collaborative agreements with local public health agencies to coordinate STD-related services, including payment for STD-related services provided to plan enrollees by public sector providers, including public STD clinics.**

Improving Training and Education of Health Care Professionals

Well-trained primary care clinicians are essential for effective STD diagnosis and treatment. The current system of clinical training for health care professionals, however, is inadequate in preparing clinicians to effectively manage patients with STDs. Inadequate professional training contributes to the widespread tendency of clinicians to oversimplify and underestimate the importance of STDs. Familiarity with population-based health promotion and disease prevention techniques, skills in evidence-based clinical decision making, and patient communication skills are all essential for every clinician. STD training programs should be expanded at the primary care level to improve clinician skills in both public and private settings to effectively prevent, diagnose, and treat patients with

STDs. Other factors that influence a clinician's ability to provide comprehensive services, including practice format constraints, also need to be addressed.

With respect to the above issues, the committee makes the following recommendation:

- **The training of primary care providers should be improved by focusing on core clinical competencies, expanding training opportunities, gaining additional federal support, and monitoring and improving STD-related education.[3]**

Improving Clinical Management of STDs

Major components of effective clinical management of STDs include screening, diagnosis and treatment, risk reduction counseling and education, identification and treatment of partners, and access to quality laboratory services for STDs. Screening allows for the detection of infected persons who would otherwise remain undetected, develop complications of STDs, and transmit the infection to their sex partners. Screening for STDs is cost-effective and sometimes cost-saving. Some screening programs, however, such as mandatory premarital testing for syphilis, are not cost-effective and contribute little to STD prevention. Therefore, screening should be appropriately focused and should be based on surveillance data and knowledge of the populations or prevalence of STDs. Screening programs for STDs such as chlamydial infection need to be expanded, because such programs can dramatically reduce rates of STD-related complications. Family planning clinics, prenatal clinics, and other settings where obstetric or gynecological care is available should screen and treat women and their partners for STDs.

With respect to the above issues, the committee makes the following recommendations:

- **All primary care providers, including managed care organizations and other health plans, should implement the recommendations of the U.S. Preventive Services Task Force and the CDC regarding clinical screening and management of STDs.**
- **States that still have laws requiring premarital syphilis testing as a condition for marriage licenses should repeal these laws.**

National treatment guidelines for STDs help promote appropriate therapy for STDs. However, because there is limited awareness of and compliance with these guidelines, especially among private sector health care professionals, such guide-

---

[3]This recommendation condenses a detailed recommendation presented in Chapter 6.

lines should be more widely disseminated. Single-dose therapy for bacterial STDs is important in preventing STDs because it averts the problems of ineffective treatment associated with the failure of infected individuals to return for subsequent treatment or to take multiple doses of drugs.

With respect to the above issues, the committee makes the following recommendations:

* **All clinicians should follow STD treatment guidelines recommended by the CDC and national medical professional organizations.**
* **Single-dose therapy for bacterial and other curable STDs should be available and reimbursable in all clinical settings where STD-related clinical care is routinely provided to populations in which treatment compliance or follow-up are problems.**

Risk reduction counseling and education of patients during routine clinical encounters and during evaluations for potential STDs is an important component of clinical management. Focused counseling in both specialized and general clinical settings has substantial potential for changing STD-related behaviors, particularly for adolescents and other high-risk groups. Major barriers that hinder clinicians from providing counseling that need to be addressed include inadequate training in counseling, lack of time allocated for counseling, and lack of reimbursement for such services.

With respect to the above issues, the committee makes the following recommendation:

* **All health care professionals should counsel their patients during routine and other appropriate clinical encounters regarding the risk of STDs and methods for preventing high-risk behaviors. Counseling for STDs, including HIV infection, should be reimbursed without copayments or other financial disincentives by Medicaid programs, managed care organizations, and other health plans.**

Current methods of partner notification are inefficient and extremely resource-intensive and should be redesigned. The optimal combination of activities that are most effective in reaching partners at risk for STDs will vary depending on the local epidemiology of STDs, available staff and other resources, and the spectrum of local health care professionals providing STD-related care. STD programs need to develop new strategies and techniques for community outreach in partnership with other professionals rather than relying solely on public sector staff.

With respect to the above issues, the committee makes the following recommendation:

• **State and local health departments, with the assistance of the CDC, should redesign current partner notification activities for curable STDs in public health clinics to improve outreach, mobilize public health staff in new ways, and enlist support from community groups or other programs that provide services to high-risk populations.**

Partner diagnosis and treatment should be provided as part of standard STD-related care, regardless of the clinical setting. The committee believes that health plans and clinicians have an ethical and public health obligation to ensure that sex partners of infected patients are appropriately identified, screened, and treated, regardless of health insurance status. This belief is based on the concept that health plans have a responsibility to improve the health of the communities from which they draw their revenue and that treating partners is in both the short- and long-term interest of the health plan. By treating partners, the health plan ensures that plan members will not be reinfected, and the reservoir of infection in the community will be reduced.

With respect to the above issues, the committee makes the following recommendations:

• **All health plans and clinicians should take responsibility for partner treatment and provide STD diagnosis and treatment to sex partners of plan members or others under their care as part of standard clinical practice. Diagnosis and treatment of partners should be reimbursable by third-party payers, including Medicaid, or by the partner's health plan if he or she is insured.**

• **Public sector laboratories should be reimbursed for STD-related laboratory tests performed on persons who have private health insurance coverage.**

1

Introduction and Background

Sex is a normal human function that can involve the expression of love and emotional feelings, and does provide a means for reproduction. Sexual intercourse, however, is not without potential harmful or unintended consequences. Two major potential health consequences of sexual intercourse are unintentional pregnancy and sexually transmitted diseases (STDs), including HIV infection. These harmful consequences can be dramatically reduced through effective prevention programs and by openly confronting these problems on a national level. A previous Institute of Medicine (IOM) report has described the national epidemic of unintentional pregnancies and recommended a strategy for prevention (IOM, 1995a). The current report focuses on the hidden epidemic of STDs in United States and presents a national strategy for how these diseases can be confronted on many levels.[1]

---

[1] The committee considers STDs to be "epidemic" (i.e., the occurrence of disease in excess of that normally expected) in the United States for the following reasons. While some STDs seemed to be declining in the last several years (e.g., gonorrhea), other STDs are increasing (e.g., genital herpes, heterosexually transmitted HIV infection) and are epidemic in the general population (Wasserheit and Aral, 1996). Rates of many STDs, especially viral STDs, are higher than they were three decades ago (CDC, DSTDP, 1996). Among the reportable diseases, five of the top ten most frequently reported diseases are STDs (CDC, 1996). In some population groups (e.g., drug users and their partners, and certain racial and ethnic groups), rates of certain STDs are clearly much higher than in the general population. In addition, if STD rates in other developed countries (i.e., western and northern European countries, Canada, Japan, and Australia) are used as the basis for comparison, then STDs are epidemic in the United States.

The genesis of this study lies in the following observations regarding STDs in the United States:

- With approximately 12 million new cases of STDs occurring annually (CDC, DSTD/HIVP, 1993), STDs are some of the most commonly reported diseases in the United States and affect all population groups (CDC, 1994). The scope of the STD epidemic, however, remains underappreciated, and the epidemic is largely hidden and excluded from public discourse.
- There is a general lack of public awareness and knowledge regarding STDs. Some STDs are initially asymptomatic but may cause serious health problems years after infection. The lag between initial infection and serious complications contributes to the lack of awareness of the impact of STDs. Surveys show that public awareness and knowledge regarding STDs, even among persons at high risk, is dangerously low (ASHA, 1995; EDK Associates, 1995). However, there has not been a comprehensive national public education campaign for STDs.
- STDs can lead to long-term health consequences that are often irreversible and are costly in both human and economic terms. Potential health consequences include serious long-term complications such as cervical and liver cancer and infertility (Holmes and Handsfield, 1994). STDs during pregnancy may result in fetal death or significant physical and developmental disabilities, including mental retardation and blindness (Brunham et al., 1990). In addition, the economic consequences of STDs are substantial (IOM, 1985; Washington et al., 1986; Washington et al., 1987; Washington and Katz, 1991), but neither the health nor economic impact of STDs is widely recognized.
- Women are particularly vulnerable to STDs because they are more biologically susceptible to certain sexually transmitted infections than men and because they are more likely to have asymptomatic infections that result in delayed diagnosis and treatment (Aral and Guinan, 1984; Cates, 1990). In addition, women develop more serious sequelae and long-term complications compared to men. The disproportionate impact of STDs on the health of women, however, is not widely understood.
- Adolescents and young adults are at greatest risk of acquiring an STD. Every year, approximately 3 million teenagers acquire an STD, and many of them will have long-term health problems as a result (CDC, DSTD/HIVP, 1993). Approximately two-thirds of persons who acquire STDs are under age 25. Despite the fact that high-risk sexual behaviors are usually initiated during adolescence, STD prevention efforts for adolescents in the United States remain unfocused and controversial.
- Campaigns to increase public awareness of STDs and behavioral interventions to promote condom use and other healthy behaviors have been implemented with varying success. Obstacles to effective prevention efforts include behavioral impediments, sociocultural taboos, and inadequate, sometimes con-

flicting, sources of public information. These barriers have not been systematically addressed and require innovative solutions.

• Prevention of STDs has important implications for HIV prevention. Studies show that STDs enhance the risk of sexually transmitted HIV infection (Cameron et al., 1989; Plummer et al., 1991; Wasserheit, 1992; Laga et al., 1993). The role and impact of improved STD prevention on HIV transmission needs to be included in national HIV prevention strategies.

• Many physicians and other health care professionals do not have adequate skills or training to obtain an accurate sexual history, diagnose and treat STDs, or counsel patients regarding high-risk sexual behavior (Stamm et al., 1982; Merrill et al., 1990; Boekeloo et al., 1991; MacKay et al., 1995). In addition, training and education programs for health care professionals in STD clinical management are inadequate.

• Many screening and treatment services for STDs are currently provided through dedicated public STD clinics that are operated by public health departments. These STD programs traditionally have been oriented towards diagnosis and treatment but not towards prevention by behavioral interventions. The focus and role of these clinics have not been reexamined in light of recent developments in the delivery of health services and the epidemiology of STDs.

• Changes in health care delivery and financing, especially the national trend towards managed care, coupled with recent initiatives to shift Medicaid populations into managed care plans, may have a significant impact on the delivery of public health services, including STD-related services. Roles and responsibilities of the public and private health sectors and of primary care professionals in providing these services need to be redefined.

In light of these developments, the IOM convened the 16-member Committee on Prevention and Control of Sexually Transmitted Diseases to examine these issues. Committee members include nationally recognized experts in one or more of the following fields: epidemiology, behavioral and social sciences, infectious diseases, public health, pediatrics, women's health, STD program management, family planning, health services administration, and health care policy. The committee was charged to "(a) examine the epidemiological dimensions of STDs in the United States and factors that contribute to the epidemic; (b) assess the effectiveness of current public health strategies and programs to prevent and control STDs;[2] and (c) provide direction for future public health programs, policy, and research in STD prevention and control.[3]"

---

[2]Although the committee examined the effectiveness of major strategies and programs in STD prevention, it did not conduct a systematic, in-depth evaluation of every STD-related program in the public and private sector. In this report, the committee focuses its discussions on effective strategies and highlights major effective programs.

[3]The terms "STD prevention" and "STD control" have been traditionally used by public health

Although public recognition of AIDS and the public health response to the disease were initially very poor (IOM, 1986), it is now probably the most recognized STD in the United States. Because HIV prevention is relatively better funded and HIV prevention efforts are more visible compared to other STDs, the committee was charged to focus its study on STDs other than HIV infection. However, because the prevention of sexually transmitted HIV infection and other STDs are inextricably linked, the committee presents information on and provides recommendations concerning HIV infection as it relates to other STDs in this report in the following areas: costs of sexually transmitted HIV infections (Chapter 2), biological and epidemiological relationship between HIV infection and other STDs (Chapter 2), prevention efforts for sexually transmitted HIV that may be relevant for other STDs (Chapter 4), coordination of STD and HIV programs (Chapter 6), and coordination of interventions related to sexually transmitted HIV infection and other STDs (Chapter 6). A comprehensive analysis and discussion of HIV prevention beyond its relationship with other STDs is outside the charge of this committee, and this issue has been addressed by other IOM committees. Readers who desire additional information regarding national policy regarding the prevention of HIV infection should consult recent studies conducted by the IOM and the National Research Council (NRC, 1990, 1991, 1993; IOM, 1991, 1994, 1995b; NRC, IOM, 1995).

STUDY METHODS

During the 18-month course of the study, the full committee met five times. To directly observe how STD-related services are delivered on the local level, the committee conducted site visits to public STD clinics and other STD programs in Atlanta and Chicago in the summer of 1995. During these visits, staff of these STD clinics and programs described their activities, provided perspectives on the adequacy and effectiveness of existing services, and suggested ways to improve current efforts against STDs.

The committee also conducted two workshops during this study. The first was a public workshop held in Washington, D.C., in July 1995 to examine the potential impact of STDs on HIV transmission. The committee invited various

---

workers without clear distinction. These terms have been commonly used to refer to behavioral interventions (e.g., counseling for behavior change), treatment of symptomatic disease, and other interventions that prevent the spread of infection (e.g., partner notification). The committee believes that most interventions for STDs both "prevent" and "control" STDs, and all prevent acquisition or transmission of STDs in a population. Essentially, effective prevention of STDs brings STDs under control. Therefore, in this report, the committee uses the term "STD prevention" rather than "STD prevention and control" to encompass all interventions, whether behavioral, curative, environmental, or otherwise, that are needed to reduce the spread of infection in a population.

experts, representing a broad array of disciplines, to present data and perspectives. The main purpose of the workshop was to examine the inextricable links between HIV infection and other STDs. Issues discussed included the biological and epidemiological relationships between other STDs and HIV infection, the potential impact of reducing STDs on HIV transmission, and integration of preventive strategies for STDs and HIV infection.

The second workshop, held in the Los Angeles area in November 1995, was a workshop to explore the potential role of managed care organizations in the prevention of STDs. The committee invited a small number of representatives from managed care organizations, public health agencies, and an employer-purchaser coalition to advise the committee on potential roles and responsibilities of the public and private health care sectors in STD prevention. Because data regarding STD-related services in managed care organizations are limited, the committee subsequently conducted a brief survey of managed care organizations to collect information regarding STD-related services.

During the course of the study, the committee identified several critical issues that were not adequately addressed by published scientific literature and other available data. Accordingly, the committee commissioned papers from several national and international experts on the economic costs of STDs, the epidemiology of substance use and STDs, the potential impact of reducing STDs on HIV transmission in the United States, and the theoretical basis for behavior change interventions. In some cases, parts of the commissioned papers were incorporated into the body of the report, and two of these papers are published as appendices to this report.

FOCUS OF REPORT

Recognizing the complexity of the STD epidemic and the fact that STDs encompass dozens of infections and syndromes, the committee chose to focus its work on fundamental, cross-cutting issues in STD prevention, that is, the underlying issues that need to be addressed in order to effectively prevent STDs. In developing this report, the committee identified the following major questions that eventually became the focus of the present report:

*   What are the health and economic impacts of STDs?
*   What are the central characteristics of the epidemic?
*   What are the underlying factors explaining why the United States has performed poorly relative to other developed countries in its efforts to contain the epidemic?
*   What tools can be used to effectively fight the epidemic?
*   What are the essential components of an effective national system for STD prevention?

• What barriers must be addressed and what specific actions can we take immediately to build an effective national and local system for prevention?

This report is not intended to be a comprehensive review of STDs or a textbook on STDs. Readers who desire more detailed biomedical information on specific STDs should consult a medical textbook on STDs (e.g., Quinn, 1992; Holmes et al., in press). Health care providers who need information on appropriate diagnosis and treatment of STDs should consult a textbook or the latest STD treatment guidelines (e.g., CDC, 1993; Celum et al., 1994). In addition, persons who need more data on reported rates of STDs should consult published national STD surveillance data (CDC, DSTDP, 1996).

The intended audience for this report is anyone who is involved directly or indirectly in STD prevention or who has an interest in general public health policy. STD prevention involves a spectrum of health- and nonhealth-related disciplines and organizations and therefore makes an excellent case study of a major public health problem whose solution requires the cooperation of the public and private sectors and various interest groups. The committee hopes to reach a multidisciplinary audience, including policymakers, public and private sector health care professionals, government agencies, epidemiologists, social scientists, allied health professionals, school health professionals, STD clinicians, health educators, employers, purchasers of health care, and health program managers. This broad audience reflects the spectrum of individuals, agencies, and organizations that are involved in various aspects of STD prevention.

FOCUS OF CHAPTERS

Chapter 2 describes the significant, but not commonly recognized, health and economic impact of STDs in the United States. The committee highlights the major health consequences of STDs, such as cervical and liver cancer and reproductive health problems. The disproportionate impact of STDs on women and infants is described. Evidence that other STDs increase the risk of HIV transmission and that reducing STDs will prevent a substantial number of HIV infections is presented. In addition, the committee presents estimates of the economic costs of STDs in the United States. The broad reach of STDs throughout the general population, especially among women and adolescents, is underscored.

In Chapter 3, the committee presents information regarding the reasons why the United States, unlike most other developed countries, has been unable to confront STDs. The committee identifies and describes biological and social factors that contribute to the STD epidemic, including the lag time from infection to complications, inadequate access to health care, and substance use. The problem of STDs among disenfranchised populations is summarized, and the public health consequences of not preventing STDs among these groups are demonstrated. From the committee's perspective, a fundamental reason for the nation's failure to successfully prevent STDs is the inability of American society to openly confront issues regarding sexuality and the adverse impact of this inability on STD prevention efforts. In the last section of the chapter, data regarding current trends in sexual behavior are presented.

Chapter 4 describes the individual factors that influence personal risk for STDs and summarizes effective interventions that, if fully exploited, offer great promise for preventing STDs. These interventions include various individual- and community-based prevention strategies that can reduce exposure to, acquisition of, and transmission of STDs. Strategies to promote healthy sexual behavior include individual-focused interventions, school-based programs, and mass media campaigns. Clinical methods for prevention include prophylaxis, partner notification and treatment, and screening. At the end of the chapter, the importance of reducing the duration of infection by early detection and treatment of STDs using appropriate diagnostic and therapeutic tools is described.

Chapter 5 addresses the assortment of STD prevention services that are currently in place in the United States. These include clinical services for STDs provided through public STD clinics, community-based programs, and private sector health care settings. There is a particular emphasis on the potential role of managed care organizations and other health plans in delivering services. The importance of disease surveillance and other information systems and of health behavior research in STD prevention is documented. The committee also describes the status of STD-related training and educational activities for health care professionals. Following that is a discussion of the pros and cons of existing and proposed funding mechanisms, including block grants, for state and local STD programs.

In Chapter 6, the committee presents its assessment of the current system of STD prevention, a vision for an effective national system, and recommendations for how an effective system can be built in the context of four major strategies. The committee begins by describing a model for an effective national system and the need to incorporate STD prevention as a strategy for HIV and cancer prevention. Under the first strategy, the committee details how barriers to the adoption of healthy sexual behaviors, including the reluctance of many Americans to openly confront issues related to sexuality and STDs, can be overcome by increasing public and health professional awareness of STDs and by a bold role for the mass media. Under the second strategy, the importance of establishing both private and public sector leadership, investing in STD prevention, and developing effective information systems are emphasized. The third strategy relates to the need to focus on preventing STDs among adolescents and underserved groups, using innovative methods. The fourth strategy involves ways for ensuring access to, and the quality of, STD-related clinical services. This strategy includes ensuring access to services at the community level, incorporating STD-related clinical services into primary care, improving dedicated public STD clinics, expanding the role and responsibilities of health plans, and improving training and education of health professionals. A central tactic of the fourth strategy also involves assurance of effective clinical management of STDs. At the end of Chapter 6, brief descriptions of how some agencies and organizations have collaborated to improve access to, and quality of, STD-related services are presented as potential models for others. The nine appendixes that follow Chapter 6 provide additional information about several major issues discussed in Chapters 2 through 6.

REFERENCES

Aral SO, Guinan ME. Women and sexually transmitted diseases. In: Holmes KK, Mårdh P-A, Sparling PF, Wiesner PJ, eds. Sexually transmitted diseases. 1st ed. New York: McGraw-Hill, Inc., 1984:85-9.

ASHA (American Social Health Association). International survey reveals lack of knowledge about STDs. STD News. A quarterly newsletter of the American Social Health Association. Fall 1995;3:1,10.

Boekeloo BO, Marx ES, Kral AH, Coughlin SC, Bowman M, Rabin DL. Frequency and thoroughness of STD/HIV risk assessment by physicians in a high-risk metropolitan area. Am J Public Health 1991;81:1645-8.

Brunham RC, Holmes KK, Embree JE. Sexually transmitted diseases in pregnancy. In: Holmes KK, Mårdh P-A, Sparling PF, Weisner PJ, Cates W Jr, Lemon SM, et al., eds. Sexually transmitted diseases. 2nd ed. New York: McGraw-Hill, Inc., 1990:771-801.

Cameron DW, Simonsen JN, D'Costa LJ, Ronald AR, Maitha GM, Gakinya MN, et al. Female to male transmission of human immunodeficiency virus type 1: risk factors for seroconversion in men. Lancet 1989; 2:403-7.

Cates W Jr. Epidemiology and control of sexually transmitted diseases in adolescents. In: Schydlower M, Shafer MA, eds. AIDS and other sexually transmitted diseases. Philadelphia: Hanly & Belfus, Inc., 1990:409-27.

CDC (Centers for Disease Control and Prevention). 1993 Sexually transmitted diseases treatment guidelines. MMWR 1993;42(No. RR-14):56-66.

CDC. Summary of notifiable diseases, United States, 1994. MMWR 1994;43:3-12.

CDC. Ten leading nationally notifiable infectious diseases—United Sates, 1995. MMWR 1996;45:883-4.

CDC, DSTD/HIVP (Division of STD/HIV Prevention). Annual report 1992. U.S. Department of Health and Human Services, Public Health Service. Atlanta: Centers for Disease Control and Prevention, 1993.

CDC, DSTDP (Division of STD Prevention). Sexually transmitted disease surveillance 1995. U.S. Department of Health and Human Services, Public Health Service. Atlanta: Centers for Disease Control and Prevention, September 1996.

Celum CL, Wilch E, Fennell C, Stamm WE. The management of sexually transmitted diseases. 2nd ed. Seattle: University of Washington, Health Sciences Center for Educational Resources, 1994.

EDK Associates. The ABCs of STDs. New York: EDK Associates, 1995.

Holmes KK, Handsfield HH. Sexually transmitted diseases. In: Isselbacher KJ, Braunwald E, Wilson JD, Martin JB, Fauci AS, Kasper DL, eds. Harrison's principles of internal medicine. 13th ed. New York: McGraw-Hill, Inc., 1994:534-43.

Holmes KK, Sparling PF, Mårdh PA, Lemon SM, Stamm WE, Piot P, Wasserheit JN, eds. Sexually transmitted diseases. 3rd ed. New York: McGraw-Hill, Inc., in press.

IOM (Institute of Medicine). New vaccine development: establishing priorities; vol. I, Diseases of importance in the United States. Washington, D.C.: National Academy Press, 1985.

IOM. Confronting AIDS: directions for public health, health care, and research. Washington, D.C.: National Academy Press, 1986.

IOM. HIV screening of pregnant women and newborns. Hardy LM, ed. Washington, D.C.: National Academy Press, 1991.

IOM. AIDS and behavior. Auerbach JD, Wypijewska C, Brodie HKH, eds. Washington, D.C.: National Academy Press, 1994.

IOM. Best intentions: unintended pregnancy and the well-being of children and families. Brown SS, Eisenberg L, eds. Washington, D.C.: National Academy Press, 1995a.

IOM. HIV and the blood supply: an analysis of crisis decisionmaking. Leveton LB, Sox HC, Stoto MA, eds. Washington, D.C.: National Academy Press, 1995b.

Laga M, Manoka A, Kivuvu M, Malele B, Tuliza M, Nzila N, et al. Non-ulcerative sexually transmitted diseases as risk factors for HIV-1 transmission in women: results from a cohort study. AIDS 1993;7:95-102.

MacKay HT, Toomey KE, Schmid GP. Survey of clinical training in STD and HIV/AIDS in the United States. Proceedings of the IDSA Annual Meeting, September 16-18, 1995, San Francisco [abstract no. 281].

Merrill JM, Laux LF, Thornby JI. Why doctors have difficulty with sex histories. Southern Med J 1990;83:613-7.

NRC (National Research Council). AIDS: the second decade. Miller HG, Turner CF, Moses LE, eds. Washington, D.C.: National Academy Press, 1990.

NRC. Evaluating AIDS prevention programs: expanded edition. Coyle SL, Boruch RF, Turner CF, eds. Washington, D.C.: National Academy Press, 1991.

NRC. The social impact of AIDS in the United States. Jonsen AR, Stryker J, eds. Washington, D.C.: National Academy Press, 1993.

NRC, IOM (National Research Council, Institute of Medicine). Preventing HIV transmission: the role of sterile needles and bleach. Normand J, Vlahov D, Moses LE, eds. Washington, D.C.: National Academy Press, 1995.

Plummer FA, Simonsen JN, Cameron DW, Ndinya-Achola JO, Kreiss JK, Gakinya MN, et al. Cofactors in male-female transmission of human immunodeficiency virus type 1. J Infect Dis 1991;163:233-9.

Quinn TC, ed. Sexually transmitted diseases. New York: Raven Press, Ltd., 1992.

Stamm WE, Kaetz SK, Holmes KK. Clinical training in venereology in the United States and Canada. JAMA 1982;248:2020-4.

Washington AE, Arno PS, Brooks MA. The economic cost of pelvic inflammatory disease. JAMA 1986;255:13:1735-8.

Washington AE, Johnson RE, Sanders LL. *Chlamydia trachomatis* infections in the United States: what are they costing us? JAMA 1987;257:2070-2.

Washington AE, Katz P. Cost of and payment source for pelvic inflammatory disease. Trends and projections, 1983 through 2000 [see comments]. JAMA 1991;266:2565-9.

Wasserheit JN. Epidemiologic synergy. Interrelationships between human immunodeficiency virus infection and other sexually transmitted diseases. Sex Transm Dis 1992; 9:61-77.

Wasserheit JN, Aral SO. The dynamic topology of sexually transmitted disease epidemics: implications for prevention strategies. J Infect Dis 1996; 174 (Suppl 2):S201-13.

2

The Neglected Health and Economic Impact of STDs

Highlights
- More than 12 million Americans, 3 million of whom are teenagers, are infected with STDs each year.
- STDs accounted for 87 percent of all cases reported among the top ten most frequently reported diseases in 1995 in the United States.
- Since 1980, eight new sexually transmitted pathogens have been recognized in the United States.
- STDs may cause serious, life-threatening complications including cancers, infertility, ectopic pregnancy, spontaneous abortions, stillbirth, low birth weight, neurologic damage, and death.
- Women and adolescents are disproportionately affected by STDs and their sequelae.
- Reducing other STDs decreases the risk of HIV transmission.
- Every year, approximately $10 billion is spent on major STDs other than AIDS and their preventable complications. This cost is shared by all Americans.

Sexually transmitted diseases (STDs) are a tremendous health and economic burden on the people of the United States. More than 12 million Americans are infected with STDs each year (CDC, DSTD/HIVP, 1993). In 1995, STDs accounted for 87 percent of all cases reported among the top ten most frequently reported diseases in the United States (CDC, 1996). Of the top ten diseases, five are STDs (i.e., chlamydial infection, gonorrhea, AIDS, primary and secondary syphilis, and hepatitis B virus infection).

Rates of "classical" STDs such as gonorrhea and syphilis are slowly declining in the United States, but rates of a number of STDs in the United States are higher than in some developing regions (Piot and Islam, 1994) and still far exceed those of every other developed country[1] (Aral and Holmes, 1991) (Figure 2-1). For example, the reported incidence of gonorrhea in 1995 was 149.5 cases per

---

[1]For the purposes of this report, defined as western and northern European countries, Canada, Japan, and Australia.

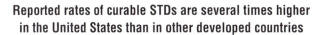

Reported rates of curable STDs are several times higher in the United States than in other developed countries

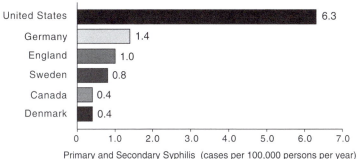

Primary and Secondary Syphilis (cases per 100,000 persons per year)

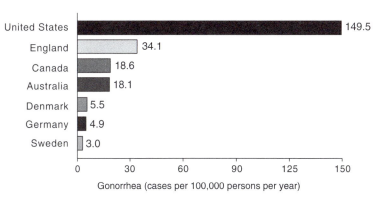

Gonorrhea (cases per 100,000 persons per year)

FIGURE 2-1 Rates of reported syphilis (primary and secondary cases) and gonorrhea in the United States and other developed countries, 1995. SOURCES: 1) Australia: Herceg A, Oliver G, Myint H, Andrews G, Curran M, Crerar S, et al. Annual report of the national notifiable diseases surveillance system, 1995. Communicable Diseases Intelligence, Commonwealth Department of Health and Family Services. October 14, 1996;20:440-464. Rates of primary and secondary syphilis not available; 2) Canada: Jo-Anne Doherty, Laboratory Center for Disease Control, Division of STD Prevention & Control, Ottawa, Ontario, Canada, personal communication, November 1996; 3) Denmark: Dr. Inga Lind, WHO Collaborating Centre for Reference and Research in Gonococci, Copenhagen, Denmark, personal communication, November 1996; 4) England: Hannah Bowers, Public Health Laboratory Services, Communicable Disease Surveillance Centre, London, England, United Kingdom, personal communication, November 1996; 5) Germany: Dr. Lyle Petersen, Robert Koch Institut, Berlin, Germany, personal communication, November 1996; 6) Sweden: Dr. Kristina Ramstedt, Swedish Institute for Infectious Disease Control, Epidemiological Department, personal communication, November 1996; 7) United States: Division of STD Prevention, Sexually transmitted disease surveillance, 1995. U.S. Department of Health and Human Services, Public Health Service. Atlanta: Centers for Disease Control and Prevention, September 1996.

100,000 persons in the United States versus 3.0 cases per 100,000 in Sweden (CDC, DSTDP, 1996; Swedish Institute for Infectious Disease Control, unpublished data, 1996). Because actual U.S. rates are estimated to be approximately twice the reported rate, the U.S. rate is 100 times the reported rate in Sweden. Similarly, the reported incidence of gonorrhea in Canada in 1995 was 18.6 cases per 100,000, or approximately 12 percent of the U.S. rate (Laboratory Centre for Disease Control, Canada, unpublished data, 1996). In addition, the rate of primary and secondary syphilis in the United States was 6.3 cases per 100,000 persons versus 0.4 cases per 100,000 persons in Canada. Therefore, rates of curable STDs, including gonorrhea, syphilis, and chancroid are many times higher in the United States than in other developed countries. The differences in rates of viral STDs between the United States and other developed countries, however, appear to be much smaller. Data for viral STDs are much more limited than for bacterial STDs, but do not suggest major differences. For example, a cohort of young Swedish women studied over a 16-year-period showed a cumulative incidence of genital herpes that was comparable to the age-specific increases in herpes simplex virus type 2 antibodies seen during the approximately the same period in U.S. women (Christenson et al., 1992; Johnson et al., 1993). Potential explanations for the observed differences between the United States and other developed countries in rates of curable STDs are presented in Chapter 3.

Further, many new STDs have been discovered or have newly arisen during the antibiotic era. Of these "modern" STDs, some, including HIV infection, human papillomavirus infection, and hepatitis B virus infection, are viral infections that are incurable and are now recognized as major preventable causes of death and disability. The bacterial STDs, such as gonorrhea and syphilis, can be easily diagnosed and successfully treated; others, such as chlamydial infection, are curable but will require a much stronger, coordinated national effort to be brought under control.

BROAD SCOPE AND IMPACT OF STDs

STDs affect persons of all racial, cultural, socioeconomic, and religious groups in the United States. Persons in all states, communities, and social networks are at risk for STDs. The estimated incidence and prevalence of major STDs are summarized in Table 2-1.

The term "STD" is not specific for any one disease but denotes the more than 25 infectious organisms that are transmitted through sexual activity and the dozens of clinical syndromes that they cause (Appendix A). With STDs, one infectious organism does not cause one syndrome; rather, there is a matrix of infectious organisms and associated syndromes. For example, some syndromes, such as pelvic inflammatory disease, can be caused by a number of organisms, including *Neisseria gonorrhoeae*, *Chlamydia trachomatis*, and other bacteria. Urethritis (inflammation of the canal leading from the urinary bladder) in men is fre-

TABLE 2-1 Estimated Annual Incidence and Prevalence of Selected Sexually Transmitted Diseases (STDs) in the United States, 1994

STD	Incidence	Prevalence
Chlamydial infection	4,000,000[a]	Not available
Gonorrhea	800,000[a]	Not available
Syphilis	101,000	Not available
Congenital syphilis	3,400	Not available
Human papillomavirus infection	500,000–1,000,000	24,000,000
Genital herpes infection	200,000–500,000	31,000,000[b]
Hepatitis B virus infection (sexually transmitted)	53,000[a]	Not available
AIDS	79,897[c]	185,000[d]
HIV infection	Not available	630,000–897,000[e]
Chancroid	3,500	Not available
Trichomoniasis	3,000,000	Not available
Pelvic inflammatory disease	>1,000,000[f]	Not available

NOTE: The Division of STD Prevention, CDC, is currently developing a process for systematically generating and updating incidence and prevalence estimates for specific STDs.

[a]Number reflects reported cases to the CDC plus estimated unreported cases.
[b]Based on Johnson RE, Nahmias AJ, Magder LS, Lee FK, Brooks CA, Snowden CB. A seroepidemiologic survey of the prevalence of herpes simplex virus type 2 infection in the United States. N Engl J Med 1989;321:7-12. However, recent data indicate a substantial recent increase in prevalence in the United States (Johnson R, Lee F, Hadgu A, McQuillan G, Aral S, Keesling S, et al. U.S. genital herpes trends during the first decade of AIDS—prevalences increased in young whites and elevated in blacks. Proceedings of the Tenth Meeting of the International Society for STD Research, August 29-September 1, 1993, Helsinki [abstract no. 22]).
[c]Reported cases to the CDC. Source: CDC. HIV/AIDS Surveillance Report. Atlanta: Centers for Disease Control and Prevention, 1995;7(2).
[d]Estimated prevalence of persons diagnosed with AIDS at the end of 1993. All AIDS cases including unreported cases.
[e]Prevalence as of January 1993. Source: Rosenberg PS. Scope of the AIDS epidemic in the United States. Science 1995;270:1372-5.
[f]Based on estimate for 1993 by Siegel (Appendix D of present report), Washington and Katz also estimated more than one million cases per year using older data (Washington AE, Katz P. Cost of and payment source for pelvic inflammatory disease. Trends and projections, 1983 through 2000 [see comments]. JAMA 1991;266:2565-9.).

PRIMARY SOURCE: CDC, DSTD/HIVP. Annual Report 1994. U.S. Department of Health and Human Services, Public Health Service. Atlanta: Centers for Disease Control and Prevention, 1995.

quently caused by gonorrhea or chlamydia but can also result from infection with ureaplasma, mycoplasma, and other organisms. Genital ulcers can result from herpes, chancroid, syphilis, or other infections. Vaginal discharge can be caused by trichomonas, bacterial vaginosis, or other infections. Syphilis and HIV infection have myriad clinical manifestations and can mimic many health conditions. In addition, common infections once considered trivial are now known to cause serious complications. For example, bacterial vaginosis, a frequent cause of vaginitis in sexually active women, was once considered to be a benign condition but has recently been shown to be associated with premature delivery, low birth weight, and pelvic inflammatory disease (Hauth et al., 1995; Hillier et al., 1995). Human papillomaviruses, originally recognized to cause warts, are now known to be important causes of several types of cancer.

Routes of Transmission

Epidemiological and other characteristics of eight common STDs are summarized in Appendix B. STDs are almost always transmitted from person to person by sexual intercourse.[2] STDs are transmitted most efficiently by anal or vaginal intercourse, and generally less efficiently by oral intercourse. A few STDs, such as scabies, can also be transmitted without sexual intercourse via direct contact with an infected site of a sex partner. Other more important blood-borne pathogens, such as hepatitis B virus, human T-cell lymphotrophic virus type I, and HIV, are transmitted among adults not only by sexual intercourse, but also by parenteral routes—particularly among intravenous drug users through contaminated injecting drug equipment. The relative contribution of parenteral versus sexual transmission varies according to the risk behaviors of the population and other factors. In addition, pregnant women with an STD may pass their infection to infants in the uterus, during birth, or through breast-feeding.

Summary of Common STDs

Human Papillomavirus Infection

Human papillomavirus is associated with the development of cervical and other genital and anal cancers (Koutsky et al., 1988; Reeves et al., 1989) and is prevalent across all socioeconomic groups in the United States. An estimated 24 million Americans already are infected with human papillomavirus, and as many as one million new human papillomavirus infections occur each year (CDC, DSTD/HIVP, 1995). In one study of female college students presenting for care at a university health center, genital human papillomavirus infections were five times more common than all other STDs combined (Laura Koutsky and King Holmes, University of Washington, unpublished data, 1995).

---

[2] The term "sexual intercourse" is used throughout this report to refer to all forms of intercourse, including vaginal, anal, and oral intercourse.

Herpes Simplex Virus Infection

Sexually transmitted herpes simplex virus infection is widespread in the United States and results in painful recurrent genital ulcers. The ulcers can be treated, but infection persists and ulcers may recur (Quinn and Cates, 1992). Herpes simplex virus can be transmitted to sex partners even when no genital ulcer is present (Mertz et al., 1992) and can also be transmitted from mother to infant during delivery. Approximately 200,000–500,000 new cases of genital herpes occur each year in the United States, and 31 million individuals already are infected (CDC, DSTD/HIVP, 1995). In 1990, the prevalence of antibodies to herpes simplex virus type 2 among persons 15–74 years of age was estimated at 21.7 percent (Johnson et al., 1993). This prevalence estimate suggests that at least one of every four women and one of every five men in the United States will become infected with herpes during their lifetime.

Viral Hepatitis

Hepatitis B virus infection is an STD with severe complications including chronic hepatitis, cirrhosis, and liver carcinoma. Of approximately 200,000 new hepatitis B virus infections in the United States each year, approximately half are transmitted through sexual intercourse (Alter and Mast, 1994; CDC, 1994b; Goldstein et al., 1996). Preliminary data from a large U.S. multisite study indicate that approximately one-third of persons with acute hepatitis B virus infections in 1995 had a history of another STD (CDC, Hepatitis Branch, unpublished data, 1996). In addition to hepatitis B, several other types of viral hepatitis can be transmitted sexually. Hepatitis A is a cause of acute hepatitis, and less than 5 percent of infections are transmitted through fecal-oral contact during sexual intercourse, mostly among men who have sex with men (CDC, 1994b; CDC, Hepatitis Branch, 1995). Hepatitis D (delta) virus is a virus that can be sexually transmitted but requires the presence of hepatitis B virus to replicate. Sexual transmission of hepatitis D virus occurs, but it is less efficiently transmitted through sexual intercourse than hepatitis B virus (Alter and Mast, 1994). Hepatitis C virus, the most common cause of non-A non-B hepatitis, causes chronic liver disease in most infected adults. The efficiency of sexual and perinatal transmission of this virus, however, seems to be low (Alter and Mast, 1994).

Syphilis

After sustaining a steady incidence rate during the 1970s and early 1980s, the rate of syphilis increased sharply from 1987 through 1990 (CDC, DSTDP, 1995), after which rates began to fall. This epidemic illustrates the ability of syphilis and other STDs to reemerge with alarming intensity in populations such as illicit drug users—particularly crack cocaine users—and their sex partners

(Farley et al., 1990; Rolfs et al., 1990). The reemergence of syphilis in this new context rendered traditional prevention efforts less effective (Andrus et al., 1990).

Gonorrhea

Gonorrhea infections in the United States are becoming increasingly resistant to routine antibiotic treatment; this has resulted in increasingly expensive treatments as effective therapeutic options become more limited. As of 1976, all gonorrhea infections were curable by penicillin (Aral and Holmes, 1991). Since then, antibiotic-resistant strains have increased steadily to 2 percent of gonorrhea infections in 1987 and to 30 percent of gonorrhea infections in 1994 (CDC, DSTDP, 1995). The Gonococcal Isolate Surveillance Project of the Centers for Disease Control and Prevention (CDC) measures national trends in gonorrhea antibiotic resistance. The proportion of isolates resistant to penicillin has increased steadily since monitoring began in 1988 (CDC, DSTDP, 1995) (Figure 2-2). In 1994, approximately 30 percent of gonococcal isolates were resistant to tetracycline, penicillin, or both; these antibiotics represent traditional, effective, low-cost treatment for gonorrhea. In addition, resistance to the newer quinolone antibiotics has been documented in the Western Pacific and Southeast Asia and in several U.S. states, indicating that some currently recommended treatment regimens may soon become inadequate (CDC, 1994a; GDHR, Epidemiology and Prevention Branch, 1995).

Chlamydial Infection

Chlamydial genital infection is the most common bacterial STD in the United States; of the more than 4 million cases estimated to occur annually, 2.6 million cases occur among women (CDC, DSTDP, 1995). As many as 85 percent of infections in women and 40 percent of infections in men may be asymptomatic and will not be identified without screening (Fish et al., 1989; Judson, 1990; Stamm and Holmes, 1990). Uncomplicated chlamydial infections can be easily treated with antibiotics (CDC, 1993); however, primarily as a result of unrecognized and untreated cervical infections, more than one million women each year develop pelvic inflammatory disease (Rolfs et al., 1992).

Impact of STDs on Women's Health

Complications of STDs are greater and more frequent among women than men for a number of reasons (Wasserheit and Holmes, 1992). Women are biologically more likely to become infected than men if exposed to a sexually transmitted pathogen. STDs are also more likely to remain undetected in women, resulting in delayed diagnosis and treatment, and these untreated infections are more likely to lead to complications.

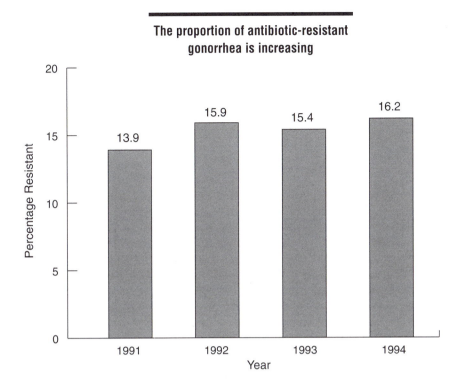

FIGURE 2-2   Percentage of isolates resistant to antibiotics, Gonococcal Isolate Surveillance Project, 1991–1994. SOURCE: CDC, DSTDP. Sexually Transmitted Disease Surveillance 1994. U.S. Department of Health and Human Services, Public Health Service. Atlanta: Centers for Disease Control and Prevention, 1995.

Many STDs are transmitted more easily from man to woman than from woman to man (Harlap et al., 1991). For example, the risk to a woman of acquiring gonorrhea from a single act of intercourse may be as high as 60 to 90 percent, while transmission from a woman to man is about 20 to 30 percent (Holmes et al., 1970; Hooper et al., 1978; Platt et al., 1983; Judson, 1990; Donegan et al., 1994). Among couples where only one partner was initially infected, the annual risk of transmission of herpes simplex virus was 19 percent from man to woman, but only 5 percent from woman to man (Mertz et al., 1992). The comparative efficiency of male-to-female versus female-to-male transmission of HIV seems to differ according to the study population (Haverkos et al., 1992). Studies in the United States (Peterman et al., 1988; Padian et al., 1991) generally have shown greater efficiency of transmission from man to woman than from woman to man, while studies in Haiti (Deschamps et al., 1996) and Europe (de Vincenzi, 1994) have shown no significant gender difference in efficiency of transmission.

STDs are often silent in women, and even when symptoms of STD occur, they may not arouse suspicion of an STD. For example, 30 to 80 percent of women with gonorrhea are asymptomatic, while fewer than 5 percent of men have no symptoms (Hook and Handsfield, 1990; Judson, 1990). Similarly, as many as 85 percent of women with chlamydial infection are asymptomatic compared to 40 percent of infected men (Fish et al., 1989; Judson, 1990; Stamm and Holmes, 1990). When an STD is suspected, it is often more difficult to diagnose in a woman because the anatomy of the female genital tract makes clinical examination more difficult (Aral and Guinan, 1984). For example, a urethral swab and a Gram stain are sufficient to evaluate the possibility of gonorrhea in men, but a speculum examination of the cervix and a specific culture for gonorrhea have been required for women (Hook and Handsfield, 1990). Thus, women with gonorrhea or chlamydial infection are often not diagnosed with an STD until complications, such as pelvic inflammatory disease, occur. Even then, symptoms of pelvic inflammatory disease due to chlamydial infection may be absent or nonspecific, resulting in as many as 85 percent of women delaying seeking medical care, thus increasing their risk for long-term complications (Hillis et al., 1993). Fortunately, the advent of newer tests for detecting gonococci and chlamydia in urine may permit testing women for these organisms without pelvic examination in the future, as described in Chapter 4.

Once infected, women are more susceptible than men to complications of certain STDs. For example, women infected with certain types of human papillomavirus are at risk for cancers of the cervix (a relatively common malignancy), as well as cancers of the vagina, vulva, and anus; whereas heterosexual men infected with these human papillomavirus types are at risk only for cancers of the penis (a relatively uncommon malignancy). Another example is the risk of infertility caused by gonorrhea or chlamydial infection, which is much higher in women than in men. Finally, pregnant women and their infants are particularly vulnerable to complications of STD during pregnancy or parturition.

Greater Risk of STDs Among Adolescents

Every year, approximately 3 million American teenagers acquire an STD (CDC, DSTD/HIVP, 1993). During the past two decades, sexual intercourse among adolescents has steadily increased, resulting in an enlarging pool of young men and women at risk for STDs (CDC, 1995c). As a result, STDs, unintended pregnancies, and other health problems that result from sexual intercourse have increased among adolescents in the United States (AGI, 1994). Adolescents (10–19 years of age) and young adults (20–24 years of age) are the age groups at greatest risk for acquiring an STD, for a number of reasons: they are more likely to have multiple sex partners; they may be more likely to engage in unprotected intercourse; and their partners may be at higher risk for being infected compared to most adults (Cates, 1990; Quinn and Cates, 1992; AGI, 1994; CDC, DSTDP,

1995). Compared to older women, female adolescents and young women are also more susceptible to cervical infections, such as gonorrhea and chlamydial infection, because the cervix of female adolescents and young women is especially sensitive to infection by certain sexually transmitted organisms (Cates, 1990). In addition, adolescents and young people are at greater risk for substance use and other contributing factors that may increase risk for STDs than older persons; these issues are discussed in Chapter 3.

Although overall rates of gonorrhea have been declining in the general population for over a decade, this decline has been less pronounced among adolescents than in other age groups. During 1993 and 1994, the gonorrhea rate for 15–19-year-old adolescents actually increased nearly 3 percent (CDC, DSTDP, 1995). The increase in gonorrhea among adolescents can be entirely attributed to increases in gonorrhea among female adolescents of all races, while rates of gonorrhea among male adolescents during this period leveled off. If one takes into account that not all teenagers are sexually active, the actual risk for acquiring an STD among sexually active teens is even higher than the rates themselves may suggest (Aral et al., 1988). Chlamydial infection has been consistently high among adolescents; in some studies, up to 30–40 percent of sexually active adolescent females studied have been infected (Toomey et al., 1987; Cates, 1990). In general, rates of chlamydia are at least two to four times higher than rates of gonorrhea in this age group (Washington et al., 1986; Shafer et al., 1987). Viral STDs also are becoming increasingly prevalent at younger ages as adolescents initiate sexual intercourse earlier (Moscicki et al., 1990). Cervical cancer rates and cohort mortality from cervical cancer (Krone et al., 1995; Kathleen Toomey, Georgia Department of Human Resources, unpublished data, 1996) are increasing among young women, undoubtedly a reflection of increased exposure to STDs such as human papillomavirus.

Other Groups at Risk

Reported STD rates in the United States vary among ethnic and racial groups (CDC, DSTDP, 1995). African Americans and Hispanic Americans have higher reported rates of chlamydial infection, gonorrhea, and syphilis than European Americans. Data on STDs among other ethnic or racial groups are more limited because of their smaller populations in the United States. Rates of certain STDs, however, among some American Indian/Alaska Native populations are high (Toomey et al., 1993). National surveillance data suggest that rates of reportable STDs, except for hepatitis B virus infection (Alter, 1991), are low among Asian Americans/Pacific Islanders compared to the general U.S. population (CDC, DSTDP, 1995).

Although national surveillance data may overrepresent cases diagnosed among some racial and ethnic groups (CDC, DSTD/HIVP, 1995), the higher prevalence of some STDs among African Americans and Hispanic Americans compared to the European American population has been confirmed by serological population surveys of markers for sexually transmitted infections (Hahn et al., 1989; Johnson et al., 1993). However, serosurvey data indicate that the differences in STD rates among racial and ethnic groups are actually smaller than those suggested by national surveillance data. The reasons for the racial and ethnic differences in STD rates are unclear and complex. Possible explanations include socioeconomic status, variability in access to and utilization of health care, differences in sexual behavior, and varying risk of STDs among sexual networks (Toomey et al., 1993). Some investigators have concluded that factors other than poverty and occupational status account for the observed differences in rates of gonorrhea and chlamydial infection and that nonbehavioral factors, such as geographic segregation, may promote a higher prevalence of these STDs in certain social networks (Ellen et al., 1995). Differences in sexual behavior also cannot entirely explain the racial gap in STD rates. African Americans, for example, are generally more likely to use condoms compared to other groups (Laumann et al., 1994; Anderson et al., 1996).

STDs are transmitted among all sexually active people, including heterosexual persons, men who have sex with men, and women who have sex with women (AMA, Council on Scientific Affairs, 1996). Men who have sex with men are at greater risk for many life-threatening STDs, including HIV infection, hepatitis B virus infection, and anal cancer compared to heterosexual men (AMA, Council on Scientific Affairs, 1996). Other STDs of concern among men who have sex with men include anal syphilis, urethritis, and a range of oral and gastrointestinal infections. While it is well established that men who have sex with men are at increased risk for STDs, including HIV infection, less is known about the risk of STD transmission among women who have sex with women (Kennedy et al., 1995). When compared to men who have sex with men and heterosexual persons, women who have sex only with women (and whose partners do likewise) are at substantially lower risk for acquisition of STDs. Studies show that some women who have sex with women and some bisexual women have high rates of risky behaviors, such as drug use and exchanging sex for drugs or money, as do some heterosexual women (Chu et al., 1990; Bevier et al., 1995). Although women who only have sex with women seem to be at less risk for some bacterial STDs compared to women who have sex with men (Robertson and Schachter, 1981), bacterial vaginosis and genital human papillomavirus infections are not uncommon in such women (Berger et al., 1995; Marrazzo et al., 1996). Most cases of HIV infection among women who have sex with women have been attributed to injection drug use or heterosexual intercourse (Chu et al., 1990, 1994; Cohen et al., 1993; Bevier et al., 1995). Female-to-female transmission of HIV infection seems to be relatively rare (AMA, Council on Scientific Affairs, 1996).

STDs as Emerging Infections

STDs are not a stationary group of infections and syndromes. Eight new sexually transmitted pathogens have been identified since 1980, bringing with them new challenges to prevention and treatment (Table 2-2). The most well-known of the recently described STDs is HIV infection. Since HIV-1 was found to be the cause of virtually all cases of AIDS in the United States in the mid-1980s, a closely related retrovirus, HIV-2, and a more distantly related pair of retroviruses, human T-lymphotrophic virus types I and II (HTLV-I, -II), have been shown to be sexually transmitted as well. In addition, in 1995, scientists confirmed and identified human herpes virus type 8 as a likely sexually transmitted virus and a possible cause of Kaposi's sarcoma and body cavity lymphomas (Chang et al., 1994). In contrast to newly recognized viral STDs, some bacterial STDs, such as syphilis and gonorrhea, have been documented for centuries and have recently reemerged in the United States along with a spectrum of barriers to prevention (Wasserheit, 1994). As demonstrated by the recent finding that bacterial vaginosis in pregnant women increases the risk for premature delivery of a low-birth-weight infant (Hauth et al., 1995; Hillier et al., 1995), the full clinical spectrum of many STDs is still being described. In addition, for many previously described pathogens, such as hepatitis B virus and cytomegalovirus, it has become evident that a major route of adult transmission—often the major route—is sexual. Further, new research shows that many common diseases of previously unknown cause, such as cervical dysplasia, are in fact caused by newly described sexually transmitted pathogens.

These examples of emerging infections (IOM, 1992) make it clear that more STDs will emerge and become established in the United States. This is because of increasing global travel and worsening ecological pressures, such as population

TABLE 2-2 Sexually Transmitted Pathogens Newly Identified or Newly Recognized as Sexually Transmitted, and Associated Syndromes, 1980–1995

Sexually Transmitted Agent (year identified or recognized)	Associated Syndromes
Human papillomaviruses (1976-present)	Genital and anal warts, dysplasias, and cancers
HTLV-I (1980)	T-cell leukemia/lymphoma; tropical spastic paraparesis
HTLV-II (1982)	Unknown
Mycoplasma genitalium (1981)	Nongonococcal urethritis
Mobiluncus sp. (1980, 1983)	Bacterial vaginosis-associated
HIV-1 (1983)	AIDS
HIV-2 (1986)	AIDS
Human herpes virus type 8 (1995)	Kaposi's sarcoma; body cavity lymphoma

growth and rural-to-urban migration, that contribute to the spread of STDs in both developed and developing countries. The advent of new techniques in bio-technology have allowed the presence of infectious organisms or genetic material from these organisms to be detected, contributing to the recognition of new sexually transmitted infections. These techniques have allowed clinicians and epidemiologists to link specific infectious organisms to the syndromes that they cause.

International Comparisons and the Global Scope of STDs

STDs are severe social, health, and economic burdens worldwide. STDs most commonly affect people who are between the ages of 15 and 44, the group that is most economically productive (Over and Piot, 1993). The World Bank estimates that STDs, excluding AIDS, are the second leading cause of healthy life lost among women between the ages of 15 and 44 in the developing world (Figure 2-3) (World Bank, 1993). STDs are severe public health problems be-cause of their potentially serious complications as well as their potential to in-crease the efficiency of HIV transmission. One study estimated that the impact of successfully treating or preventing one hundred cases of syphilis among a group at high risk for STDs would prevent 1,200 HIV infections that would otherwise be linked to those one hundred syphilis infections during a 10-year period (Over and Piot, 1993). Over and Piot (1996) also found that, in developing countries, targeting groups with the highest rates of sex partner change markedly improves the cost-effectiveness of HIV and other STD prevention efforts.

The World Health Organization (WHO) Global Programme on AIDS re-cently estimated regional and global incidence rates for four curable STDs—gonorrhea, chlamydial infection, syphilis, and trichomoniasis (WHO, 1996). Us-ing a database of country-specific prevalence rates and estimated regional prevalence rates for each curable STD, WHO estimated that there were 333 million new cases of the four curable STDs worldwide in 1995 among adults 15–49 years of age. Prevalence rates for other STDs for which estimates are not available, such as human papillomavirus and herpes simplex virus type 2 infec-tions, are much higher, and the number of adults infected is likely to exceed one billion. In addition, in the last few years, STDs have rapidly become epidemic in some areas of the world, such as certain countries of the former Soviet Union. These epidemics have relevance for the United States because Americans are increasingly traveling abroad, and some will have high-risk sexual intercourse during their stay (Moore et al., 1995). With increasing access to international travel and easing of travel restrictions, it is now possible for persons with infec-tious diseases to spread their infection to others around the world in a matter of hours or days.

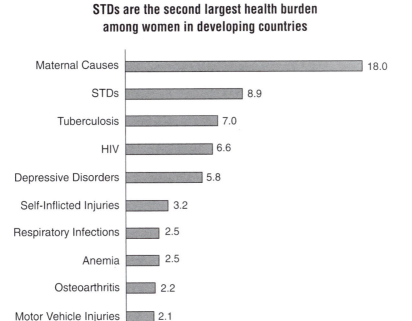

STDs are the second largest health burden among women in developing countries

Maternal Causes	18.0
STDs	8.9
Tuberculosis	7.0
HIV	6.6
Depressive Disorders	5.8
Self-Inflicted Injuries	3.2
Respiratory Infections	2.5
Anemia	2.5
Osteoarthritis	2.2
Motor Vehicle Injuries	2.1

Percentage of Total DALYs lost

FIGURE 2-3   Top 10 health burdens among women in developing countries by total DALYs lost, 1990. NOTE: STDs included syphilis, chlamydial infection, gonorrhea, and pelvic inflammatory disease; DALY = disability-adjusted life year. SOURCE: World Bank. World development report, 1993: investing in health. New York: Oxford University Press, 1993.

HEALTH CONSEQUENCES OF STDs

The general population is largely unaware of the health consequences of STDs for three reasons. First, many STDs are often asymptomatic and thus go undetected (Fish et al., 1989; Judson, 1990; Stamm and Holmes, 1990). Second, major health consequences, such as infertility, various cancers, and other chronic diseases, occur years after the initial infection, so that there is a lack of awareness of any link to the original STD (the exception is the public awareness of the connection of AIDS to HIV infection). Third, the stigma associated with having an STD has inhibited public discussion and health education concerning the consequences of STDs and frequently even prevents clinicians from educating their patients regarding STDs as discussed in Chapter 3. Many sexually transmitted infections can persist for years without evidence of infection until life-threatening complications are recognized. In particular, viral STDs often result in lifelong infection for which there is currently no curative treatment. The serious long-term complications of STDs affecting millions of women, infants, and men in the United States each year are summarized in Table 2-3.

Cancers Caused by STDs

Several sexually transmitted pathogens cause cancer. The direct role of STDs in causing genital cancers has been largely unrecognized. Certain types of sexually acquired human papillomavirus are now considered to be a cause of most cancers of the cervix, vagina, vulva, anus, and penis. Hepatitis B virus, which is usually transmitted either by sexual contact or by intravenous drug use among adults in the United States, is a cause of hepatocellular carcinoma, one of the world's most common forms of cancer. Human T-cell lymphotrophic virus type I (HTLV-I), sexually transmitted among adults and transmitted to infants especially by breast-feeding, causes certain malignancies, including T-cell leukemia and lymphoma. Human herpes virus type 8 (HHV8) is a newly discovered virus, probably sexually transmitted, that may cause Kaposi's sarcoma and certain forms of lymphoma. Epstein-Barr virus (EBV), transmitted among adults by intimate contact, including kissing and sexual intercourse, is associated with other types of lymphoma and with nasopharyngeal (nasal cavity and pharynx) carcinoma.

Cervical Cancer

Carcinoma of the uterine cervix, particularly among women of reproductive age, is now known to be strongly associated with certain oncogenic types of human papillomavirus (NIH, 1996). Of more than 70 types of human papillomavirus that have been identified, several oncogenic forms, such as types 16, 18, 31, and 45, have the strongest association with cervical cancer. Both biological and epidemiological data suggest that human papillomavirus is a dominant etiologic factor for cervical cancer. Studies show that cervical infection with oncogenic types of human papillomavirus is associated with at least 80 percent of invasive cervical cancer cases (NIH, 1996) and that women with human papillomavirus infection of the cervix are 10 times more likely to develop invasive cervical cancer compared to women without human papillomavirus infection (Schiffman, 1992).

Much of the cervical cancer burden related to human papillomavirus infection may be averted by preventing high-risk sexual behaviors (Brinton, 1992), especially avoiding unprotected sex with multiple male partners, some of whom may have chronic genital infection with oncogenic human papillomavirus types. Screening with the Pap smear is currently the best available method for reducing incidence of, and mortality associated with, invasive cervical cancer, but this is not being widely applied among certain population groups (NIH, 1996). Approximately 4,900 American women will die from cervical cancer in 1996 (ACS, 1996). Cervical cancer is the second most common cancer among women worldwide, with more than 450,000 new cases estimated to occur each year (Paavonen et al., 1990). It is the most frequently detected cancer among women in many countries in Africa, Asia, Central America, and South America, where case fatality rates are much higher than those in the United States. In this country, approximately 16,000 new cases of cervical cancer are diagnosed each year, placing it third among reproductive tract cancers in women and seventh among all cancers in women (ACS, 1996).

Although these morbidity and mortality statistics are clearly significant by themselves, they do not capture the physical, mental, or psychosocial trauma experienced by the hundreds of thousands of women who develop precancerous cervical lesions. For example, approximately 5 percent of the 50 million Pap smears performed each year are associated with findings consistent with cervical dysplasia (Kurman et al., 1994). These abnormalities result in enormous anxiety among women and their partners and require diagnostic and treatment procedures, including surgery, that are painful, invasive, and expensive.

An especially disturbing recent finding is the increasing incidence of invasive cervical cancer among European American women under age 50 in the last few years (Krone et al., 1995). This new, ominous trend may be related to the high prevalence of human papillomavirus infection recently reported among young women. In one study, nearly half of female college students tested had evidence of genital human papillomavirus infection (Bauer et al., 1991).

Other STD-Related Cancers

Although carcinomas of the vulva, vagina, anus, and penis each occur considerably less frequently than cervical carcinoma, aggregate numbers of vulvar, vaginal, anal, and penile carcinomas equal nearly half the total numbers of cases of cervical cancer in the United States. These cancers are also strongly associated with human papillomavirus infection. Approximately 60 to 90 percent of cancers at these sites are associated with human papillomavirus, particularly types 16 and 18 (Paavonen et al., 1990). Infection with HIV also may increase the risk that human papillomavirus infection will progress to cancer of the cervix or to the other sites mentioned above.

Reproductive Health Problems

STDs represent a serious threat to the reproductive capability of couples, largely because of the impact of STDs on women. A variety of women's health problems all result from unrecognized or untreated STDs. Reproductive health complications include both short-term (e.g., pelvic inflammatory disease, pregnancy complications, epididymitis) and long-term consequences (e.g., infertility and ectopic pregnancy).

Pelvic Inflammatory Disease

One of the most serious threats to the reproductive capability of women is infection of the upper genital tract, referred to as pelvic inflammatory disease (McCormack, 1994). Most cases of this disease are associated with chlamydial infection and gonorrhea (Jossens et al., 1994), which initially involve the cervix, but in some women disease can spread up into the uterus and through the fallopian tubes into the pelvis and abdominal cavity. Pelvic inflammatory disease is a preventable complication of these sexually transmitted infections (Washington et al., 1991).

Each year, more than one million U.S. women experience an episode of pelvic inflammatory disease (Washington and Katz, 1991; Rolfs et al., 1992). Some cases of acute pelvic inflammatory disease result in abscesses involving the ovaries and fallopian tubes, which require surgical intervention. At least one-quarter of women with acute pelvic inflammatory disease will experience serious long-term sequelae, the most common and important of which are ectopic pregnancy (the development of a fetus outside the uterus) and tubal-factor infertility. Other complications include chronic pelvic pain and pain during intercourse caused by scarring in the pelvis.

The above health problems are all recognized consequences of symptomatic pelvic inflammatory disease. Perhaps even more devastating to women's reproductive health is the more recently described "atypical pelvic inflammatory disease" (Cates et al., 1993). Women with this syndrome experience only mild symptoms, unrecognized symptoms, or possibly, in many cases, no symptoms ("silent pelvic inflammatory disease") (Wolner-Hanssen, 1995). This more indolent but insidious form of pelvic inflammatory disease is less likely to be detected compared to symptomatic pelvic inflammatory disease, thus placing unsuspecting women at increased risk of disease sequelae (Morell, 1995). Because these cases of atypical pelvic inflammatory disease are also associated with chlamydial and gonococcal infection in women, prevention of these STDs will result in reductions in morbidity of pelvic inflammatory disease heretofore unrecognized, with accompanying decreases in cost and human suffering.

Ectopic Pregnancy

Ectopic pregnancy usually results from partial tubal blockage due to pelvic inflammatory disease. After an episode of pelvic inflammatory disease, a woman is six to ten times more likely to have an ectopic pregnancy compared to women who do not have pelvic inflammatory disease (Marchbanks et al., 1988). Approximately 9 percent of women with laparoscope-confirmed pelvic inflammatory disease experience an ectopic pregnancy for their first pregnancy subsequent to their episode of pelvic inflammatory disease (Weström et al., 1992). In 1992, the estimated number of ectopic pregnancies was 108,800, or 1 in 50 pregnancies (CDC, 1995a). In addition, in the same year, approximately 9 percent of all pregnancy-related deaths were a result of ectopic pregnancy (NCHS, 1994), making ectopic pregnancy one of the leading and most preventable causes of maternal death during pregnancy (Marchbanks et al., 1988). In fact, ectopic pregnancy is the leading cause of first-trimester deaths among African American women (CDC, DSTD/HIVP, 1995).

Infertility

Infertility can occur when the fallopian tubes become blocked or damaged by STDs. Of all infertile American women, at least 15 percent are infertile because of tubal damage caused by pelvic inflammatory disease. This type of infertility is treated by tubal microsurgery (which attempts to repair the damaged tubes) or by in vitro fertilization (in which an egg is surgically removed from the ovary, mixed with sperm and fertilized outside the body, and then placed directly into the uterus, thus bypassing the blocked fallopian tubes). Of all women infertile because of tubal damage, no more than one-half have previously been diagnosed and treated for acute pelvic inflammatory disease. The remaining half have also had pelvic inflammatory disease but had symptoms that were presumably so mild or atypical that they were never treated for the disease. A large prospective study of women who had laparoscopy because of clinical evaluation for pelvic inflammatory disease showed that approximately 16 percent of women with abnormal laparoscopic findings consistent with this disease tried but failed to conceive during the follow-up period, compared to 3 percent of women with normal laparoscopic findings (Weström et al., 1992). Eleven percent of women with abnormal laparoscopic findings became infertile as a result of tubal factor infertility (5 percent were infertile because of other reasons). After one episode of laparoscope-confirmed pelvic inflammatory disease, approximately 8 percent of women developed tubal-factor infertility, with the risk increasing with the severity of the episode. Each subsequent episode roughly doubled the rate of tubal-factor infertility (20 percent after two episodes and 40 percent after three or more episodes). Ectopic pregnancy also substantially increases the risk of tubal-factor infertility. STDs rarely produce infertility in men.

Health Consequences for Pregnant Women and Infants

STDs are associated with multiple acute complications for pregnant women and their infants (Brunham et al., 1990) (Table 2-3). Pregnant women with STDs may transmit the infection to the fetus, newborn, or infant through the placenta

TABLE 2-3 Major Sequelae of STDs

Health Consequence	Women	Men	Infants
Cancers	Cervical cancer Vulva cancer Vaginal cancer Anal cancer Liver cancer T-cell leukemia Kaposi's sarcoma Body cavity lymphoma	Penile cancer Anal cancer Liver cancer T-cell leukemia Kaposi's sarcoma Body cavity lymphoma	
Reproductive health problems	Pelvic inflammatory disease Infertility Ectopic pregnancy Spontaneous abortion	Epididymitis Prostatitis Infertility	
Pregnancy-related problems	Preterm delivery Premature rupture of membranes Puerperal sepsis Postpartum infection		Stillbirth Low birth weight Conjunctivitis Pneumonia Neonatal sepsis Acute hepatitis Neurologic damage Congenital abnormalities
Neurologic problems	HTLV-associated myelopathy (paralysis) Neurosyphilis	HTLV-associated myelopathy (paralysis) Neurosyphilis	Cytomegalovirus-, herpes- simplex- virus-, and syphilis-associated neurologic problems Group B strep meningitis
Other common health consequences	Chronic liver disease Cirrhosis	Chronic liver disease Cirrhosis	Chronic liver disease Cirrhosis

(congenital infection), during passage through the birth canal (perinatal infection), or after birth as a result of breast-feeding or close direct contact. Common sexually transmitted infections that have been shown to cause adverse health effects among pregnant women and their infants include chlamydial infection, gonorrhea, syphilis, cytomegalovirus infection, genital herpes, and HIV infection. Other sexually transmitted pathogens transmitted from the mother to the fetus, newborn, or infant may produce mainly delayed manifestations that may appear only after years (e.g., human papillomavirus) or even decades (e.g., hepatitis B virus, human T-cell lymphotrophic virus type I).

Active sexually transmitted infection during pregnancy may result in spontaneous abortion, stillbirths, premature rupture of membranes, and preterm delivery. For example, up to 80 percent of pregnancies associated with untreated early syphilis result in stillbirth or clinical evidence of congenital syphilis in the newborn (Schulz et al., 1990). Preterm delivery accounts for approximately 75 percent of neonatal deaths not caused by congenital malformations (Main and Main, 1991). A recent study confirmed that bacterial vaginosis in pregnant women is associated with premature delivery of a low-birth-weight infant; women with bacterial vaginosis are 40 percent more likely to deliver a premature infant compared to women without this condition (Hillier et al., 1995).

Health Consequences for Infected Infants

Sexually transmitted pathogens that have serious consequences among adults tend to cause even more severe, potentially life-threatening health conditions in the fetus or newborn, whose immune system is immature. Damage to the brain, spinal cord, and the organs of special senses (especially the eyes and the auditory nerves) are of particular concern with many sexually transmitted infections in the fetus or infant. Infections with cytomegalovirus, herpes simplex virus, HIV, and human T-cell lymphotropic virus type I, as well as syphilis and gonococcal and chlamydial infection, all can produce one or more of the above complications. Severe, permanent central nervous system manifestations or fetal or neonatal death can result from congenital syphilis. Infection of the fetus with cytomegalovirus may result in growth retardation, destruction of portions of the central nervous system, auditory nerve deafness, low IQ, and damage to other organs. Similarly, severe neurological damage resulting in mental retardation, other manifestations of severe brain damage, or death can result from herpes simplex virus infections.

Currently, essentially all transmission of HIV to young children in the United States is attributable to mother-to-infant transmission. HIV infection progresses more rapidly in infants than in adults; more than 80 percent of untreated infants will develop symptoms of infection by 18–24 months of age (Pizzo et al., 1995). Survival models suggest that there are two distinct groups of HIV-infected infants with regard to survival: the median age at death for the first group, who have a high probability of dying within four years, is 5–11 months, and the median age at death for the second group is more than five years (Byers et al., 1993). Human T-cell lymphotropic virus type 1, a retrovirus that is transmitted sexually among adults, is also transmitted perinatally or postnatally from mother to infant and may result in T-cell malignancies and a progressive form of paralysis known as HTLV-1-associated myelopathy later in life. Ophthalmia neonatorum, an eye infection in newborns, results when infants of women with vaginal gonorrhea or chlamydial infection are infected during delivery. Gonococcal ophthalmia neonatorum often produces severe initial inflammation of the tissues around the eye, which may result in corneal ulcers and eventual blindness. Chlamydial pneumonia is also a common illness among infants born to mothers with chlamydial cervical infection. Hepatitis B virus infection, when acquired during birth, becomes a chronic infection in as many as 90 percent of infected newborn infants and may lead to cirrhosis of the liver or liver cancer during midlife in a large proportion of those infected perinatally.

Health Consequences for Infected Pregnant Women

Pregnant women are at increased risk for complications of STDs. Vaginal and cervical infections with STD pathogens can lead to inflammation of the placenta or fetal membranes, resulting in maternal fever during or after delivery, to wound and pelvic infections after Cesarean section, and to postpartum infection of the uterus that may result in infertility (Brunham et al., 1990). As mentioned previously, ectopic pregnancy caused by previous pelvic inflammatory disease is one of the leading causes of maternal death during pregnancy.

Health Consequences for Men

In the United States, HIV infection is currently much more common among men than among women. Acute health consequences of some STDs (e.g., syphilis) are similar in both men and women. Human papillomavirus is associated with cancer of the penis and anus in men; these cancers, however, are less common than cervical cancer in women. Certain STDs, such as gonorrhea and chlamydial infection, produce complications that are unique or more severe in women than in men. However, both gonorrhea and chlamydial infection produce epididymitis in men and chlamydial infection is associated with Reiter's Syndrome, which seems to be more common among men than among women (Berger, 1990). Urethral stricture is a late manifestation of gonorrhea or chlamydial urethritis and is common in developing countries. Infertility seems to be a rare complication of STDs in men. The role of STDs in prostatitis (inflammation of the prostate gland) is uncertain (Colleen and Mårdh, 1990). Over and Piot (1993) compared the health impact of STDs in men and women and have reported that the health burden attributed to five STDs (i.e., chancroid, chlamydial infection, gonorrhea, HIV infection, and syphilis) in men was also high.

Deaths Associated with STDs

AIDS-associated deaths, which account for the largest number of STD-related deaths, have received considerable attention. Of 513,486 persons with AIDS reported in the United States through December 1995, more than 62 percent (319,849) have died (CDC, 1995b). As indicated above, many other STDs cause potentially fatal complications in adults as well as in the fetus or infant. The largest number of deaths related to STDs other than AIDS are caused by cervical and other human papillomavirus-related cancers; liver disease (e.g., chronic liver disease and liver cancer) caused by hepatitis B virus; pelvic inflammatory disease and ectopic pregnancy; and various pregnancy, fetal, and neonatal complications.

In a recent study completed by investigators at the CDC, more than 150,000 deaths were directly attributed to STDs, including AIDS, from 1973 through 1992 among American women 15 years of age and older (Ebrahim et al., 1995). According to this report, the three leading causes of STD-related deaths in 1992 among these women were cervical cancer (57 percent of deaths), AIDS (29 percent), and hepatitis B and C virus infection (10 percent), all of which are related to viral STDs (Figure 2-4). From 1972 through 1984, the annual number of these STD-related deaths declined by 24 percent; but from 1984 through 1992, STD-related deaths increased by 31 percent, largely as a result of AIDS-related deaths.

In developing countries, the impact of STDs on health also is very substantial. Even when deaths caused by human papillomavirus and hepatitis B virus were not considered, five other STDs (HIV infection, chlamydial infection, gonorrhea, syphilis, and chancroid) ranked among the top 20 causes of loss of productive life in a sub-Saharan African country (Over and Piot, 1993).

IMPACT OF STDs ON HIV TRANSMISSION

The evidence that "ulcerative" STDs, such as chancroid, syphilis, and genital herpes, and "inflammatory" STDs, such as gonorrhea, chlamydia, and trichomoniasis, increase the risk of HIV infection has developed incrementally over the past decade. Although the proportion of HIV infections that could be prevented in the United States by preventing other STDs has not yet been well defined, current estimates suggest that much—perhaps most—of the heterosexually transmitted HIV infection could be prevented by reducing other underlying STDs.

Epidemiological Evidence

The earliest cross-sectional studies found an association between genital

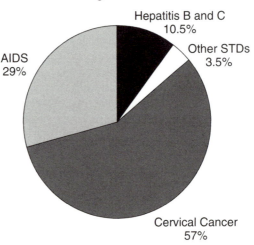

**Cervical cancer is the most common
cause of STD-related deaths
among U.S. women**

FIGURE 2-4 Causes of STD-related deaths among U.S. women, 1992. SOURCE: Ebra-him SH, Peterman TA, Zaidi AA, Kamb ML. Mortality related to sexually transmitted diseases in women, U.S., 1973-1992. Proceedings of the Eleventh Meeting of the International Society for STD Research, August 27-30, 1995, New Orleans, LA [abstract no. 343].

ulcers and HIV infection (Kreiss et al., 1986; Greenblatt et al., 1988), but cohort studies were required to assess the temporal relationship between STDs and acquisition of HIV infection and to prospectively obtain other data that might explain away the apparent association. An extensive 1991 review article (Wasserheit, 1992) found that, of 15 studies that had prospectively analyzed the association between STDs and HIV infection, 3 (Cameron et al., 1989; Plummer et al., 1991; Laga et al., 1993) were designed to allow both accurate ascertainment of the occurrence of an STD prior to HIV infection and adjustment for potential confounding by sexual behaviors and condom use.

As summarized in Table 2-4, three prospective cohort studies in Africa have demonstrated increased risk of HIV infection following genital ulcer disease among heterosexual men (Cameron et al., 1989) and among female sex workers[3]

---

[3] The term "sex worker" is commonly used by public health workers to refer to persons who exchange sex for drugs, money, or other goods. This term is preferable to the term "prostitute."

(Plummer et al., 1991; Nyange et al., 1994). Although the magnitude of the increased risk of transmission attributable to genital ulcers in these studies was expressed as risk ratios ranging from 3.3 to 4.7, Hayes and others (1995) have estimated that genital ulcer disease may increase the per exposure risk of transmission by a factor of 10 to 50 for male-to-female transmission and by a factor of 50 to 300 for female-to-male transmission. Boily and Anderson (1996) also have recently demonstrated that published cohort studies are very likely to underestimate the true magnitude of the increased risk of sexual transmission of HIV conferred by other STDs. Some of these studies have also found that gonorrhea of the cervix (Plummer et al., 1991; Laga et al., 1993; Nyange et al., 1994), chlamydial infection of the cervix (Laga et al., 1993) and vaginal trichomoniasis (Laga et al., 1993), all increase the risk of subsequent HIV infection. Although Laga and others initially reported no increase in HIV infection following genital ulcer disease among female sex workers (Laga et al., 1993), a later study involving the same study population did find such an association (Laga et al., 1994).

In the United States, the multicenter AIDS cohort study found no association between herpes simplex virus type 2 antibody and subsequent HIV infection among men who have sex with men (Kingsley et al., 1990). However, an earlier retrospective cohort study in gay men found that herpes simplex virus type 2 infection was a risk factor for HIV infection (Holmberg et al., 1988). In addition, a study of heterosexual men attending an STD clinic in New York showed that men presenting with chancroid were more likely to become infected with HIV than were men presenting with other STDs (Telzak et al., 1993).

Explaining the Association Between STDs and HIV Infection

The above prospective studies establish the temporal relationship of exposure to STD prior to HIV infection. The observed associations between STDs and HIV infection are compatible with three possible explanations, other than the confounding factors addressed by the study designs:

1. *STDs increase infectivity of HIV.* Persons who have both an STD and HIV infection may be more likely to transmit HIV to others due to the effects of the STD on HIV infectivity, such as increased shedding of HIV.

2. *STDs increase susceptibility to HIV.* Persons with an STD may be more susceptible to a subsequent exposure to HIV, since the STD may compromise the mucosal or cutaneous surfaces of the genital tract that normally act as a barrier against HIV.

3. *The association between STDs and HIV remains confounded by sexual behavior and/or by immune suppression in persons with sexually acquired HIV.* HIV-infected persons may be more likely than uninfected persons to have another STD due to high-risk sexual behavior or because HIV-related immune suppression predisposes to active STD (e.g., by reactivating genital ulcers or by

TABLE 2-4 Results of Major Epidemiological Studies Regarding the Risk of Subsequent HIV Infection Among Persons with Specific Existing STDs

Reference	Study Site: Population	Relative Risk or Odds Ratios (95% confidence intervals)					
		Genital Ulcerative Disease	Syphilis	Herpes Simplex Virus type 2	Gonorrhea	Chlamydial Infection	Trichomoniasis
Cameron et al., 1989	Nairobi: Male STD patients	4.7 (1.3, 17)					
Plummer et al., 1991	Nairobi: Female sex workers	3.3 (1.2, 10.1)				2.7 (0.9, 7.8)	
Laga et al., 1993	Kinshasa: Female sex workers	a			4.8 (2.4, 9.8)	3.6 (1.3, 11.0)	1.9 (0.9, 4.1)
Telzak et al., 1993	New York: Male STD patients	3.3[b] (1.1, 10.1)					
Kingsley et al., 1990	U.S.: Men who have sex with men			1.0 (0.3, 2.9)			
Nyange et al., 1994	Mombasa: Female sex workers		6.5 (1.5, 27.9)		1.8 (1.0, 9.9)		

NOTE: The studies in this table represent prospective cohort or cohort-nested case-control studies that were designed to demonstrate temporal relationships between STDs and HIV infection. In this context, relative risks and odds ratios indicate the likelihood of an outcome (HIV infection) in a person with a specific STD compared to a person without that STD. For example, in the first study, men with genital ulcerative disease were almost five times as likely as those without genital ulcerative disease to become subsequently infected with HIV.

[a]Genital ulcerative disease did not significantly increase the risk for HIV infection in this study, but did increase the risk for HIV infection in a subsequent analysis (Laga et al., 1994).

[b]Odds ratio is for chancroid, based on laboratory or clinical diagnosis.

SOURCES:

Cameron DW, Simonsen JN, D'Costa LJ, Ronald AR, Maitha GM, Gakinya MN, et al. Female to male transmission of human immunodeficiency virus type 1: risk factors for seroconversion in men. Lancet 1989;2:403-7.

Kingsley LA, Armstrong J, Rahman A, Ho M, Rinaldo CR Jr. No association between herpes simplex virus type-2 seropositivity or anogenital lesions and HIV seroconversion among homosexual men [see comments]. J Acquir Immune Defic Syndr 1990; 3:773-9.

Laga M, Alary M, Nzila N, Manoka AT, Tuliza M, Behets F, et al. Condom promotion, sexually transmitted diseases treatment, and declining incidence of HIV-1 infection in female Zairian sex workers. Lancet 1994;344:246-8.

Laga M, Manoka A, Kivuvu M, Malele B, Tuliza M, Nzila N, et al. Non ulcerative sexually transmitted diseases as risk factors for HIV-1 transmission in women: results from a cohort study. AIDS 1993;7:95-102.

Nyange P, Martin H, Mandaliya K, Jackson D, Ndinya-Achola JO, Ngugi E, et al. Cofactors for heterosexual transmission of HIV to prositutes in Mombasa Kenya. Ninth International Conference on AIDS and STD in Africa, December 10-14, 1994, Kampala, Uganda.

Plummer FA, Simonsen JN, Cameron DW, Ndinya-Achola JO, Kreiss JK, Gakinya MN, et al. Co-factors in male-female transmission of human immunodeficiency virus type 1. J Infect Dis 1991;163:233-9.

Telzak EE, Chiasson MA, Bevier PJ, Stoneburner RL, Castro KG, Jaffe HW. HIV-1 seroconversion in patients with and without genital ulcer disease. A prospective study. Ann Int Med 1993;119:1181-6.

making ulcerative disease harder to cure). Therefore, at any given level of sexual activity, persons exposed to an HIV-infected person may also be exposed to another STD.

Although the third explanation may account for at least some of the association of STDs with subsequent HIV infection, there are strong data to support the concept that STDs increase HIV infectivity and HIV susceptibility. An effect on HIV infectivity is strongly supported by the presence of HIV in genital ulcers (Plummer et al., 1991; Kreiss et al., 1994); by the increased rate of detection of HIV DNA (cell-associated HIV) in cervical swab specimens among women with cervical inflammation (Clemetson et al., 1993; Kreiss et al., 1994; John et al., 1996; Gys et al., 1996; Mostad et al., 1996); by the increased prevalence of HIV DNA in swab specimens from men with gonococcal urethritis (Moss et al., 1995); and by increased concentrations of cell-free HIV RNA in semen from men with gonococcal urethritis (Hoffman et al., 1996). The impact of genital shedding of HIV on sexual or perinatal transmission has yet to be precisely measured but is likely a critical factor in transmission. An effect of other STDs on susceptibility to HIV is supported by studies of couples where one partner was HIV-positive and the other was not. HIV-negative partners who developed genital infections were more likely to become subsequently infected with HIV than were those HIV-negative partners who did not have genital infections (de Vincenzi, 1994; Deschamps et al., 1996).

Evidence of Effect of STD Prevention on HIV Prevention

Several studies provide evidence that early detection and treatment of STDs can have a major impact on sexual transmission of HIV. Moss and colleagues (1995) found that the rate of detection of HIV DNA in urethral specimens among men with gonococcal urethritis fell by half within one to two weeks after curative treatment. It remains unclear if urethral shedding of cell-associated HIV is a good surrogate for HIV infectivity. Moreover, Hoffman and colleagues (1996) recently reported that the concentration of cell-free HIV RNA in semen fell significantly in men after treatment of gonococcal urethritis.

Laga and others (1994) demonstrated that monthly laboratory testing and treatment for STDs reduced the incidence of HIV infection among female sex workers in Zaire. An increasing proportion of visits for STD-related care significantly reduced the incidence of HIV infection over time, among both regular and inconsistent condom users. Nonetheless, such time-series analyses remain subject to participation bias, despite adjusting for frequency of unprotected sex. For example, those with less frequent visits may have had higher-risk partners or riskier behaviors that were not measured. A randomized controlled trial remains essential to prove that STD screening and treatment decrease susceptibility of women to acquisition of HIV.

The strongest data demonstrating that improved STD management reduces sexual transmission of HIV are from the findings of a large, prospective, randomized controlled trial recently completed in Tanzania (Grosskurth et al., 1995a, 1995b). Six pairs of communities were each randomized to receive either improved syndromic management of STDs at the primary care level or the standard management for STDs. Improved syndromic management was developed through extensive training and supervision of primary health center workers, provision of antimicrobials, and educational activities to improve health-care seeking behavior for symptoms of STDs. Sentinel cohorts of one thousand persons per community were followed for two years to measure the incidence of new HIV infections. Overall, the incidence of HIV infection was 42 percent lower in communities with improved management of STDs compared to control communities, and each community with improved STD management experienced a lower incidence of HIV infection compared to the paired control community. The prevalence and incidence of symptomatic urethritis in men and serologic evidence of active syphilis in the sentinel cohorts also were significantly lower in the intervention communities (Hayes et al., 1996). The investigators hypothesized that the reduction of HIV incidence among communities with improved syndromic management of STDs resulted from shortening the duration of STD syndromes among infected persons. These findings suggest that large reductions in STD incidence or prevalence are not necessary to influence HIV transmission. It is possible that greater reductions in STD rates might have produced even greater reductions in HIV incidence.

Estimating the Impact of STDs on HIV Transmission

Estimating the impact of preventive interventions on the transmission of STDs in a population is extremely complex. Static epidemiological models that depend upon relative risks and attributable risks to estimate the contribution of causal factors to noncommunicable disease incidence are not sufficient to estimate the impact of causal factors on communicable diseases, including STDs or HIV (Aral et al., 1996). One also needs to consider partner selection patterns that lead to exposure of uninfected to infected individuals in the population; the prevalence of the causal factor at the point where infected and uninfected individuals mix; and the existence of threshold levels of transmission required to sustain the infection in population subgroups (Anderson and May, 1991).

Retrospective cohort studies in the United States have suggested that other STDs do increase sexual transmission of HIV among men who have sex with men (Darrow et al., 1987; Holmberg et al., 1988). The rapid decline of HIV incidence among these men during the early 1990s was accompanied by rapid declines in STDs such as gonorrhea and syphilis. Declining rates of STDs, along with changing sexual practices, may have contributed to the rapid decline in incidence of HIV infection. However, the strongest evidence for the link between

STD and HIV transmission in the United States is related to heterosexual transmission of HIV. In the United States, heterosexual transmission represents the fastest growing proportion of AIDS cases (CDC, 1994c). Studies indicate that heterosexual transmission of HIV is currently most common among age, ethnic, and socioeconomic groups that have the highest incidence of traditional STDs, such as gonorrhea and syphilis (Ellerbrock et al., 1992; Johnson et al., 1993; Edlin et al., 1994; Levine et al., 1995; Shakarishvili et al., 1995). In addition, increases in syphilis incidence in specific areas throughout the United States have preceded increases in HIV prevalence among prenatal women by about two years (St. Louis et al., 1995). For example, the geographic distribution of reported gonorrhea and syphilis in the United States corresponds closely with the distribution of areas with the highest prevalence of HIV among pregnant women (Figure 2-5).

In the absence of prospective studies or formal trials of strengthened STD interventions to reduce sexual transmission of HIV in the United States (which may not be feasible), mathematical modeling may be essential to assess the potential impact of reducing STDs on HIV transmission. Such models are very complex and dependent on many assumptions related to sexual behaviors, the natural history and epidemiology of STDs, and the interactions between STDs and HIV. Robinson and colleagues (1995) predicted that a 50 percent reduction in the duration of STDs in Uganda could decrease HIV transmission by 43 percent—a prediction remarkably close to that observed in the intervention trial in nearby Tanzania. A number of approaches have been used to model the impact of various determinants on the spread of HIV and other STDs and the influence of other STDs on the HIV epidemic (Appendix C).

Boily has developed a model using published data on the distribution of sexual activity in the United States; estimates of the prevalence and duration of chlamydial infection; the effect of chlamydia on the efficiency of HIV transmission (including effects on infectivity and susceptibility to HIV); assumptions on the patterns of sexual mixing of the U.S. population; and demographic parameters (Appendix C). Given parameter assumptions, the model showed that HIV infection could not be established in the general U.S. heterosexual population in the absence of chlamydial infection (or other STDs with comparable effects on HIV transmission).

The work of Over and Piot (1993) also supports the concept that reducing STDs could have a significant impact on sexually transmitted HIV infections. As mentioned previously, they estimated that successfully treating or preventing one hundred cases of syphilis among high-risk groups for STDs would prevent 1,200 HIV infections that would be linked to those one hundred syphilis infections during a 10-year period.

57

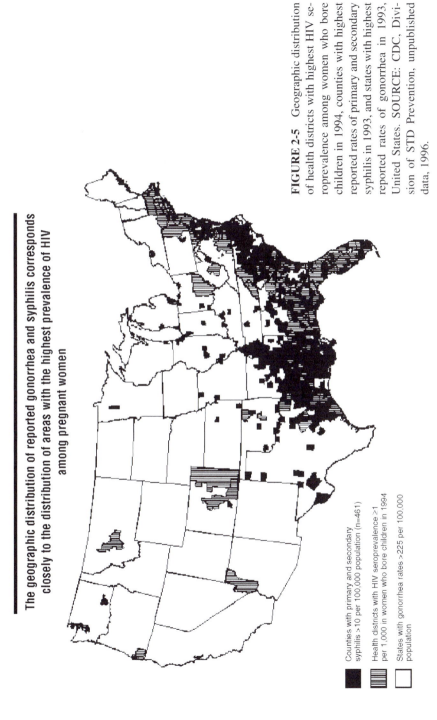

The geographic distribution of reported gonorrhea and syphilis corresponds closely to the distribution of areas with the highest prevalence of HIV among pregnant women

Counties with primary and secondary syphilis >10 per 100,000 population (n=461)

Health districts with HIV seroprevalence >1 per 1,000 in women who bore children in 1994

States with gonorrhea rates >225 per 100,000 population

FIGURE 2-5 Geographic distribution of health districts with highest HIV seroprevalence among women who bore children in 1994, counties with highest reported rates of primary and secondary syphilis in 1993, and states with highest reported rates of gonorrhea in 1993, United States. SOURCE: CDC, Division of STD Prevention, unpublished data, 1996.

ECONOMIC CONSEQUENCES OF STDs

While the substantial morbidity caused by STDs is now being more widely recognized, little attention has been paid to what they cost. Limited resources and current competing health care needs, however, are forcing consideration of the economic consequences of STDs as a pivotal criterion for determining the relative urgency of this problem. By this measure also, STDs rank as a formidable health problem.

Estimating STD-Associated Costs

The economic burden of STDs is associated with both direct and indirect cost. Direct costs refer to expenditures for health care and represent the value of goods and services that actually were used to treat STDs or associated sequelae. These direct health care expenditures may be for either medical or nonmedical services and materials. Examples of STD-related direct costs include costs for health professionals' services (i.e., physicians, nurses, and technicians), costs of laboratory services, and cost of hospitalizations for STD (i.e., hospital accommodations and operating room). Resources used for transportation, residential care, special education, and other similar purposes are also considered direct costs. In contrast, indirect costs refer to lost productivity and represent the value of output forgone by individuals with STDs and associated disability. Indirect costs include these lost wages due to not working and/or value of household management that is not performed because of STD-related illnesses. Lost wages due to premature deaths are also considered indirect costs.

The costs of a few STDs have been estimated (IOM, 1985; Washington et al., 1987; Washington and Katz, 1991), but no comprehensive, current analysis of the direct and indirect costs of STDs is available. Such information is vital to accurately depict the full magnitude of the STD problem. Moreover, only with complete STD cost data can the true benefits of investments in STD prevention be assessed. Therefore, the committee commissioned a paper to provide the basis for estimating the economic burden of STDs. Results from this analysis (conducted by Joanna Siegel at the Harvard School of Public Health) are summarized below (Table 2-5) and described in more detail in Appendix D.

Total costs for a selected group of common STDs and related syndromes are estimated to be approximately $10 billion in 1994 dollars (Table 2-5). Important to note is that this rough, conservative estimate does not capture the economic consequences of several other STDs and associated syndromes such as vaginal bacteriosis, trichomoniasis, nongonococcal urethritis, mucopurulent cervicitis, lymphogranuloma venereum, molluscum contagiosum, scabies, and pediculosis pubis. Nor does this estimate include the annual cost of sexually transmitted HIV/ AIDS-related illness, which is estimated to be $6.7 billion (Table 2-5). Inclusion of these costs raises the overall cost of sexually transmitted illnesses in the United

TABLE 2-5 Estimated Costs of Selected STDs and Associated Sequelae in the United States, 1994

STD	Direct Cost (1994$ millions)	Total Cost[a] (1994$ millions)
Bacterial[b]		
Chlamydial infection	1,513.9	2,013
Gonorrhea	790.6	1,051
Pelvic inflammatory disease	3,118.8	4,148
Syphilis	79.4	106
Chancroid	0.7	1
Viral		
Herpes simplex virus infection[b]	178.3	237
Human papillomavirus infection[c]	2,877.5	3,827
Hepatitis B virus infection[d]	117.0	156
Cervical cancer[a]	554.0	737
Subtotal STDs (excluding HIV/AIDS)	7,484.4[e]	9,954[e]
Sexually transmitted HIV/AIDS[f]	5,025.0	6,683
Total (including HIV/AIDS)[a]	12,509.4	16,638

[a]Total cost assumes a direct to indirect cost ratio of 3:1 (total cost = direct cost × 1.33); this is based on computed ratios for chlamydia of 1:1 (Washington AE, et al., 1987; see above); pelvic inflammatory disease of 2:1 (Washington AE, Katz P. Cost of and payment source for pelvic inflammatory disease. Trends and projections, 1983 through 2000 [see comments]. JAMA 1991;266:2565-9), and hepatitis B of 1:1 (Hepatitis Branch, CDC, unpublished data, 1996).

[b]Bacterial STD, herpes simplex virus infection, and cervical cancer direct costs estimates from Joanna E. Siegel, Sc.D., Harvard School of Public Health (Appendix D of the present report). Estimate assumes 70 percent of cervical cancer is STD-related.

[c]Human papillomavirus direct cost estimate provided by Laura Koutsky, Ph.D., Center for AIDS and STD, University of Washington, Seattle, based on data from Medicaid and other sources. Cost estimate excludes cost of HPV-related cervical cancer.

[d]Hepatitis B virus infection direct costs based on unpublished data from the Hepatitis Branch, Centers for Disease Control and Prevention, Atlanta. Assumes half of estimated cases are sexually transmitted.

[e]Estimate assumes that the non-pelvic-inflammatory-disease-related costs for chlamydia are approximately $462 million, or approximtely 30.5 percent of total chlamydial costs (Washington AE, Johnson RE, Sanders LL. *Chlamydia trachomatis* infections in the United States: what are they costing us? JAMA 1987;257:2070-2), and the non-pelvic-inflammatory-disease-related costs for gonorrhea are $96.4 million or the cost of just primary treatment for gonorrhea (Appendix D of present report).

[f]HIV/AIDS estimates provided by James G. Kahn, M.D., M.P.H., Institute for Health Policy Studies, University of California, San Francisco, based on data in Hellinger FJ. The lifetime cost of treating a person with HIV. JAMA 1993;270:474-8; CDC. HIV/AIDS surveillance report. Atlanta: Centers for Disease Control and Prevention, 1995;7(2); and Rosenberg PS. Scope of the AIDS epidemic in the United States. Science 1995;270:1372-5. Does not reflect costs of more recently recommended therapeutic regimes for this infection.

States to nearly $17 billion in 1994. These cost estimates underscore the enormous burden of STDs on the U.S. economy. They also represent compelling evidence of the need for effective STD prevention programs, especially in light of the fact that a sizable proportion of the direct costs of STDs results from failure to detect and effectively manage STDs in the initial, acute stage. For example, nearly three-fourths of the $1.5 billion cost of chlamydial infections is due to preventable consequences of untreated, initially uncomplicated infections (Washington et al., 1987; Appendix D).

Sources of Payment for STD-Related Costs

There are limited data regarding who pays for the costs associated with STDs. A study of payment sources for pelvic inflammatory disease from 1983 through 1987 found that private insurance and public payment sources covered 41 and 30 percent, respectively, of the direct costs associated with this STD (Washington and Katz, 1991). During the study period, the proportion of payments from private insurance decreased from 54 to 41 percent. Another study in a Midwest county hospital in 1984 and 1985 showed that 54 percent of total charges associated with pelvic inflammatory disease were not reimbursed by a third-party payer or by county funding to the hospital (Nettleman and Jones, 1989).

CONCLUSIONS

STDs affect persons of all racial, cultural, socioeconomic, and religious groups in the United States. Persons of all sexual orientations and sexually active persons in all states, communities, and social networks are at risk for STDs. These diseases are a tremendous health and economic burden on the people of the United States. STDs predominantly affect otherwise healthy youth and young adults, but the consequences can be lifelong. This impact is largely unrecognized by the public and even some health care professionals. Severe complications of STDs include cancer, reproductive health problems, neurologic diseases, and sometimes death. Women and their infants bear a disproportionate burden of these STD-associated complications. The committee estimates that the total annual cost associated with major STDs is approximately $10 billion, which rises to $17 billion when sexually transmitted HIV infections are included. The large number of STD-related deaths and morbidity, and the high costs of managing STDs and their complications, in the United States underscores the importance of effective prevention programs for STDs. Many cases of cancer, infertility, spontaneous abortions, low birth weight, STD-related deaths, and other STD-related conditions are clearly preventable. These data justify investing in effective STD prevention programs to both reduce human suffering and contain health care costs.

The impact of STDs on women's health is substantial. STDs disproportionately impact women because women are more susceptible to infection, they are more likely to have undetected infections, and they are more likely to have STD-related complications compared to men. Adolescents and young adults are at greatest risk for acquiring STDs. Female adolescents appear to be particularly susceptible to several STDs. As described in Chapter 3, adolescents and young adults are also likely to lack information regarding STDs, lack health insurance, and use intoxicating drugs; these factors significantly increase risk for STDs.

Many STDs increase an individual's risk for acquiring and transmitting HIV infection. Therefore, reducing STDs would decrease the incidence of HIV infection in the population. Given the strong association between certain STDs and cervical, liver, and other cancers, cancer prevention programs need to incorporate STD prevention strategies as means for preventing such cancers. As emerging and reemerging infections, new sexually transmitted infections appear on a regular basis and are likely to continue to do so as long as rates of risky sexual behaviors remain high and global economic and demographic factors continue to promote emergence of new STDs. STDs are major international health problems, and all nations will have to contribute to prevention efforts on a global scale.

REFERENCES

ACS (American Cancer Society). Cancer facts and figures—1996. Atlanta: American Cancer Society, 1996.

AGI (Alan Guttmacher Institute). Sex and America's teenagers. New York: AGI, 1994.

Alter MJ. Heterosexual transmission of hepatitis B and implications for vaccine prevention strategies. Can J Infect Dis 1991;2(suppl A):13A-17A.

Alter MJ, Mast EE. The epidemiology of viral hepatitis in the United States. Gastroenterol Clin of North Am 1994;23:437-55.

AMA (American Medical Association), Council on Scientific Affairs. Health care needs of gay men and lesbians in the United States. JAMA 1996;275:1354-9.

Anderson JE, Brackhill R, Mosher WD. Condom use for disease prevention among unmarried U.S. women. Fam Plann Perspect 1996;28:25-28, 39.

Anderson RM, May RM. Infectious diseases of humans: dynamics and control. Oxford, England: Oxford University Press, Inc., 1991.

Andrus JK, Fleming DW, Harger DR, Chin MY, Bennet DV, Horan JM, et al. Partner notification: can it control epidemic syphilis [see comments]? Ann Intern Med 1990;112:539-43.

Aral SO, Guinan ME. Women and sexually transmitted diseases. In: Holmes KK, Mårdh P-A, Sparling PF, Wiesner PJ, eds. Sexually transmitted diseases. 1st ed. New York: McGraw-Hill, Inc., 1984:85-9.

Aral SO, Holmes KK. Sexually transmitted diseases in the AIDS era. Sci Am 1991;264:62-9.

Aral SO, Holmes KK, Padian NS, Cates W Jr. Overview: individual and population approaches to the epidemiology and prevention of sexually transmitted diseases and human immunodeficiency vrus infection. J Inf Dis 1996;174(Suppl 2):S127-33.

Aral SO, Schaffer JE, Mosher WD, Cates W Jr. Gonorrhea rates: what denominator is most appropriate [see comments]? Am J Public Health 1988;78:702-3.

Bauer HM, Ting Y, Greer CE, Chambers JC, Tashiro CJ, Chimera J, et al. Genital human papillomavirus infection in female university students as determined by a PCR-based method. JAMA 1991;265:472-7.

Berger RE. Acute epididymitis. In : Holmes KK, Mårdh P-A, Sparling PF, Weisner PJ, Cates W Jr, Lemon SM, et al., eds. Sexually transmitted diseases. 2nd ed. New York: McGraw-Hill, Inc., 1990:641-51.

Berger BJ, Kolton S, Zenilman JM, Cummings MD, Feldman J, McCormack SM. Bacterial vaginosis in lesbians: a sexually transmitted disease. Clin Inf Dis 1995;21:1402-5.

Bevier PJ, Chiasson MA, Hefferman RT, Castro KG. Women at a sexually transmitted disease clinic who reported same-sex contact: their HIV seroprevalence and risk behaviors. Am J Public Health 1995;85:1366-71.

Boily M-C, Anderson RM. Human immunodeficiency virus transmission and the role of other sexually transmitted diseases: measures of association and study design. Sex Transm Dis 1996;23:312-30.

Brinton LA. Epidemiology of cervical cancer—overview. In: Munoz N, Bosch FX, Shah KV, Meheus A, eds. The epidemiology of cervical cancer and human papillomavirus. Lyon, France: IARC, 1992:3-23.

Brunham RC, Holmes KK, Embree JE. Sexually transmitted diseases in pregnancy. In: Holmes KK, Mårdh P-A, Sparling PF, Weisner PJ, Cates W Jr, Lemon SM, et al., eds. Sexually transmitted diseases. 2nd ed. New York: McGraw-Hill, Inc., 1990:771-801.

Byers B, Caldwell B, Oxtoby M, Pediatric Spectrum of Disease Project. Survival of children with perinatal HIV infection: Evidence for two distinct populations. Proceedings of the Ninth International Conference on AIDS, June 5-11, 1993, Berlin [abstract no. WS-C10-6].

Cameron DW, Simonsen JN, D'Costa LJ, Ronald AR, Maitha GM, Gakinya MN, et al. Female to male transmission of human immunodeficiency virus type 1: risk factors for seroconversion in men. Lancet 1989; 2:403-7.

Cates W Jr. Epidemiology and control of sexually transmitted diseases in adolescents. In: Schydlower M, Shafer MA, eds. AIDS and other sexually transmitted diseases. Philadelphia: Hanly & Belfus, Inc., 1990:409-27.

Cates W Jr, Joesoef MR, Goldman MB. Atypical pelvic inflammatory disease: can we identify clinical predictors? Am J Obstet Gynecol 1993;169:341-6.

CDC (Centers for Disease Control and Prevention). 1993 Sexually transmitted diseases treatment guidelines. MMWR 1993;42(No. RR-14):56-66.

CDC. Decreased susceptibility of *Neisseria gonorrhoeae* to fluoroquinolones—Ohio and Hawaii, 1992-1994. MMWR 1994a;43:325-7.

CDC. Hepatitis surveillance report no. 55. Atlanta: Centers for Disease Control and Prevention, 1994b:36.

CDC. Heterosexually acquired AIDS—United States, 1993. MMWR 1994c;43:9:156-60.

CDC. Ectopic pregnancy—United States, 1990-1992. MMWR 1995a;44:46-8.

CDC. HIV/AIDS surveillance report. Atlanta: Centers for Disease Control and Prevention, 1995b;7(2).

CDC. Trends in sexual risk behavior among high school students—United States, 1990, 1991, and 1993. MMWR 1995c;44:124-5, 131-2.

CDC. Ten leading nationally notifiable infectious diseases—United Sates, 1995. MMWR 1996;45:883-4.

CDC, DSTD/HIVP (Division of STD/HIV Prevention). Annual report 1992. U.S. Department of Health and Human Services, Public Health Service. Atlanta: Centers for Disease Control and Prevention, 1993.

CDC, DSTD/HIVP. Annual report 1994. U.S. Department of Health and Human Services, Public Health Service. Atlanta: Centers for Disease Control and Prevention, 1995.

CDC, DSTDP (Division of STD Prevention). Sexually transmitted disease surveillance 1994. U.S. Department of Health and Human Services, Public Health Service. Atlanta: Centers for Disease Control and Prevention, 1995.

CDC, DSTDP. Sexually transmitted disease surveillance 1995. U.S. Department of Health and Human Services, Public Health Service. Atlanta: Centers for Disease Control and Prevention, September 1996.

CDC, Hepatitis Branch. Epidemiology and prevention of viral hepatitis A to E: an overview. U.S. Department of Health and Human Services, Public Health Service. Atlanta: Centers for Disease Control and Prevention, 1995. [slide set]

Chang Y, Cesarman E, Pessin MS, Lee F, Culpepper J, Knowles DM, et al. Identification of herpesvirus-like DNA sequences in AIDS-associated Kaposi's sarcoma. Science 1994;266:1865-9.

Christenson B, Bottiger M, Svensson A, Jeansson S. A 15-year surveillance study of antibodies to herpes simplex virus types 1 and 2 in a cohort of young girls. J Infect 1992;25:147-54.

Chu SY, Buehler JW, Fleming PL, Berkelman RL. Epidemiology of reported cases of AIDS in lesbians: United States 1980-1989. Am J Public Health 1990;80:1380-1.

Chu SY, Conti L, Schable BA, Diaz T. Female-to-female sexual contact and HIV transmission. JAMA 1994;272:433.

Clemetson DB, Moss GB, Willerford DM, Hensel M, Emonyi W, Holmes KK, et al. Detection of HIV DNA in cervical and vaginal secretions. Prevalence and correlates among women in Nairobi, Kenya. JAMA 1993;269:2860-4.

Cohen H, Marmor M, Wolfe H, Ribble D. Risk assessment of HIV transmission among lesbians. J Acquir Immune Defic Syndr 1993;6:1173-4.

Colleen S, Mårdh PA. Prostatitis. In : Holmes KK, Mårdh P-A, Sparling PF, Weisner PJ, Cates W Jr, Lemon SM, et al., eds. Sexually transmitted diseases. 2nd ed. New York: McGraw-Hill, Inc., 1990:653-61.

Darrow WW, Echenberg DF, Jaffe HW, O'Malley PM, Byers RH, Getchell JP, et al. Risk factors for human immunodeficiency virus (HIV) infections in homosexual men. Am J Public Health 1987;77:479-83.

Deschamps MM, Pape JW, Hafner A, Johnson WD. Heterosexual transmission of HIV in Haiti. Ann Intern Med 1996;125:324-30.

de Vincenzi I. A longitudinal study of human immunodeficiency virus transmission by heterosexual partners. European Study Group on Heterosexual Transmission of HIV [see comments]. N Engl J Med 1994; 331:341-6.

Donegan SP, Jani DB, Flaherty EE, Heeren TC, Rice PA. The male to female transmission of Neisseria gonorrhoeae is influenced by level of antibody to gonococcal reduction modifiable protein (Rmp) or protein III. In: Conde-Glez CJ, Morse S, Rice P, Sparling PF, Calderon E, eds. Pathobiology and immunology of Neisseriaceae. National Institute of Public Health, Cuernavaca, Mexico, 1994 p. 645.

Ebrahim SH, Peterman TA, Zaidi AA, Kamb ML. Mortality related to sexually transmitted diseases in women, U.S., 1973-1992. Eleventh Meeting of the International Society for STD Research, August 27-30, 1995, New Orleans, LA [abstract no. 343].

Edlin BR, Irwin KL, Faruque S, McCoy CB, World C, Seranno Y, et al. Intersecting epidemics—crack cocaine use and HIV infection among inner-city young adults. Multicenter Crack Cocaine and HIV Infection Study Team. N Engl J Med 1994;331:1422-7.

Ellen JM, Kohn RP, Bolan GA, Shiboski S, Krieger N. Socioeconomic differences in sexually transmitted disease rates among black and white adolescents, San Francisco, 1990 to 1992. Am J Public Health 1995;85:1546-8.

Ellerbrock TV, Lieb S, Harrington PE, Bush TJ, Schoenfisch SA, Oxtoby MJ, et al. Heterosexually transmitted human immunodeficiency virus infection among pregnant women in a rural Florida community. N Engl J Med 1992;327:1704-9.

Farley TA, Hadler JL, Gunn RA. The syphilis epidemic in Connecticut: relationship to drug use and prostitution. Sex Transm Dis 1990;17:163-8.

Fish AN, Fairweather DV, Oriel JD, Ridgeway GL. Chlamydia trachomatis infection in a gynecology clinic population: identification of high-risk groups and the value of contact tracing. Eur J Obstet Gynecol Reprod Biol 1989;31:67-74.

GDHR (Georgia Department of Human Resources), Epidemiology and Prevention Branch. Fluoro-quinolone resistant *Neisseria gonorrhoeae* in Georgia. Georgia Epideml Rep 1995;11:2-3.

Goldstein S, Alter M, Moyer L, Kaluba J, Mahoney F, et al. The incidence and epidemiology of acute hepatitis B in the United States; 1989-1994. Ninth Triannual International Symposium on Viral Hepatitis and Liver Disease, April 21-25, 1996, Rome [abstract no. A234].

Greenblatt RM, Lukehart SA, Plummer FA, Quinn TC, Critchlow CW, Ashley RL, D'Costa LJ, Ndinya-Achola JO, Corey L, Ronald AR, Holmes KK. Genital ulceration as a risk factor for human immunodeficiency virus infection. AIDS 1988;2:47-50.

Grosskurth H, Mosha F, Todd J, Mwijarubi E, Klokke A, Senkoro K, et al. Impact of improved treatment of sexually transmitted diseases on HIV infection in rural Tanzania: randomized controlled trial [see comments]. Lancet 1995a;346:530-6.

Grosskurth H, Mosha F, Todd J, Senkoro K, Newell J, Klokke A, et al. A community trial of the impact of improved STD treatment on the HIV epidemic in rural Tanzania: 2. Baseline survey results. AIDS 1995b;9:927-34.

Gys PD, Fransen K, Diallo MO, Ettiegne-Traore V, Maurice C, Hoyi-Adansou YM, et al. The association between cervico-vaginal HIV-1 shedding and STD, immunosuppression, and serum HIV-1 load in female sex workers in Abidjan, Côte D'Ivoire. Eleventh International Confer-ence on AIDS, July 7-12, 1996, Vancouver [abstract no. WeC 332].

Hahn RA, Magder LS, Aral SO, Johnson RE, Larsen SA. Race and the prevalence of syphilis seroreactivity in the United States population: a national sero-epidemiologic study. Am J Pub-lic Health 1989;79:467-70.

Harlap S, Kost K, Forrest JD. Preventing pregnancy, protecting health: a new look at birth control choices in the United States. New York: Alan Guttmacher Institute, 1991.

Hauth JC, Goldenberg RL, Andrews WW, Dubard MD, Copper RL. Reduced incidence of preterm delivery with metronidazole and erythromycin in women with bacterial vaginosis. N Engl J Med 1995;333:1732-6.

Haverkos HW. Female-to-male transmission of HIV [letter]. JAMA 1992;268:1855.

Hayes R, Mwijarubi E, Grosskurth H, Heiner J, Fosha F, Mayaud P, et al. Improved STD treatment significantly reduces prevalence of syphilis and symptomatic urethritis in rural Tanzania. Elev-enth International AIDS Conference, July 7-12, 1996,Vancouver [abstract no. LB.C.6062].

Hayes RJ, Schulz KF, Plummer FA. The cofactor effect of genital ulcers on the per exposure risk of HIV transmission in sub-Saharan Africa. J Trop Med Hyg 1995;98:1-8.

Hillier SL, Nugent RP, Eschenbach DA, Krohn MA, Gibbs RS, Martin DH, et al. Association between bacterial vaginosis and preterm delivery of a low birth-weight infant. N Engl J Med 1995;333:1737-42.

Hillis SD, Joesoef R, Marchbanks PA, Wasserheit JN, Cates W Jr, Westrom L. Delayed care of pelvic inflammatory disease as a risk factor for impaired fertility. Am J Obstet Gynecol 1993;168:1503-9.

Hoffman I, Maida M, Royce R, Costello-Daly C, Kazembe P, Vernazza P, et al. Effects of urethritis therapy on the concentration of HIV-1 in seminal plasma. Eleventh International Conference on AIDS, July 7-12, 1996, Vancouver [abstract no. mo.C.903].

Holmberg SD, Stewart JA, Gerber AR, Byers RH, Lee FK, O'Malley PM, et al. Prior herpes simplex virus type 2 infection as a risk factor for HIV infection. JAMA 1988;259:1048-50.

Holmes KK, Johnson DW, Trostle HJ. An estimate of the risk of men acquiring gonorrhea by sexual contact with infected females. Am J Epidemiol 1970;91:170-4.

Hook EW III, Handsfield HH. Gonococcal infections in the adult. In: Holmes KK, Mårdh PA, Sparling PF, Weisner PJ, Cates W Jr, Lemon SM, et al., eds. Sexually transmitted diseases. 2nd ed. New York: McGraw-Hill, Inc., 1990:149-65.

Hooper RR, Reynolds GH, Hones OG, Zaid A, Weisner PJ, Latimer KP, et al. Cohort study of venereal disease. I: The risk of gonorrhea transmission from infected women to men. Am J Epidemiol 1978;108:136-44.

IOM (Institute of Medicine). New vaccine development: establishing priorities; vol. I, Diseases of importance in the United States. Washington, D.C.:National Academy Press, 1985.

IOM. Emerging infections: microbial threats to health in the United States. Washington, D.C.: National Academy Press, 1992.

John G, Nduati R, Mbori-Ngacha D, Overbaugh J, Welch M, Richardson B, et al. Cervico-vaginal HIV-1 DNA in pregnancy. Eleventh International Conference on AIDS, July 7-12, 1996, Vancouver [abstract no. We.C. 331].

Johnson R, Lee F, Hadgu A, McQuillan G, Aral S, Keesling S, et al. U.S. genital herpes trends during the first decade of AIDS—prevalences increased in young whites and elevated in blacks. Proceedings of the Tenth Meeting of the International Society for STD Research, August 29-September 1, 1993, Helsinki [abstract no. 22].

Jossens MO, Schachter J, Sweet RL. Risk factors associated with pelvic inflammatory disease of differing microbial etiologies. Obstet Gynecol 1994;83:989-97.

Judson FN. Gonorrhea. Med Clin North Am 1990;74:1353-67.

Kennedy MB, Scarlett MI, Duerr AC, Chu SY. Assessing HIV risk among women who have sex with women: scientific and communication issues. J Am Med Wom Assoc 1995;50:103-7.

Kingsley LA, Armstrong J, Rahman A, Ho M, Rinaldo CR Jr. No association between herpes simplex virus type-2 seropositivity or anogenital lesions and HIV seroconversion among homosexual men [see comments]. J Acquir Immune Defic Syndr 1990; 3:773-9.

Koutsky LA, Galloway DA, Holmes KK. Epidemiology of genital human papillomavirus infection. Epidemiol Rev 1988;10:122-63.

Kreiss JK, Koech D, Plummer FA, Holmes KK, Lightfoote M, Piot P, et al. AIDS virus infection in Nairobi prostitutes. Spread of the epidemic to East Africa. N Engl J Med 1986;314:414-8.

Kreiss JK, Willerford DM, Hensel M, Emonyi W, Plummer F, Nkinya-Achola J, et al. Association between cervical inflammation and cervical shedding of human immunodeficiency virus DNA. J Infect Dis 1994;170:1597-601.

Krone MR, Kiviat NB, Koutsky LA. The epidemiology of cervical neoplasms. In: Luesley D, Jordan J, Richart RM, eds. Intraepithelial neoplasia of the lower genital tract. New York: Churchill Livingston, Inc., 1995: 49.

Kurman RJ, Henson DE, Herbst AL, Nolter KL, Schiffman MH, for the 1992 National Cancer Institute Workshop. Interim guidelines for the management of abnormal cervical cytology. JAMA 1994;271:1866-9.

Laga M, Alary M, Nzila N, Manoka AT, Tuliza M, Behets F, et al. Condom promotion, sexually transmitted diseases treatment, and declining incidence of HIV-1 infection in female Zairian sex workers. Lancet 1994;344:246-8.

Laga M, Manoka A, Kivuvu M, Malele B, Tuliza M, Nzila N, et al. Non ulcerative sexually transmitted diseases as risk factors for HIV-1 transmission in women: results from a cohort study. AIDS 1993;7:95-102.

Laumann EO, Gagnon JH, Michael RT, Michaels S. The social organization of sexuality: Sexual practices in the United States. Chicago: University of Chicago Press, 1994.

Levine WC, Hughes E, Turner N, et al. Dual epidemics of syphilis and HIV infection among adolescent African-American women in Houston, 1988-1993. Eleventh Meeting of the International Society for STD Research, August 27-30, 1995, New Orleans, LA [abstract no. 51].

Main DM, Main EK. Preterm birth. In: Gabbe SG, Niebyl JR, Simpson JL, eds. Obstetrics: normal and problem pregnancies. 2nd ed. New York: Churchill Livingstone, Inc., 1991:829-80.

Marchbanks PA, Annegers, JF, Coulam CB, Strathy JH, Kurland LT. Risk factors for ectopic pregnancy. A population-based study. JAMA 1988;259:1823-7.

Marrazzo JM, Stine K, Handsfield HH, Kiviat NB, Koutsky LA. Epidemiology of sexually transmitted diseases and cervical neoplasia in lesbian and bisexual women. 18th Conference of the National Lesbian and Gay Health Association, July 13-16, 1996, Seattle, WA [abstract no. C2483]

McCormack WM. Pelvic inflammatory disease [see comments]. N Engl J Med 1994;330:115-9.

Mertz GJ, Benedetti J, Ashley R, Selke SA, Corey L. Risk factors for the sexual transmission of genital herpes. Ann Intern Med 1992;116:197-202.

Moore J, Beeker C, Harrison JS, Eng TR, Doll LS. HIV risk behavior among Peace Corps volunteers. AIDS 1995;9:95-9.

Morell V. Attacking the causes of "silent" infertility. Science 1995;269:775-7.

Moscicki AB, Palefsky J, Gonzales J, Schoolnik GK. Human papillomavirus infection in sexually active adolescent females: prevalence and risk factors. Pediatr Res 1990;28:507-13.

Moss GB, Overbaugh J, Welch M, Reilly M, Bwayo J, Plummer FA, et al. Human immunodeficiency virus DNA in urethral secretions in men: association with gonococcal urethritis and CD4 depletion. J Infect Dis 1995; 172:1469-74.

Mostad S, Welch M, Chohan B, Reilly M, Overbaugh J, Mandaliya K, et al. Cervical and vaginal HIV-1 DNA shedding in female STD clinic attenders. Eleventh International Conference on AIDS, July 7-12, 1996, Vancouver [abstract no. WeC 333].

NCHS (National Center for Health Statistics). Advanced report of final mortality statistics, 1992. U.S. Department of Health and Human Services, Public Health Service, Centers for Disease Control and Prevention, Hyattsville, MD, 1994. Monthly vital statistics report 43(6 Suppl).

Nettleman MD, Jones RB. Proportional payment for pelvic inflammatory disease: who should pay for chlamydial screening? Sex Transm Dis 1989;16:36-40.

NIH (National Institutes of Health). Consensus Development Conference statement on cervical cancer. National Institutes of Health, Bethesda, MD, April 1-3, 1996.

Nyange P, Martin H, Mandaliya K, Jackson D, Ndinya-Achola JO, Ngugi E, et al. Cofactors for heterosexual transmission of HIV to prostitutes in Mombasa Kenya. Ninth International Conference on AIDS and STD in Africa, December 10-14, 1994, Kampala, Uganda.

Over M, Piot P. HIV infection and sexually transmitted disease. In: Jamison DT, Mosley WH, Measham AR, Bobadilla JL, eds. Disease control priorities in developing countries. New York: Oxford University Press, 1993:455-527.

Over M, Piot P. Human immunodeficiency virus infection and other sexually transmitted diseases in developing countries: public health importance and priorities for resouce allocation. J Infect Dis 1996; 174 (Suppl 2):S162-75.

Paavonen J, Koutsky LA, Kiviat N. Cervical neoplasia and other STD-related genital and anal neoplasias. In: Holmes KK, Mårdh P-A, Sparling PF, Weisner PJ, Cates W Jr, Lemon SM, et al., eds. Sexually transmitted diseases. 2nd ed. New York: McGraw-Hill, Inc., 1990:561-92.

Padian N, Shiboski SC, Jewell NP. Female-to-male transmission of human immunodeficiency virus. JAMA 1991;266:1664-7.

Peterman TA, Stoneburner RL, Allen JR, Jaffee HW, Curran JW. Risk of human immunodeficiency virus transmission from heterosexual adults with transfusion-associated infections [published erratum appears in JAMA 1989;262:502]. JAMA 1988;259:55-8.

Piot P, Islam MQ. Sexually transmitted diseases in the 1990s. Global epidemiology and challenges for control. Sex Transm Dis 1994;21(2 Suppl):S7-S13.

Pizzo PA, Wilfert CM, Pediatric AIDS Siena Workshop II. Markers and determinants of disease progression in children with HIV infection. Report of a consensus workshop June 4-6, 1993, Siena, Italy. J Acquir Immune Defic Syndr Hum Retrovirol 1995;8:30-44.

Platt R, Rice PA, McCormack WM. Risk of acquiring gonorrhea and prevalence of abnormal adnexal findings among women recently exposed to gonorrhea. JAMA 1983;250:3205-9.

Plummer FA, Simonsen JN, Cameron DW, Ndinya-Achola JO, Kreiss JK, Gakinya MN, et al. Cofactors in male-female transmission of human immunodeficiency virus type 1. J Infect Dis 1991;163:233-9.

Quinn TC, Cates W Jr. Epidemiology of sexually transmitted diseases in the 1990s. Adv Host Defen Mech 1992; 8:1-37.

Reeves WC, Rawls WE, Brinton LA. Epidemiology of genital papillomaviruses and cervical cancer. Rev Infect Dis 1989;11:426-39.

Robertson P, Schachter J. Failure to identify venereal disease in a lesbian population. Sex Transm Dis 1981;8:75-6.

Robinson NJ, Mulder DW, Auvert B, Hayes RJ. Modeling the impact of alternative HIV intervention strategies in rural Uganda. AIDS 1995; 9:1263-70.

Rolfs RT, Galaid EI, Zaidi AA. Pelvic inflammatory disease: trends in hospitalizations and office visits, 1979 through 1988. Am J Obstet Gynecol 1992;166:983-90.

Rolfs RT, Goldberg M, Sharrar RG. Risk factors for syphilis: cocaine use and prostitution. Am J Public Health 1990;80:853-7.

Rosenberg PS. Scope of the AIDS epidemic in the United States. Science 1995;270:1372-5.

Schiffman MH. Recent progress in defining the epidemiology of human papillomavirus infection and cervical neoplasia. J Natl Cancer Inst 1992;84:394-8.

Schulz KF, Murphy FK, Patamasucon P, Meheus AZ. Congenital syphilis. In: Holmes KK, Mårdh P-A, Sparling PF, Weisner PJ, Cates W Jr, Lemon SM, et al., eds. Sexually transmitted diseases. 2nd ed. New York: McGraw-Hill, Inc., 1990:821-42.

Shafer MA, Prager V, Shalwitz J, Vaughan E, Moscicki B, Brown R, et al. Prevalence of urethral *Chlamydia trachomatis* and *Neisseria gonorrhoea* among asymptomatic, sexually active adolescent boys. J Infect Dis 1987;156:223-4.

Shakarishvili A, Groseclose SL, Hadgu A, Johnson RE, Hayman CR, Miller CA, et al. Chlamydia trachomatis genital infection in disadvantaged young women across the United States: findings from the U.S. Job Corps. Eleventh Meeting of the International Society for STD Research, August 27-30, 1995, New Orleans, LA [abstract no. 23].

Stamm WE, Holmes KK. Chlamydia trachomatis infections in the adult. In: Holmes KK, Mårdh P-A, Sparling PF, Weisner PJ, Cates W Jr, Lemon SM, et al., eds. Sexually transmitted diseases. 2nd ed. New York: McGraw-Hill, Inc., 1990:181-93.

St. Louis ME, Gwinn M, Nakashima A, Davis S, Steinberg S, Wasserheit JN, et al. Covariation of HIV infection among childbearing women with other sexually transmitted diseases in the United States. Eleventh Meeting of the International Society for STD Research, August 27-30, 1995, New Orleans, LA [abstract no. 50].

Telzak EE, Chiasson MA, Bevier PJ, Stoneburner RL, Castro KG, Jaffe HW. HIV-1 seroconversion in patients with and without genital ulcer disease. A prospective study. Ann Int Med 1993;119:1181-6.

Toomey KE, Moran JS, Raffety MP, Beckett GA. Epidemiological considerations of sexually transmitted diseases in underserved populations. Infect Dis Clinics N Am 1993;7:739-52.

Toomey KE, Rafferty MP, Stamm WE. Unrecognized high prevalence of *Chlamydia trachomatis* genital infection in an isolated Alaskan Eskimo population. JAMA 1987;258:53-6.

Washington AE, Cates W Jr, Wasserheit JN. Preventing pelvic inflammatory disease [see comments]. JAMA 1991;266:2574-80.

Washington AE, Johnson RE, Sanders LL. *Chlamydia trachomatis* infections in the United States: what are they costing us? JAMA 1987;257:2070-2.

Washington AE, Johnson RE, Sanders LL, Barnes RC, Alexander ER. Incidence of Chlamydia trachomatis infections in the United States: using reported *Neisseria gonorrhoea* as a surrogate. In: Oriel D, Ridgeway HG, Schachter J, et al., eds. Chlamydia infections. Cambridge, England: Cambridge University Press, 1986:487-90.

Washington AE, Katz P. Cost of and payment source for pelvic inflammatory disease. Trends and projections, 1983 through 2000 [see comments]. JAMA 1991;266:2565-9.

Wasserheit JN. Epidemiologic synergy. Interrelationships between human immunodeficiency virus infection and other sexually transmitted diseases. Sex Transm Dis 1992; 9:61-77.

Wasserheit JN. Effect of changes in human ecology and behavior on patterns of sexually transmitted diseases, including human immunodeficiency virus infection. Proc Natl Acad Sci 1994;91:2430-5.

Wasserheit JN, Holmes KK. Reproductive tract infections: challenges for international health policy, programs, and research. In: Germain A, Holmes KK, Piot P, Wasserheit JN, eds. Reproductive tract infections: global impact and priorities for women's health. New York: Plenum Press, 1992.

Weström L, Joesoef R, Reynolds G, Hagdu A, Thompson SE. Pelvic inflammatory disease and fertility. A cohort study of 1,844 women with laparoscopically verified disease and 657 control women with normal laparoscopic results. Sex Transm Dis 1992;19:185-92.

WHO (World Health Organization), Global Programme on AIDS. Global prevalence and incidence of selected curable sexually transmitted diseases: overview and estimates. Geneva: WHO, 1996.

Wolner-Hanssen P. Silent pelvic inflammatory disease: is it overstated? Obstet Gynecol 1995;86:321-5.

World Bank. World development report, 1993: Investing in health. New York: Oxford University Press, 1993.

3

Factors That Contribute to the Hidden Epidemic

Highlights

- One-quarter of adolescents and young adults in high-risk age groups for STDs do not have health care coverage.
- Only 11 percent of teenagers surveyed reported getting most of their information regarding STDs from their parents or other family members.
- Among prime-time network television shows, there is only 1 portrayal of protective behavior or comment regarding STDs for every 25 instances of sexual behavior shown.
- Nearly 70 percent of students in the twelfth grade have had sexual intercourse and 27 percent of twelfth-grade students have had sex with four or more partners.
- Knowledge and awareness of STDs among the public is poor; almost two-thirds of women 18–60 years of age surveyed knew nothing or very little about STDs other than AIDS.

STDs are behavior-linked diseases that result from unprotected sex. Behavioral, biological, and social factors contribute to the likelihood of contracting an STD. Wasserheit (1994) has described how microenvironments, including microbiological, hormonal, and immunologic factors, influence individual susceptibility and transmission potential for STDs. These microenvironments are partially determined by an individual's sexual practices, substance use, and other health behaviors. These health behaviors, in turn, are influenced by socioeconomic, epidemiologic, and other macroenvironmental factors. In this chapter, the committee examines biological factors contributing to the spread of STDs and shows how both broad and specific social factors affect exposure to STDs and create obstacles to STD prevention. In Chapter 4, the committee examines behavioral factors contributing to risk of STDs.

BIOLOGICAL FACTORS

In Chapter 2, several biological factors that affect the risk of acquiring or transmitting STDs, such as gender and other preexisting or concurrent STDs including HIV infection, were discussed. Other biological factors that contribute to the spread of STDs include the lack of conspicuous signs and symptoms manifested by infected persons, the long lag time from initial infection to signs of severe complications, and the propensity of STDs to more easily infect young women and female adolescents than men. In addition, the committee summarizes the potential impact of male circumcision, vaginal douching, risky sexual practices, and other factors on the spread of STDs or risk of sequelae.

Asymptomatic Infections

As discussed in Chapter 2, many STDs either do not produce acute symptoms or clinical signs of disease or do not produce symptoms sufficiently severe for an infected individual to seek medical attention. For example, as many as 85 percent of women with chlamydial infection are asymptomatic (Fish et al., 1989; Judson, 1990; Stamm et al., 1990). A study of college women seen for routine gynecological examinations found that 79 percent of those who tested positive for chlamydia had no symptoms of disease (Keim et al., 1992). Asymptomatic infection also contributes to the spread of viral STDs including HIV infection, hepatitis B virus infection, genital herpes, and human papillomavirus infection. HIV infection is a prime example of how certain STDs that may go unrecognized for many years allow wide dissemination of infection before it is detected and treated. Lack of awareness that most cases of certain STDs are asymptomatic or otherwise unrecognized leads many susceptible persons to falsely believe that it is possible to tell whether a potential partner is infected with an STD, and similarly explains why many infected asymptomatic persons fail to take precautions to avoid transmitting their infection. Even when symptoms are present, many STDs have nonspecific signs and symptoms, making them difficult to diagnose without laboratory tests. Asymptomatic infection, therefore, is an extremely important biological factor that reduces the likelihood that infected individuals will seek health care and/or receive appropriate diagnoses. This hinders detection and treatment of the infection, increases the period of infectiousness, and thereby promotes the spread of the infection.

Lag Time to Complications

Another biological factor that contributes to the STD epidemic is the long period of time (sometimes years or decades) from initial infection until the appearance of clinically significant problems. The best examples of sexually transmitted pathogens and complications that have long lag times are (a) human papillomavirus and cervical cancer and (b) hepatitis B virus and liver cancer. In both instances, the initial phase of the infection is often asymptomatic and creates obstacles to detection and treatment, as noted above. In addition, the clinical signs of the associated life-threatening cancers usually do not appear until years or decades after the initial infection. Because of this phenomenon, many cases of STD-related cancers and other long-term complications are not attributed to a sexually transmitted infection. At both individual and population levels, the lack of a perceived connection between sexually transmitted infections and these serious complications reduces both the perceived significance of STDs and the motivation to undertake preventive action. Although the lag time between exposure to HIV and development of clinical symptoms of AIDS likewise can be quite long, there is greater awareness of the link between unprotected sex and the risk of acquiring HIV, and ultimately AIDS, compared to other STDs.

Increased Susceptibility of Women and Female Adolescents

Age and gender may influence risk for an STD. Specifically, as mentioned in Chapter 2, young women and female adolescents are more susceptible to STDs compared to their male counterparts because of the biological characteristics of their anatomy (Cates, 1990). This is because in puberty and young adulthood, specific cells (columnar epithelium) that are especially sensitive to invasion by certain sexually transmitted organisms, such as chlamydia and gonococcus, extend from the inner cervix out over the vaginal surface of the cervix, where they are unprotected by cervical mucus. These cells eventually recede into the inner cervix with age.

In addition to biological factors, women and female adolescents may also find it more difficult than men to implement protective behaviors, partly because of the power imbalance between men and women (Elias and Heise, 1994; IOM, 1994). For example, condoms are the most effective protection against STDs for sexually active persons, but the decision whether to use a condom is ultimately up to the male partner, and negotiating condom use may be difficult for women (Rosenberg and Gollub, 1992). The determinants of condom use are discussed in Chapter 4.

Other Biological Factors

Other biological factors that may increase risk for acquiring, transmitting, or developing complications of certain STDs include presence of male penile foreskin, vaginal douching, risky sexual practices, use of hormonal contraceptives or intrauterine contraceptive devices, cervical ectopy, immunity resulting from prior sexually transmitted or related infections, and nonspecific immunity conferred by normal vaginal flora.

Lack of male circumcision seems to increase the risk of acquiring and perhaps transmitting certain STDs. A review of 30 published epidemiological studies that examined the relationship between HIV infection and male circumcision concluded that most studies found a statistically significant association between lack of circumcision and increased risk for HIV infection (Moses et al., 1994). In a prospective study of men at high risk for STDs, those who were not circumcised were 8 times as likely to become infected with HIV than circumcised men (Cameron et al., 1989). Another study of gay men suggested that uncircumcised men were twice as likely to be infected with HIV compared to circumcised men (Kreiss and Hopkins, 1993). As a result of these studies, some have proposed that male circumcision be considered an intervention to prevent HIV infection. Several studies have found associations between lack of circumcision and other STDs, including chancroid (Aral and Holmes, 1990). It has been hypothesized that lack of circumcision increases risk for STDs because (a) the cells that line the fold of skin that is removed by circumcision are prone to trauma or infection, (b) this fold of skin may serve as a reservoir for pathogens, and (c) this fold of skin may increase the likelihood that infections will go undetected (Aral and Holmes, 1990).

Vaginal douching seems to increase risk for pelvic inflammatory disease (Forrest et al., 1989; Wolner-Hanssen, Eschenbach DA, Paavonen J, Stevens CE, et al., 1990;). In one study, compared to women who did not douche, women who douched during the previous 3-month period were twice as likely to have clinical pelvic inflammatory disease (Scholes et al., 1993). The risk for pelvic inflammatory disease seems to increase with greater frequency of douching (Wolner-Hanssen, Eschenbach DA, Paavonen J, Stevens CE, et al., 1990; Scholes et al., 1993).

Certain sexual practices such as receptive rectal intercourse predispose to STDs. As mentioned in Chapter 2, STDs such as HIV infection and hepatitis B virus infection are more easily acquired by rectal intercourse than by vaginal intercourse. This may be because the bleeding and tissue trauma that can result from rectal intercourse facilitate invasion by pathogens. Other sexual practices, such as sex during menses and "dry sex," also predispose to acquisition of an STD.

The influence of hormonal contraceptives on acquisition and transmission of STDs is not fully defined. However, several studies have found oral contraceptive use to be associated with increased risk of acquiring chlamydial infection (Critchlow et al., 1995) but with decreased risk of developing pelvic inflammatory disease among women with chlamydial infection (Wolner-Hanssen P, Eschenbach DA, Paavonen J, Kiviat N, et al., 1990; Kimani et al., 1996). Some, but not all, studies have found an association of oral contraceptives with increased risk of HIV acquisition (Cates, in press). A recent study in Kenya has demonstrated that use of oral contraceptives or injectable progesterone among women with HIV-1 infection is associated with increased shedding of HIV-1 DNA from the cervix (Mostad et al., 1996). In one animal model study, monkeys with progesterone implants were several times more likely to become infected with the simian immunodeficiency virus than monkeys who did not have such implants (Marx et al., 1996). More study is indicated, but these data raise the possibility that hormonal contraceptives may increase the likelihood of infectious genital tract secretions in HIV-infected women and/or increase susceptibility to HIV infection.

Cervical ectopy (extension of columnar epithelial cells present in the adult endocervix onto the exposed portion of the cervix within the vagina) has also been found to be a risk factor for HIV infection (Moss et al., 1991). Among women attending an STD clinic and among college women, cervical ectopy was positively associated with use of oral contraceptives and with chlamydial infection; ectopy disappeared with increasing age (Critchlow et al., 1995).

As previously discussed, other STDs can increase risk for acquiring or transmitting HIV infection. However, prior infection with certain STDs can provide specific immunity against reinfection with the same pathogen (Plummer et al., 1989; Brunham et al., 1994). Cross-immunity (protection conferred by prior infection with a different pathogen) also occurs. For example, a prospective study of women found that asymptomatic shedding of herpes simplex virus type 2 occurs more often during the first three months after acquisition of primary type 2 disease (Koelle et al., 1992). Among persons with herpes simplex virus type 2 infections, previous infection with type 1 virus was associated with a lower rate of asymptomatic viral shedding. This observation suggests that, as prevalence of herpes simplex virus type 1 infections in childhood decline, the risk of herpes simplex virus type 2 infection may be increased when this STD is encountered by a sexually active adult. Nonspecific immunity may make some individuals more resistant to certain STDs even though they have never experienced prior STDs or related infections. For example, the normal vaginal flora contains hydrogen-peroxidase-producing bacteria that have antimicrobial activity. Recent data suggest that women with bacterial vaginosis who lack hydrogen-peroxidase-producing bacteria (lactobacilli) are at increased risk of gonorrhea (Sharon Hillier and King Holmes, University of Washington, unpublished data, 1996; Martin et al., 1996).

SOCIAL FACTORS

On a population level, preventing the spread of STDs is difficult without addressing social issues that have a tremendous influence on transmission of STDs. Some fundamental societal problems such as poverty, lack of education, and social inequity indirectly increase the prevalence of STDs in certain populations. In addition, lack of openness and mixed messages regarding sexuality create obstacles to STD prevention for the entire population and contribute to the hidden nature of the STDs. In the following discussion, the committee highlights several social problems that directly affect the spread of STDs in subpopulations and shows how societal norms regarding sexuality impede prevention of STDs. In Chapter 4 the committee describes interventions that can be used to lessen the adverse impact of these social problems on STDs, even if these dilemmas are not solved directly.

Poverty and Inadequate Access to Health Care

Health insurance coverage enables individuals to obtain professional assistance in order to prevent potential exposures to sexually transmitted infections and to seek care for suspected STDs. Uninsured persons delay seeking care for health problems longer than those who have private insurance or Medicaid coverage (Freeman et al., 1987; Donelan et al., 1996). Those with private health insurance who are living at or near poverty level have limited access to health care because of copayments and deductibles that are typically part of private insurance coverage (Freeman and Corey, 1993). Medicaid coverage is often less effective than private health insurance coverage since many physicians refuse to treat Medicaid beneficiaries, thereby restricting access to comprehensive health services (Schwartz et al., 1991).

Private health insurance generally provides the most comprehensive coverage with the greatest access to physicians and other health care professionals. However, not all plans offer adequate coverage for STD-related services. Little information is available on coverage for STD-related services in the private health care sector. A recent study of how women pay for reproductive health care suggests that many health plans either do not cover some important STD-related preventive reproductive health services or require copayments and deductibles for these services (WREI, 1994). STD-related diagnostic and treatment services are covered under general clinical care. However, the study found that only about half of all health plans cover preventive care such as routine gynecological examinations that may be important in detection of asymptomatic sexually transmitted infections.

Managed care organizations may provide better coverage for certain STD-related services than do many indemnity health plans, but they pose different challenges to the prevention of STDs, particularly for many Medicaid beneficiaries enrolled in managed care. Most managed care organizations require their enrollees to obtain all their health services from the plan's network of providers. This disrupts established patterns of STD care for many women on Medicaid by denying patients access to their preferred providers. A recent study found that neither the federal government nor the states had taken steps to ensure that Medicaid beneficiaries enrolled in managed care organizations could obtain services from family planning programs or public STD clinics (Rosenbaum et al., 1995). A number of family planning programs have taken the initiative to develop contracts with managed care organizations that serve Medicaid clients, thus both avoiding the problem of nonreimbursed out-of-plan use and retaining an important source of revenue for their program (Orbovich, 1995). This is an especially important policy issue as states increasingly encourage or require Medicaid beneficiaries to enroll in managed care organizations. The role of managed care organizations and other health plans in STD prevention is further discussed in Chapter 5.

Health insurance coverage influences where people obtain STD services. A recent study found that uninsured women and those covered by Medicaid were far more likely to obtain reproductive health services from a public or community-based clinic rather than a private physician's office, compared to women who were covered by either a managed care organization or other private health insurance (Sonenstein et al., 1995). Even those with adequate insurance coverage may be reluctant to obtain care for potential STDs from their regular health care providers because of the social stigma associated with these infections. A significant number of persons with private insurance are reluctant to bring STD exposures to the attention of their family doctor or health plan and prefer the anonymity of a public STD clinic or other public clinic (Celum et al., 1995).

In 1993, 40.9 million Americans, or 18.1 percent of the nonelderly population, were not covered by any public or private health insurance coverage, up from 39.8 million or 17.8 percent of the nonelderly population in 1992 (EBRI, 1995b). Further analysis of these data revealed that of the 1.1 million increase in uninsured persons from 1992 to 1993, 900,000 or 81.8 percent of the newly uninsured population were children and youth under 18 years of age (EBRI, 1995a).

The age and ethnic groups with the highest rates of STDs are also the groups with the poorest access to health services. One-third of persons in high-risk age groups are uninsured or covered by Medicaid (UCLA Center for Health Policy Research, unpublished data, 1996). Among persons 15–29 years of age, 25 percent are completely uninsured (Figure 3-1), including one in every five persons 15–20 years old and at least one in every four persons 21–29 years old. One in every nine persons 15–29 years old depends on Medicaid or other publicly sponsored insurance for health care access. In addition, Hispanic and African Americans are most likely to lack insurance coverage.

Poverty and other socioeconomic factors also contribute to STD risk in other ways. Even if a person in poverty perceives himself or herself to be at risk for an STD, he or she may not practice preventive behaviors if there are other risks that appear more imminent or more threatening or both (Mays and Cochran, 1988; Ramos et al., 1995). Mays and Cochran (1988:951) point out that poor women of certain ethnic groups face continual danger and have few resources to deal with them: "Competition for these women's attention includes more immediate survival needs, such as obtaining shelter for the night, securing personal safety or safety of their children, or interfacing with the governmental system in order to obtain financial resources." Traditional cultural values associated with passivity and subordination also diminish the ability of many women to adequately protect themselves (Amaro, 1988; Stuntzner-Gibson, 1991).

One of every four adolescents and young adults does not have health insurance coverage

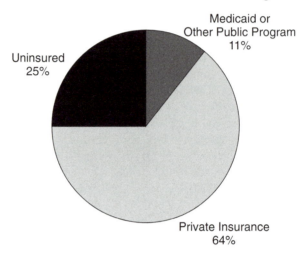

FIGURE 3-1 Distribution of 15–29-year-old persons in the United States by health insurance coverage, 1993. SOURCE: UCLA Center for Health Policy Research, unpublished data, 1996.

Substance Use

Substance use, especially drugs and alcohol, is associated with STDs at both population and individual levels.[1] At the population level, rates of STDs are high in geographic areas where rates of substance use are also high, and rates of substance use and STDs have also been shown to co-vary temporally (Greenberg et al., 1991). At the individual level, persons who use substances are more likely to acquire STDs (Marx et al., 1991; Anderson and Dahlberg, 1992; Shafer et al., 1993). There are several possible reasons for this association. One is that underlying social and individual factors lead both to higher rates of STDs and to greater use of substances. Social factors such as poverty, lack of economic and educational opportunities, and weak community infrastructure may contribute to both outcomes. Individual factors, such as risk-taking and low self-efficacy, could similarly contribute to both outcomes.

---

[1]Much of the following discussion of substance use and STDs was based on the following paper: Beltrami JF, Wright-DeAgüero LK, Fullilove MT, St. Louis ME, Edlin BR. Substance abuse and the spread of sexually transmitted diseases. Commissioned paper for the IOM Committee on Prevention and Control of STDs.

Use of substances may also directly contribute to risk of STD infection by undermining an individual's cognitive and social skills, thus making it more difficult to take actions needed to protect themselves against STDs. For example, at low doses cocaine can decrease inhibitions and heighten sexuality, leading to increased numbers of sexual encounters and partners and to increased high-risk sexual behaviors (Marx et al., 1991). In addition, drug users may be at greater risk for STDs as a result of the practice of trading sex for drugs; in these situations, drug users have a large number of high-risk partners (Marx et al., 1991). Those who are involved in frequent and sustained use of substances are most likely to be at risk for STDs.

Data from the National Household Survey on Drug Abuse indicate that, in 1994, approximately 54 percent of the U.S. population age 12 and over and 63 percent of those age 18–25 used alcohol in the prior month (SAMHSA, 1995). In addition, approximately 6 percent of the U.S. population used an illicit drug in the prior month, and there were approximately 500,000 crack cocaine users during the year.

To illustrate the broad impact of substance use on STD transmission, the committee focused on the association of STDs with use of two substances: crack cocaine, often used by disenfranchised groups, and alcohol, which is commonly used by most Americans, especially adolescents. In the following sections, the committee describes the evidence for the association between substance use/ abuse and STDs.

Impact of Crack Cocaine on STD Transmission

Numerous studies show that drug use is associated with increased risk of STDs, including HIV infection. Marx and colleagues (1991) reviewed 16 epidemiologic studies that examined drug use, sexual behavior, and STDs. Crack use paralleled the trends for syphilis, gonorrhea, chancroid, and HIV infection, both temporally and among the groups most affected. For example, a study at an STD clinic in 1990 in Trenton, New Jersey, evaluated the relationship between syphilis and behavior related to sexual activity and drug use (Finelli et al., 1993). The study showed that in addition to crack use and lack of condom use within the past three months, a high number of sex partners, drug-using partners, and partners exchanging sex for drugs increased the risk for syphilis, especially for women.

The association of syphilis and crack cocaine may lead to concentrations of the disease in specific social networks and in crack houses. For example, in 1991 and 1992, a series of syphilis outbreaks in four rural towns in Texas were linked to crack users exchanging sex for drugs (Schulte et al., 1994). Three outbreaks were concentrated in neighborhoods where crack cocaine dealers worked and where exchange of sex for drugs or money was common. All 26 cases in one outbreak were linked to a single sex worker. In a second outbreak, all 34 cases were among people frequenting a crack house, 3 of whom were sex workers. In the third and fourth outbreaks, 12 percent and 50 percent of infected persons, respectively, reported exchanging sex for drugs or money.

Crack cocaine use is associated with high-risk sexual behaviors such as multiple partners and unprotected sex. McCoy and Inciardi (1993) found that in a sample of women who did not inject drugs, crack was found to be the strongest predictor of high-risk sexual behavior. Edlin and others (1994) reported in a multisite study that crack smokers were at greater risk for HIV infection compared to persons who did not smoke crack. In addition, male crack users are more likely than those who do not use crack to choose high-risk partners (Seidman et al., 1994). Compared with heroin users, men who used crack also are more likely to have a greater number of sex partners and to receive money or drugs for sex (Hudgins et al., 1995).

How Drug Use Increases STD Transmission

How does substance use increase STD transmission on a population level? Examining the population-wide impact of crack cocaine may provide answers. Crack cocaine appears to play a central role in the transmission of STDs within various social networks. The transmission and persistence of STDs in a population or social network are dependent on the rate of partner change, the probability of transmission of infection from an infected individual to a susceptible individual, and the duration of infectiousness (May and Anderson, 1987). The rate of partner change can be considered to be a function of a complex set of interactions involving social and sexual networks, sex partner mixing patterns, and other parameters. The rate of partner change is influenced by the exchange of sex for drugs that results from crack cocaine use (Marx et al., 1991; Edlin et al., 1994). The probability of infection per sexual encounter is influenced both by the type of sexual contact and by specific sexual practices and is strongly affected by the use of condoms. The urgency to use crack may overwhelm any consideration of condom use. Because crack use in persons with STDs discourages health-care-seeking behavior (Webber et al., 1993) and modifies social norms with respect to behavior such as engaging in unprotected sex (Finelli et al., 1993) or having multiple sex partners (Greenberg et al., 1992), the duration of infectiousness in these persons may be lengthened. In addition, explosive bursts of new partner acquisition, particularly in crack houses or other settings where addicted persons trade sex for drugs, represent a potentially powerful mechanism for amplifying and maintaining chains of transmission of genital ulcer diseases among crack users. Crack also appears to influence health-care-seeking behavior among pregnant women infected with STDs, resulting in late or absent prenatal care (Warner et al., 1995); frequent changes in prenatal care providers may complicate appropriate follow-up for positive serologic tests.

Association Between Alcohol Use and STDs

Although some studies have failed to find a correlation between alcohol use and unprotected heterosexual intercourse (Leigh and Stall, 1993; Leigh et al., 1994), most studies show that both average and extreme alcohol use are associated with greater risk of STDs. From 1988 to 1990, 2,896 adults completed the General Social Survey, a nationally representative household survey of U.S. adults (Anderson and Dahlberg, 1992). Respondents who reported that they sometimes drink "more than they should" were more likely to have had the following three outcome variables compared to those who did not: sexual intercourse with two or more partners, intercourse with five or more partners, and intercourse with a stranger in the past year. A household survey in the San Francisco Bay area showed that having ever had an STD was associated with nonmonogamous behavior; with having more than five sex partners in the last five years; and, at a minimum with, three kinds of drinking behavior: going to a bar at least monthly, getting drunk at least annually, and having five or more drinks at one sitting in the last year (Ericksen and Trocki, 1992). In addition, a large nationwide survey in 1991 and 1992 showed that persons who occasionally drank five or more drinks at one sitting were significantly more likely to have multiple partners, be nonmonogamous, and participate in other high-risk sexual activities (Caetano and Hines, 1995).

A number of studies have reported that for men who have sex with men, drug and alcohol use are risk factors for relapse into unsafe sexual behaviors (Stall et al., 1986; Siegel et al., 1989). Alcohol use among adolescents has also been found to be associated with high-risk sexual behaviors (Hingson et al., 1990; Shafer et al., 1993; Lowry et al., 1994). In addition, alcohol use has been found to be a risk factor for HIV-related sexual behaviors among runaway youth (Koopman et al., 1994), the mentally ill (Kalichman et al., 1994), and seronegative female partners of HIV-seropositive men (Kennedy et al., 1993). In a survey of attendees at an STD clinic, drug and alcohol use was found to correlate with unprotected sex during their most recent sexual intercourse (CDC, 1990). In a multiple logistic regression analysis controlling for age, race, income, number of sex partners, and other variables, failure to use condoms was significantly associated with drug and alcohol use at the last sexual encounter for heterosexual men.

Sexual Abuse and Violence

Sexual violence against women and sexual abuse of children are societal problems of enormous consequences. Approximately 500,000 women were raped annually in 1992 and 1993 in the United States (U.S. Department of Justice, 1994), and studies suggest that approximately one in three young girls and one in six young boys may experience at least one sexually abusive episode by the time they reach adulthood (Guidry, 1995). Women who have been sexually abused during childhood are twice as likely to have gynecological problems, including STDs, compared to women who do not have such a history (Plichta and Abraham, 1996). In addition, women with a history of involuntary sexual intercourse are more likely to have voluntary intercourse at an earlier age (a risk factor for STDs) and to have subsequent psychological problems (Miller et al., 1995).

Transmission of STDs as the result of sexual abuse is particularly salient among prepubescent children and very young adolescents. STDs among children presenting for care after the neonatal period almost always indicate sexual abuse (AAP, Committee on Child Abuse and Neglect, 1991; Gutman et al., 1991; CDC, 1993). Sexually abused children may have severe and long-lasting psychological consequences, may become sexual abusers themselves, and may abuse children (Guidry, 1995). In addition, they may engage in a pattern of high-risk behavior that often puts them at risk for further abuse and subsequent STDs. Guidelines for the clinical management of children with STDs as a result of suspected abuse have been published (CDC, 1993; AAP, Committee on Child Abuse and Neglect, 1991).

Many women who are subjected to sexual violence may not be able to implement practices to protect against STDs or pregnancy (O'Leary and Jemmott, 1995; Plichta and Abraham, 1996). A phenomenon that also may impede protective behaviors among women is the pairing of older men with young women. The age discrepancy between older men and younger, sometimes adolescent, females may predispose to power imbalances in the relationship, thus increasing the potential for involuntary intercourse, lack of protective behavior, and exposure to STDs (Finkelhor and Associates, 1986). In addition, early initiation of sexual intercourse among adolescent males with an older female partner has been shown to increase the number of sex partners later in life (Weber et al., 1992).

STDs Among Disenfranchised Populations

STDs, like most communicable diseases in the United States, disproportionately affect disenfranchised groups and persons who are in social networks where high-risk health behaviors are common. These groups are often of low priority to policymakers since they possess little political power or influence and, without publicly sponsored health services, would not have access to STD-related services. In addition, these groups are difficult to reach, difficult to teach, and difficult to treat (Donovan, 1996). However, they are important from an STD prevention perspective because they represent "core" transmitters of STDs in the population (Thomas and Tucker, 1996). In this section, the committee describes several examples of populations at high risk for STDs that require special attention.

Sex Workers

Sex workers and their clients represent traditional "core" transmitters of STDs (Plummer and Ngugi, 1990). Extremely high rates of STDs, including HIV infection, have been reported among sex workers in the United States (Darrow, 1992). For example, in a national study of more than 1,300 female sex workers, 56 percent had serological evidence of past or current hepatitis B virus infection (Rosenblum et al., 1992). Studies in the late 1970s and early 1980s found that up to 22 percent of sex workers screened in some U.S. cities were infected with gonorrhea (Plummer and Ngugi, 1990). As mentioned previously, exchanging sex for drugs is a major factor in the recent upsurge in syphilis infections in several large cities. In addition to unprotected sex with multiple partners, female sex workers also are likely to have other factors that increase their risk for STDs, such as intravenous drug use, a history of being victims of sexual abuse and violence, and inadequate access to health care (Rosenblum et al., 1992).

Policies related to sex workers have ranged from punitive interventions such as criminalizing prostitution, as in the United States, to legalizing and controlling it, as is the case in many European countries. In those European countries, sex workers must submit to periodic health examinations and testing for STDs (Plummer and Ngugi, 1990). Studies indicate that screening and treatment programs to reduce the prevalence of STDs among sex workers, while ignoring the legal and moral debates regarding prostitution, may be effective in controlling outbreaks of treatable STDs, such as syphilis and chancroid, but less effective for untreatable STDs or STDs that are more widespread in the general population (Plummer and Ngugi, 1990). More recent approaches combine peer health educators, promotion of barrier methods, screening and treatment, and counseling (CDC, 1996a).

Homeless Persons

Estimates of the number of runaway and homeless adolescents in the United States vary from hundreds of thousands to millions (AMA, Council on Scientific Affairs, 1989). Adolescents living on the streets are at risk for many health problems, including STDs (Sherman, 1992). One study showed that approximately one-third of runaways in Los Angeles detention facilities had an STD at the time of detention (Manov and Lowther, 1983). Runaways and homeless adolescents are at increased risk for STDs because they tend to be more sexually active than other adolescents (Hein et al., 1978); have multiple high-risk sexual behaviors that include trading sex for drugs or money (AMA, Council on Scientific Affairs, 1989; Sugerman et al., 1991; Sherman, 1992; Forst, 1994); have high levels of substance use (Manov and Lowther, 1983; Sugerman et al., 1991; Sherman, 1992); and are frequently sexually and physically abused by others (AMA, Council on Scientific Affairs, 1989). A survey of states regarding pregnancy prevention and family planning policy found that only eight states had a written policy on sexuality education for youths in out-of-home care (i.e., family foster care, group homes, and residential care) (Mayden, 1996).

STDs are also a major problem among homeless adults. For example, a study of homeless women in Chicago seeking gynecological care revealed that 26 percent had trichomoniasis, 6 percent had gonorrhea, and 5 percent had pelvic inflammatory disease (Johnstone et al., 1993). Another study of homeless persons in Baltimore found that 8 percent of men and 11 percent of women had positive gonorrhea or syphilis tests and nearly one-third reported a prior STD (Breakey et al., 1989).

Adolescents in Detention

Adolescents in detention facilities have higher rates of risky sexual and substance use behaviors than do other adolescents (Shafer et al., 1993; Shafer, 1994). Adolescents in detention facilities may represent "core" transmitters of STDs since they have problems, such as high rates of drug and alcohol use and poor access to health care, that place them at continuing risk for STDs (Shafer, 1994). Compared to other adolescents, those in detention facilities tend to have engaged in sexual intercourse earlier and more frequently; have engaged in unsafe sexual practices more often; and have higher rates of STDs (Bell et al., 1985; DiClemente et al., 1991; Weber et al., 1992; Oh et al., 1994). Of 966 sexually experienced male adolescents examined in an Alabama detention center, 48 percent became sexually active before age 13; age at first intercourse ranged from 5 to 17 years (Oh et al., 1994). In a study of 1,580 male adolescents in juvenile detention in rural Florida, 27 percent were sexually active by age 11 (Weber et al., 1992). Multivariate models show that inconsistent condom use, multiple partners, and frequent alcohol use appear to increase the risk of STDs (Shafer et al., 1993). These same factors are likely to play a role in the larger population as well. Although condom use is low among adolescents in detention, those who communicate with their partners regarding their sexual history and who know someone with AIDS are more likely to use condoms (Rickman et al., 1994).

Both male and female adolescents in detention facilities have high rates of STDs. A 1994 national survey of state and local juvenile detention facilities found that the rate of gonorrhea was, respectively, 152 and 42 times greater among confined male and females adolescents than among their counterparts in the general population (CDC, 1996b). In a study of 414 sexually active male adolescents in a San Francisco detention center, 15 percent were diagnosed with at least one STD and 34 percent reported a history or had current evidence of an STD at the time of entry into the facility (Shafer et al., 1993). Twelve percent of male adolescents tested in an Alabama detention center for gonorrhea, chlamydial infection, and syphilis were positive for at least one of the three STDs (Oh et al., 1994). In addition, almost a third of the female adolescents in a King County,

Washington, detention facility, many of whom were sex workers, tested positive for chlamydia, gonorrhea, or both (Bell et al., 1985).

In detention facilities, if STD education is provided, it is usually incorporated into HIV education programs. In 1994, approximately 57 percent of state juvenile detention facilities provided instructor-led HIV education and 7 percent provided peer-led education programs (CDC, 1996b). Only one county correctional system reported making condoms available in its juvenile detention facilities (i.e., Alameda County, California) (Widom and Hammett, 1996).

Adults in Detention

The number of prisoners in the United States is at record levels. A total of 1,104,074 persons were in state or federal prisons in June 1995 (U.S. Department of Justice, 1995). From 1990 through 1995, the number of prisoners grew at an annual rate of 7.9 percent. Inmates in correctional facilities have high levels of communicable diseases, including tuberculosis, hepatitis B virus infection, and HIV infection and other STDs (Glaser and Greifinger, 1993). A study of 6,309 men at the main jail facility for men in Los Angeles County used a rapid test for syphilis to show that the rate of infectious syphilis was 507 cases per 100,000 persons. This was more than 11 times higher than the rate in the general county population (Cohen et al., 1992). Results of routine testing for STDs between 1993 and 1994 show that up to 17 percent of inmates were infected with syphilis, up to 32.5 percent were positive for gonorrhea, and up to 4.4 percent were positive for chlamydia (Hammett et al., 1995). Female detainees are at high risk of STDs because many are involved with drugs and exchange sex for drugs or money. For example, among women prisoners at Rikers Island in New York, 57 percent were jailed because of drug-related offenses and 80 percent had cocaine in their urine at the time of their arrest (Holmes et al., 1993). In 1988, 35 percent of a sample of female inmates at Rikers Island were positive for human papillomavirus (9 percent had abnormal Pap smears) (Bickell et al., 1991); 27 percent had positive cultures for chlamydia; 16 percent were serologically positive for syphilis; and 8 percent had positive cultures for gonorrhea (Holmes et al., 1993).

The prevalence of HIV infection among incarcerated persons in the United States, like other STDs, is many times higher than in the general population (Hammett et al., 1995; CDC, 1996b). Comparing the HIV seroprevalence among entrants into 10 federal and state prisons to the seroprevalence among first-time blood donors, the prevalence among male and female detainees is more than 50 and 130 times, respectively, the rate among blood donors (CDC, 1992b). Anonymous serosurveys of inmates throughout the United States indicate that anywhere from less than 1 percent to as high as 25.6 percent of inmates are HIV-positive and that female inmates often have higher infection rates compared to men (Hammett et al., 1995).

The prevalence of STDs among incarcerated persons reflects both the high prevalence of STDs in the social networks from which they come and the transmission of STDs among prisoners (Moran and Peterman, 1989). Within prisons, unprotected sex, intravenous drug use, and tattooing are potential modes of transmission of STDs, including HIV infection (Doll, 1988; Dolan et al., 1995; Hammett et al., 1995). A wide range of unprotected consensual and nonconsensual sexual activity occurs among prisoners and between prisoners and staff (Mahon, 1996). Although transmission of STDs has been documented among prisoners (Moran and Peterman, 1989; Mutter et al., 1994), it is unclear if prisoners in correctional facilities are more likely to acquire STDs, including HIV infection, during incarceration or outside in the community (Dolan et al., 1995). While it is possible that the frequency of unprotected sexual intercourse or injecting drug use among prisoners is typically higher while they are not in confinement (Decker et al., 1984; Horsburg et al., 1990), some prisoners have high rates of risky behaviors while incarcerated. For example, one study of male Tennessee prisoners showed that 37 percent of prisoners reported using intravenous drugs while not incarcerated compared to 28 percent who reported such use while in prison, and 7 percent reported engaging in same-sex intercourse while not incarcerated compared to 18 percent who reported such intercourse in prison (Decker et al., 1984).

Correctional systems are more focused on HIV education than for other STD educational programs. A 1994 survey revealed that 75 percent of state and federal correctional systems and 62 percent of city and county systems reported providing instructor-led HIV education (Hammett et al., 1995; CDC, 1996b). In addition, 35 percent of state and federal correctional systems and 7 percent of city and county systems reported peer-led educational programs in at least one facility. In contrast, 49 percent of state and federal systems and 48 percent of city and county systems reported instructor-led STD education.

The National Commission on Correctional Health Care recommends that all inmates be screened for STDs and that a comprehensive education program and "appropriate protective devices" to reduce the risk of HIV/STDs be provided (NCCHC, 1992, 1994). In 1994, 82 percent of state and federal systems and 34 percent of city and county systems reported policies for screening all incoming inmates for syphilis, gonorrhea, and/or chlamydial infection (Hammett et al., 1995). Screening and follow-up treatment of prisoners for STDs are difficult because of the rapid turnover of inmates, and innovative screening programs are needed. An example of such a program for rapid screening and treatment for syphilis is presented in Box 3-1.

Very few correctional facilities provide access to condoms. Facility administrators commonly cite the potential use of condoms as weapons or to conceal drugs or contraband as a reason for denying access (Hammett et al., 1995). In addition, some prison administrators are concerned that providing condoms contradicts official policies that prohibit sexual activity among prisoners. Two state correctional systems (Mississippi and Vermont) and four local jail systems (New

---

BOX 3-1
An Effective Screening and Treatment Protocol for
Syphilis in a Correctional Facility

A rapid screening and treatment protocol for syphilis was recently evaluated in New York City's major facility for medical screening of female inmates at time of admission. The protocol's strength lies in its ability to accurately identify inmates needing syphilis treatment and to provide that treatment at the time of the obligatory medical evaluation. This service, piloted by the New York City Department of Health, introduced the use of a quick screening test for syphilis (STAT RPR) and the New York City Syphilis and Reactor Registry (which includes syphilis serologic results and treatment history of New York City residents), in addition to the routine medical evaluation data (which includes pregnancy testing), to make on-site treatment decisions. Information from the STAT RPR test and from the Syphilis Registry are available to clinicians at the time of the medical evaluation. Under the protocol, treatment is recommended for women with reactive STAT RPRs (unless this individual completed treatment within the last three weeks); with evidence in the registry of previously untreated syphilis, regardless of current STAT RPR status; and, in cases of pregnancy, with registry documentation of syphilis (unless treatment was completed within the last week). This protocol resulted in an improvement of syphilis treatment rates from 7 percent of seropositive women prior to implementing the protocol to 87 percent of seropositive women and 94 percent of pregnant seropositive women after implementing the protocol (Blank et al., 1994). The protocol also resulted in treatment for women whom the New York City Department of Health had been unable to locate for treatment in the past.

SOURCE: Margaret Hamburg, M.D., New York City Department of Health, unpublished data, 1996.

York City, Philadelphia, San Francisco, and Washington, D.C.) make condoms available to inmates (CDC, 1996b). Among correctional systems with condom availability programs, there have been few or no problems with the use of condoms as weapons or to smuggle contraband (Hammett et al., 1995). Most correctional systems have a policy for notifying partners of inmates who test positive for a treatable STD if the partner is a fellow inmate. The high annual rate of turnover among prisoners, 800 and 50 percent in jails and prisons, respectively, is a major barrier to screening and follow-up treatment for STDs (Glaser and Greifinger, 1993). Follow-up of released detainees who test positive for STDs and notification of partners who are not inmates are considered to be rare.

Migrant Workers

STDs, including HIV infection, are major health problems among migrant workers (Jones et al., 1991; CDC, 1992a). In addition, lack of condom use and other high-risk sexual behaviors are common among these workers (Jones et al.,

1991). Migrant workers tend to be young, uneducated, and from developing countries. They and their families have limited access to health care because of their frequent relocation, language and cultural barriers, and limited economic resources (Bechtel et al., 1995). Traditionally, there have been distinct patterns of movement for migrant workers: north and south along the East and West Coasts and from Texas up through the Midwest. Currently, however, many migrant workers do not follow these patterns but criss-cross the country seeking work (Dougherty, 1996). Among migrant workers, men who are single or not accompanied by their families are at greatest risk for STDs. In some areas, it is common practice for sex workers to visit migrant camps for men and have sex with many men (Oscar Gomez, East Coast Migrant Health Project, personal communication, March 1996). STDs persist in migrant populations because of cultural influences against open discussion of sex and STDs, language barriers, lack of access to health care, and general lack of understanding of disease transmission (Smith, 1988; Bechtel et al., 1995). Social and cultural taboos make discussion of STDs uncomfortable for many migrant workers. For example, there is a reluctance to use condoms or request the use of a condom among migrant workers because there is an implied aspersion that the partner is not trustworthy (Bobbi Ryder, National Center for Farm Worker Health, personal communication, March 1996).

SECRECY AS A CONTRIBUTING FACTOR

Many of the obstacles to prevention of STDs at both individual and population levels are directly or indirectly attributable to the social stigma associated with STDs. It is notable that although there are consumer-based political lobbies and support groups for almost every disease and health problem, there are few individuals who are willing to admit publicly to having an STD. STDs are stigmatized because they are transmitted through sexual behaviors. Although sex and sexuality pervade many aspects of our culture, and sexuality is a normal aspect of human functioning, sexual behavior is a private—and secret—matter in the United States.

The committee uses the word "secrecy" in this report to describe certain aspects of sexuality in the United States. By the word "secrecy," the committee includes both the passive by-product of the inherent difficulties of discussing intimate aspects of life and the ongoing efforts by some groups to prevent open dissemination of information regarding sexuality and its health consequences. In this section, the committee summarizes the basis for the stigma surrounding STDs, the reticence to deal openly with sexual behaviors, and the impact of these two factors on preventing STDs.

Sexuality and Secrecy in the United States

Perhaps more than any other aspect of life, sexuality reflects and integrates biological, psychological, and cultural factors that must be considered when delivering effective health services and information to individuals. Sexuality is an integral part of how people define themselves. It influences how, with whom, and with what level of safety people engage in sexual behaviors. However, sexuality is a value-laden subject that makes people—including health care professionals, researchers, educators, and the public—feel anxious and uncomfortable talking about it. The resulting inability to address issues of sexuality places individuals at risk of STDs. The discomfort that many Americans feel discussing sexual behavior is reflected in a recent nationwide survey that showed that, including married couples, approximately one of four women and one of five men surveyed had no knowledge of their partner's sexual history (EDK Associates, 1995).

Sexuality has been described in many ways. The common denominator in all definitions is the recognition that sexuality is an intrinsic part of one's being. It is much more than the sexual act and encompasses more than the anatomy, physiology, and biochemistry of the sexual response system. It is the quality of being human—all that we are as men and women (Hogan, 1980). Sexuality is also an energy, a life force, that is an important aspect of individual behavior and includes personal roles, identity, thoughts, feelings and emotions, and relationships. In addition, sex is entwined with ethical, spiritual, and moral issues and is influenced by sociocultural values and norms, religion, family, and economic status (Chilman, 1978).

It is helpful to examine the origins of secrecy regarding sexuality to understand why it has had such a significant impact on STDs in the United States. STDs were considered to be a threat to the late Victorian social system, which valued discipline, restraint, and homogeneity (Brandt, 1988). Advocates of repressive sexuality perceived that social structure and traditional morality were in danger and wanted to restore order and morality to American society (Sokolow, 1983). During this time, societal sexual mores dictated that sexual intercourse was only acceptable within the context of marriage. The Victorian code of ethics considered all discussion of sexuality and STDs to be inappropriate. According to these ethics, sexuality should be disciplined, not only by law but also by shame, and then concealed by silence (Kosovich, 1978). This code was upheld by key groups and opinion leaders in the community. For example, some physicians hid diagnoses of STDs from their patients and families and did not talk about the "medical secret" (Brandt, 1988). The press also contributed to this code of secrecy by refusing to print any explicit articles regarding STDs. When public health officials were finally able to conduct educational campaigns regarding STDs during the first few decades of the twentieth century, these campaigns emphasized the dangers of sexual activity rather than disease prevention. By focusing on the "loathsome" and disfiguring aspects of STDs, these early campaigns may have contributed to the stigma associated with STDs and encouraged discrimination against persons with STDs (Brandt, 1988). The historical phenomenon of secrecy surrounding sexuality and STDs in the United States offers some insight into why Americans are reluctant to openly discuss STDs, but some other industrialized societies (e.g., Scandinavia) are not.

The depiction of sexuality has been paradoxical within modern American culture. On the one hand, there is the saturation and sensationalism of sexual images and messages in the mass media, and the public is fascinated with sexual subjects. On the other hand, sexuality remains an extremely private and uniquely complex sphere of human behavior with sociocultural taboos and rules of behavior that make talking openly and comfortably about sexuality difficult. For some individuals, opposition to research in sexual behavior can represent very deep-seated fears and doubts about the role and significance of sexuality in personal life and the appropriateness of addressing this issue in public (di Mauro, 1995). The paradoxical nature of sexuality in the United States is further illustrated by a mass media culture that portrays casual sexual activity as the norm, while data show that most Americans disapprove of adult women having premarital sexual intercourse (Klassen et al., 1989). It is interesting to note that American society has had difficulty in openly discussing many health issues other than sexuality and STDs. For example, public discussion of health problems such as cancer, alcoholism, and mental illness are relatively recent phenomena. This observation provides optimism that sexuality and STDs will eventually be part of public discourse.

Secrecy surrounding sexuality is reflected in individual values, attitudes, and beliefs regarding sexuality that impede a person's ability or willingness to communicate regarding sex (Hyde, 1994). Additionally, this secrecy has a negative impact upon both sexual behavior and the ability to take protective action against STDs. The United States has a diverse population, and people develop their sexual value system based on their culture, religion, family, social status, and community (Woods, 1979). The secrecy regarding sexuality is perpetuated and supported by influences that include the family, partners, peers, and religion (Jemmott and Jemmott, 1992a). If social norms do not support open discussion of sex and sexuality, then the individual is unlikely to do otherwise.

Impact of Secrecy on STD Prevention

An examination of the social history of STDs in the United States is informative. Historically, a moralistic approach to STDs has directly hindered the ability of public health officials and programs to successfully control the epidemic (Brandt, 1985; Cutler and Arnold, 1988). For example, in the 1930s, many hospitals refused admission of patients with STDs and private physicians were reluctant to treat them because persons with STDs were viewed as immoral or not deserving of care (Brandt, 1985). Coupled with the high costs of syphilis treatment, this led many infected persons to turn to quacks and over-the-counter "cures." This practice quickly led to a growing number of untreated individuals and an escalating epidemic. Unwillingness to confront issues regarding sexuality, and the judgmentalism that often accompanies it, had a detrimental effect on efforts to prevent STDs as early as the nineteenth century. Reflecting on America's efforts around syphilis during the last century, Martensen (1994:269) wrote:

> For the predominant voices in the late 19th-century US medicine and society, humans were divided into good (celibate and on the way to being married and monogamous) or not good (the intentionally single and/or unmarried but sexually active). . . . Such cultural bifurcations of innocence and evil presented few barriers to *T pallidum* [the cause of syphilis], and they made it difficult to develop consistent policies for the treatment and containment of venereal contagion.

The portrayal of STDs as symbols of immoral behavior continues today. This phenomenon was especially evident during the early stages of the AIDS epidemic when some in society considered this epidemic to be a symbol of deviant sexual behavior and lapse in societal moral values. In his book on the social history of STDs, Brandt (1985:186) writes:

> Medical and social values continue to define venereal disease as a uniquely sinful disease, indeed, to transform the disease into an indication of moral decay. . . . Behavior—bad behavior at that—is seen as the cause of venereal disease [STDs]. These assumptions may be powerful psychologically, and in some cases they may influence behavior, but so long as they are dominant—so long as disease is equated with sin—there can be no magic bullet.

Changing sexual behaviors that spread STDs is an important component of prevention. But in order to establish preferred behavior or to change risky behaviors, parents must feel comfortable talking to their children, individuals must be able to discuss sex with their sex partners, and educators and health professionals must be able to communicate with their students and patients. In this section, the committee describes how the constraints on acknowledgment and open discussion of sexuality adversely impact sexuality education programs for adolescents, open communication between parents and their children and between sex partners, balanced messages from the mass media, education and counseling activities of health care professionals, and community activism for STDs.

Impact on Sexuality Education for Adolescents

Traditionally, sexual behavior has been regarded as a personal issue and involvement by schools or health care professionals has been seen as intrusive. Debates regarding access of adolescents to sexuality education in public schools, family planning services, and abortion services have raised questions about who has jurisdiction in matters related to sexual behavior. Although there is widespread agreement that parents should be the major source of information and guidance for their children with regard to sexual behavior, communication does not occur if parents are uncomfortable in discussing sexuality or lack the requisite knowledge or skills for such discussion. Parents may also deny the possibility that their child is or will be sexually active. Conversations regarding healthy sexual behaviors and STDs do not take place when parents deny that their children are sexually active or that adolescents have sexual drives. Children in these families are unable to seek information from their parents about such issues.

The denial or fear that their children are sexually active may lead some parents to oppose those, including the educational system, providing sexuality education to their children. Opponents of school-based sexuality education and condom availability programs argue that such programs lead to premarital sex and promiscuity. However, there is no scientific evidence that this occurs. Sexuality education appears to make students more tolerant of the attitudes and behavior of others, but it has not been found to increase premarital sex or promiscuity. Numerous evaluations of the ability of school-based education programs to reduce sexual risk behaviors have found no association between having had sexuality education and the probability of initiating sexual activity (Zelnik and Kim, 1982; Furstenberg et al., 1985; Kirby et al., 1994). In fact, there is evidence that responsible sexuality education may have a number of desirable effects in increasing AIDS-related knowledge and promoting positive changes in attitudes and risk-related behavior (Jemmott et al., 1992; Kirby et al., 1994). This issue is discussed further in Chapter 4.

Where do children get their information regarding sex? Relatively few children obtain essential information regarding STDs from their parents. A 1995 survey showed that only 11 percent of teenagers got most of their information regarding STDs from parents and other family members (Figure 3-2). Even parents who attempt to teach their children about sex may do so through general and diffused admonitions that do not recognize or end their child's interest in sex, but rather contribute to concealment and subsequent guilt. Because many parents do not talk to their children about sex, children are more likely to learn about sex through clandestine and secretive exchanges with peers that result in a massive amount of misinformation (Smith and Lanthrop, 1993). Guilty knowledge develops and children learn to keep sexuality a secret, especially from those they love (Hogan, 1980), thus perpetuating the cycle. Effective school-based programs and other means to educate children regarding sexuality might be less important if all parents discussed these issues with their children. Children who do not have open information exchange with their parents or others regarding sexuality may be less likely to communicate openly with their sex partners in the future, and thus be less likely to implement protective behaviors than others.

Impact on Communication Between Sex Partners

In addition to hindering communication between parents and their children, many societal barriers prevent sex partners from talking to each other about sex.

Only 11 percent of teenagers get most of their information regarding STDs from parents and other family members

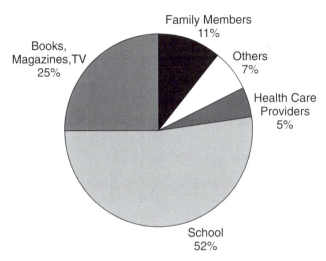

FIGURE 3-2   Distribution of U.S. teenagers by primary source of information regarding STDs, 1995. SOURCE: ASHA (American Social Health Association). Teenagers know more than adults about STDs, but knowledge among both groups is low. STD News. A quarterly newsletter of the American Social Health Association. Winter 1996;3:1,5.

Ironically, it may require greater intimacy to discuss sex than to engage in it. The kind of communication that is necessary to explore a partner's sexual history, establish STD risk status, and to plan for protection against STDs is made difficult by the taboos that surround sex and sexuality. As Lear (1995:1313) notes, individuals rarely engage in explicit discussions about sex: "The existing discourse on sex is marked by a lack of vocabulary. . . . Sexual encounters, at least early in a relationship, often involve very little spoken communication; communication is rather non-verbal and coded." Barriers to open discussion include gender roles, modesty, and cultural, family or religious beliefs. For instance, the "good woman" or the "modest woman" is not supposed to know about sex, so it is inappropriate for her to bring up subjects like HIV and condoms. Many studies have shown that both adolescents and adult women who are uncomfortable about their sexuality and who have high levels of guilt regarding sexual behavior are less effective in their use of contraceptives than others (Herold et al., 1979; Gerrard, 1982, 1987). Narrow attitudes towards sexuality and sex roles can make it difficult to initiate a conversation regarding sex and safer sex strategies with one's partner. Two factors that influence women's abilities to communicate with current or new sex partners are their level of confidence in being able to initiate the conversation and perception of their partner's reaction to the conversation. The importance of perceived partner reaction may be related to the woman's level of dependence on her partner, including emotional and financial dependency.

The ability to communicate with sex partners is a critical element for protective behaviors such as condom use. Secrecy hinders an individual's ability to develop skills and ways to normalize condom use. One way to facilitate condom use is to eroticize their use and make them fun and pleasurable for partners (Jemmott and Jemmott, 1992b). To do so, however, requires feeling comfortable about sexuality and having open communication regarding sexual behaviors.

Impact on Mass Media Messages

Americans, especially adolescents, receive unbalanced mass media messages about sexuality, sexual behavior, and sexual responsibility. Premarital sex, cohabitation, and nonmarital relationships are depicted as the norm for adults (Lichter et al., 1994). However, the media provide little frank and informed advice about STDs, sexuality, contraception, or the harsh realities of early pregnancy and parenting. The portrayal of widespread casual sex is contrasted with messages that adolescents receive from other sources of information that premarital sex is not acceptable. American society is ambivalent about sex, and mixed messages from mass media contribute to the confusion and communication problems of many adolescents.

Television is currently the most significant mass media influence for adolescents (Strasburger, 1990). About one-third of an American's free time is spent watching television. That is more time than is spent on the next 10 most popular leisure activities combined (Gerbner, 1993). Children spend more time watching television than they do in school (Dietz and Strasburger, 1991). Television is an important source of information regarding sexual behavior (Strasburger, 1995): 37 percent and 41 percent of men and women surveyed, respectively, cite television talk shows as a primary source of information regarding STDs (STD Communications Roundtable,1996).

A recent study found an average of 10 incidents of sexual behavior per hour on network television during prime time (Lowry and Schidler, 1993). When the content of promotions for upcoming shows is added, the number of such incidents increases. Analysis of multiple episodes of 11 top Nielsen-rated television talk shows found that topics related to sexual activity were discussed in 34 percent of episodes screened, sexual infidelity in 18 percent, and sexual orientation in 11 percent (Greenberg et al., 1995). Soap operas also have strong sexual content (Lowry and Towles, 1989); the most popular ones have more than six incidents of sexual behavior per hour and only six references to safer sex or contraception in 50 episodes studied (Greenberg and Busselle, 1994). Most music videos and rock music lyrics, which frequently target adolescents, have strong sexual content (Sherman and Dominick, 1986; Strasburger, 1989). Other forms of media, including cable television, movies, and videotapes, also frequently portray sexual incidents (Brown and Steele, 1996).

Although sex is frequently portrayed on television, protective behavior is rarely shown and references to adverse consequences are rare; casual unprotected intercourse is presented as the norm. Lowry and Shidler (1993) found that there were approximately 25 instances of sexual behavior portrayed on prime-time television for every one instance of protective behavior shown or comment regarding STDs or unintended pregnancy. In addition, the references to protective behavior were portrayed in a nonserious manner. Another study estimated that the average teenager will be exposed to almost 14,000 television messages associated with sex annually, but less than 1 percent of these messages will deal with contraception, refraining from sex, or STDs (Harris and Associates, 1988). There is some evidence that producers may be starting to decrease the sexual content of some television shows (Lowry and Schidler, 1993; Olson, 1994).

In addition to serving as a source of information, mass media may influence social attitudes, and sometimes social behavior. For example, depictions of violence in the mass media have been shown to be a significant factor in real-life violence (Strasburger, 1995). The ability of sexual content in mass media to directly affect sexual behavior is unclear because appropriate longitudinal studies have not been conducted (Strasburger, 1995), but such content has been shown to influence adolescents' attitudes and beliefs regarding sex (Strasburger, 1992, 1995; Buerkel-Rothfuss and Strouse, 1993; Greenberg et al., 1993; Strouse and Buerkel-Rothfuss, 1993). One study found an association between frequent viewing of television programs with strong sexual content and early onset of sexual intercourse among adolescents, but it was not possible to distinguish which factor came first (Brown and Newcomer, 1991). Another recent study that examined the influence of mass media on eight potentially risky behaviors, including sexual intercourse, found that adolescents who had engaged in more risky behaviors listened to radio and watched music videos and movies on television more frequently than those who had engaged in fewer risky behaviors, independent of demographic factors (Klein et al., 1993).

The reluctance and past refusal of mass media to become involved in the dissemination of information regarding STDs and other sexual issues is not new. In his book on the social history of STDs, Brandt (1985) writes about an incident in November 1934. The Columbia Broadcast Company scheduled a live radio broadcast with Thomas Parran, Jr., then New York State Commissioner of Health, to talk about the major public health problems of the time. Just before airtime, Parran was told that he could not mention syphilis or gonorrhea by name. In response, Parran abruptly canceled his appearance and never delivered his talk. He went on to criticize the hypocritical standards in radio broadcasting that prevented him from mentioning the names of STDs yet allowed "the veiled obscenity permitted by Columbia in the vaudeville acts of some of their commercial programs." More than 60 years later, this hypocrisy still exists among most major television broadcasters and other mass media. Promoting condom use or even mentioning the word "condom" on television is deemed inappropriate for young viewers, but it is accepted practice for young viewers to be exposed to shows and movies that portray persons practicing high-risk sexual behaviors. Similarly, while condom advertisements are not acceptable for prime-time television, it is common for advertisers to sell their products using sexually suggestive advertisements (Kilborne, 1993).

Advertisers and other sponsors have historically exerted considerable control over the content of television programming and magazines because the sponsors represent the major source of income for these media (Brown and Steele, 1995). Advertisers have implicitly supported sexual content in programming but have generally refused to support the incorporation of explicit information regarding protective behaviors for STDs for fear of offending viewers (Strasburger, 1989; Lebow, 1994; Brown and Steele, 1995). Opinion polls, however, show that most Americans support incorporating information regarding STDs and contraceptives in mass media (Harris and Associates, 1987; EDK Associates, 1994), including advertising of condoms on television (Buchta, 1989). Advertisers and sponsors commonly use sexual appeals to sell their products, but until recently the television networks had strictly forbidden advertisements for contraceptives (Lebow, 1994). Condom advertisements on television have been controversial ever since the first such advertisement in 1975 (Lebow, 1994). It was not until 1986 that the word "condom" was first used on prime-time television (Lichter et al., 1994). Recently, the Centers for Disease Control and Prevention (CDC) had to fight to use the word "condom" in its HIV prevention public service announcements (Hall, 1994). Despite agreeing to air the recent HIV prevention announcements promoting condoms, the networks have restricted showing the messages to non-prime-time hours (Hall, 1994). Primarily as a result of the HIV epidemic, in 1991 the Fox Broadcasting Company became the first national television network to run a condom commercial (Elliot, 1991), and some network-owned stations recently have begun to accept condom advertisements with certain restrictions and as long as they are in "good taste" (Lebow, 1994). Some networks, such as Fox and MTV, are less restrictive in accepting condom advertisements.

Despite the current lack of involvement of mass media in promoting messages regarding healthy sexual behaviors, the mass media can be an extremely powerful ally in efforts to prevent STDs. HIV prevention messages delivered through mass media have been effective in increasing knowledge and changing behavior (Flora et al., 1995). This issue is discussed in further detail in Chapter 4. In addition, a nationwide survey of women found that 83 percent of women surveyed agreed that STDs would be more likely to be prevented if these diseases were more frequently discussed in public (i.e., on television, on the radio, and in print media) (EDK Associates, 1994). In an effort to address the lack of accurate information regarding STDs in the mass media, the STD Communications Roundtable was formed in 1995. This ad hoc committee of public health experts, communications professionals, and mass media executives met to discuss ways of assisting the mass media in producing and incorporating messages supporting healthy sexual behavior. Building on these discussions, they recently produced a resource guide for media executives (STD Communications Roundtable, 1996). This roundtable, however, does not have plans to reconvene. In addition, the Media Project[2] has been working with television producers and writers to improve the content of sexual messages in television shows and to increase the promotion of healthy sexual behaviors. A coalition of organizations with an interest in sexuality education, the National Coalition to Support Sexuality Education, recently issued a consensus statement and suggested guidelines for incorporating information regarding healthy sexual behavior and STDs into the mass media (Box 3-2).

Impact on Clinical Preventive Services

STD-related risk assessment and counseling are not routinely performed by most primary care clinicians. A 1994 nationwide survey of 450 physicians and 514 other primary care providers showed that 60 percent of physicians and 51 percent of other primary care providers do not routinely evaluate all or most new adult patients for STDs (ARHP and ANPRH, 1995). In addition, only 30 percent of physicians and 34 percent of other primary care providers reported collecting information regarding their patients' sexual activity.

Health care providers have two major hurdles to effective communication with their patients regarding sexuality issues. One is their own comfort level in talking about sex and sexual health issues, and the other is reserving time in their schedule to do it. The reluctance to discuss sexual health issues with patients can be partially attributed to the discomfort and embarrassment of some health care professionals in discussing these issues (Risen, 1995). A physician survey found that embarrassment was perceived to be a major reason physicians did not take sexual histories (Merrill et al., 1990). If clinicians are not comfortable talking to their patients about STDs, assessing their patients' risk behavior, and providing information on STD prevention, patients may detect this discomfort and decide not to raise questions or concerns regarding sex with their health care provider. The reluctance of clinicians to discuss sexual health issues may be especially problematic among older clinicians and gay patients (Matthews et al., 1986; Lewis and Freeman, 1987; Lewis and Montgomery, 1990). In order to address

---

[2] The Media Project is a program supported by the Advocates for Youth to supply writers, producers, and network executives with information and services related to sexuality.

BOX 3-2
Media Recommendations for More Realistic, Accurate Images Concerning Sexuality

The National Coalition to Support Sexuality Education recommends that the media use their influence to convey more realistic, medically accurate, and health-promoting ideas and images concerning sexuality.

It has long been recognized that the media help shape the attitude of the public—particularly young people—on a myriad of topics. The media play a major role in educating Americans about sexuality, gender roles, and sexual behaviors.

Sexual images and references may be commonplace in the media, but sexuality is much broader than the media typically portray. Human sexuality encompasses the sexual knowledge, beliefs, attitudes, values, and behaviors of individuals. It deals with one's roles, identity, personality; with individual thoughts, feelings, behaviors, and relationships as well as one's body. Sexual health encompasses sexual development and reproductive health, as well as such characteristics as the ability to develop and maintain meaningful interpersonal relationships, to appreciate one's own body, to interact with both genders in respectful and appropriate ways, and to express affection, love, and intimacy in ways consistent with one's own values.

Becoming a sexually healthy adult is a key developmental task of adolescence. The media can enhance adolescent sexual health by communicating accurate information and portraying realistic situations. The media provide opportunities for adolescents to gain clearer insights into their own sexuality and to make more responsible decisions about their behavior.

We, the undersigned members of the National Coalition to Support Sexuality Education, strongly encourage writers, producers, film makers, programming executives, performers and program hosts, reporters, advertising professionals, Internet access providers, and others to incorporate the following into their work whenever possible:

Sexually Healthy Behavior

• When possible and appropriate, include the portrayal of effective communication about sexuality and relationships between children and their parents or other trusted adults.

• Present the choice of abstinence from sexual intercourse from the point of view of characters knowledgeable and comfortable with their sexuality, but clear about their decision to postpone this sexual behavior for reasons of health, emotional maturity, or personal ethics. Portray young people refusing unwanted sexual advances in order to maintain their decision about abstinence.

• Show typical sexual interactions between people as verbally and physically respectful, non-exploitive and promoting gender equity.

• Suggest intimate behaviors other than intercourse to inform the public about the possibility of alternative, pleasurable, consensual, and responsible sexual activity.

- Recognize and show that the healthier sexual encounters are anticipated events, not spur-of-the moment responses to the heat of passion. Model communication about upcoming sexual encounters, including expressions of partners' wishes and boundaries.
- When describing, alluding to, or portraying sexual intercourse, include steps that should be taken for prevention, such as using contraceptives and condoms to prevent unwanted pregnancy and information about the full spectrum of sexually transmitted diseases.
- When an unprotected sexual encounter results in negative consequences, realistically portray or refer to the possible, specific, short- and long-term repercussions of the individual's decision-making process.

Sensitivity to Diversity

- Eliminate stereotypes and prejudices about sexuality and sexual behaviors; for example, eliminate the notion that only "beautiful people" have sexual relationships, that sexual interaction always leads to intercourse, or that all adolescents have intercourse.
- Provide diverse and positive representations of the scope of people who express their sexuality in caring, consensual, and responsible ways; for example, when possible and appropriate, include disabled adults, older adults, adolescents, gay men, and lesbians.
- Provide more and positive views of a diverse range of body types and sizes.

Accurate Information

- Lift barriers to contraceptive and condom product advertising.
- Promote responsible sexual adolescent behavior by using articulate characters that teens can identify with in order to highlight success stories where teens take appropriate actions, make healthy decisions, and follow through with them such as exercising self-control, and making plans and setting goals for their lives.
- Provide ways for young people to obtain additional information about sexuality and related issues, such as by listing addresses and telephone numbers of public health organizations and support groups in such places as public service announcements; trailers at the end of sitcoms, daytime television programs, music videos, and news programs; mailing inserts in magazines and age-appropriate comic books; computer e-mail or subject-related bulletin boards; and toll-free phone numbers before, during, or after subject-related programming.

Signed April 1996 by:
AIDS Action Council
Advocates for Youth
American Association of Sex Educators, Counselors, and Therapists
American Counseling Association
American Jewish Congress-Commission for Women's Equality
American Medical Association-Department of Adolescent Health

continued on next page

BOX 3-2 Continued

American Orthopsychiatric Association
American Psychological Association
American School Health Association
American Social Health Association
Association for the Advancement of Health Education
Association for Sex Education and Training
Association of Reproductive Health Professionals
Association of State and Territorial Health Officials
AVSC, International
Catholics for a Free Choice
Federation of Behavioral, Psychological, and Cognitive Sciences
Gay and Lesbian Medical Association
Girls, Incorporated
Hetrick-Martin Institute
Human Rights Campaign
National Abortion Federation
National Abortion and Reproductive Rights Action League
National Asian Women's Health Organization
National Association of School Psychologists
National Council of the Churches of Christ
National Education Association-Health Information Network
National Lesbian and Gay Health Association
National Minority AIDS Council
National Native American AIDS Prevention Center
National Resource Center for Youth Services
National Women's Law Center
Planned Parenthood Federation of America
Parents, Family and Friends of Lesbians and Gays
Presbyterians Affirming Reproductive Options
Religious Coalition for Reproductive Choice
Sexuality Information and Education Council of the United States
Society for the Scientific Study of Sex
The Alan Guttmacher Institute
Unitarian Universalist Association
University of Pennsylvania, Graduate School of Education
Zero Population Growth, Incorporated

REPRINTED FROM: SIECUS Report. Sexuality in the media: Part 1. New York: Sexuality Information and Education Council of the United States, 1996:24:22–23.

this issue, the American Medical Association's Council on Scientific Affairs has recently released guidelines for providing STD-related care to gay and lesbian patients (AMA, Council on Scientific Affairs, 1996).

Limited time and resources also constrain clinicians from communicating with their patients regarding STDs and sexuality. If STDs are not seen as a high priority, clinicians, who typically have limited time to evaluate patients, will be hesitant to commit the necessary time and resources to STD prevention. This may be reinforced by clinicians' discomfort in dealing with the issues related to their patients' sexuality. Clinicians may not feel that dealing with sexuality is their responsibility. For example, while some consider sexuality to be within the physicians' province, medical training continues to reflect the predominant opinion of society that sexual health issues are private issues; therefore, such training has ignored sexuality (Lief and Karlen, 1976). As further discussed in Chapter 5, medical students learn little beyond the anatomy and physiology of the sexual reproductive system; they are not trained to deal with patients' sexual problems, and many feel uncomfortable with their lack of preparation (Merrill et al., 1990). Moreover, every clinician has biases, beliefs, and preferences related to sexuality, based on his or her own experiences and judgment, that should be recognized.

Health care professionals may subconsciously rebuke those whose sexuality differs from their own and provide services in a superficial or judgmental manner. Clinicians need to develop an awareness of their values in order to avoid unwittingly imposing them on patients or letting their values affect clinical judgment and management (Lief and Karlen, 1976; AMA, Council on Scientific Affairs, 1996). The individual's comfort level with sexuality influences the interaction between the health care professional and patient, and between the health educator and student, in subtle ways that are not always readily perceivable (Woods, 1979). This points to the need for educational and training efforts that will facilitate open and clear discussions of sex and sexuality between health care professionals and their patients (Woods, 1979; Hogan, 1980; Lewis and Freeman, 1987; Poorman and Albrecht, 1987).

Impact on Community Activism

The stigma associated with STDs hinders public discourse and, as a result, community activism for STDs other than HIV infection. Because having an STD is still socially unacceptable, there are few if any patient-based constituent groups who advocate publicly or lobby for STD-related programs. In contrast, persons with cancer and other common diseases have successfully advocated for additional funding for their causes. There also has been good advocacy for HIV infection. In considering why there is a difference in how HIV infection and other STDs are publicly viewed, the committee speculates that the following factors may help explain the disparity: (a) the stakes are higher for HIV infection than other STDs since it is a fatal disease, (b) the HIV epidemic initially spread within an organized and largely educated community (gay men) with a substantial social support network and infrastructure, and (c) HIV infection occurred among and was publicly acknowledged by highly visible opinion leaders such as persons in the arts and entertainment industry.

Experiences of Other Countries

An examination of the social policies and experiences of other developed countries regarding sexuality underscores the adverse impact of the secrecy surrounding sexuality on STD prevention in the United States. For example, the Scandinavian countries have comparable levels of sexual activity, but their rates of many STDs and unintended pregnancy are much lower than in the United States (Piot and Islam, 1994; IOM, 1995). These differences may be largely a result of differences in how sexuality issues are dealt with in these countries. For example, lower rates of STDs and unintended pregnancies in northern and western European countries compared to the United States have been attributed to the pragmatic, rather than moralistic, approach to sexuality issues in these countries. In Denmark, for example, information regarding sexuality and STDs is provided freely in the media and sex education is mandated for all students beginning no later than third grade (age 9) (David et al., 1990). Because school-based sexual health education, mass media interventions, and public discussion regarding sexual health issues are much more common in many other developed countries, it follows that private communication regarding these issues—between parents and children, and between couples—is also more common in those societies than in the United States.

Another major factor that may explain the observed differences in STD rates is universal access to health services in other developed countries. As mentioned previously, a substantial proportion of young people at high risk for STDs in the United States do not have health insurance coverage. The positive impact of better access to clinical services for STDs on STD rates is supported by the observation that the differences in viral STD rates between the United States and other developed countries are much smaller than for curable STDs. In addition, the higher rates of drug use, such as crack cocaine use, in the U.S. population compared to some other developed countries contribute to the higher rates of STDs in the U.S. It is also possible that structural or policy differences play a role. For example, in some developed countries sex workers are licensed and screened and treated for STDs to prevent transmission to others. Another potential contributing factor is the higher level of "conforming" health behaviors (e.g., health-care-seeking behavior for STDs) in many other developed countries compared to the United States. While many factors may be responsible for the observed differences in rates of STDs between the United States and other developed countries, it seems that more appropriate social norms around discussion and education regarding sexual health issues and universal access to health care in other developed countries are major factors.

Research and Training Issues in Sexuality

For the past decade, behavioral research regarding sexuality has been driven largely by public health efforts to decrease HIV transmission. In the absence of a comprehensive research agenda to study sexual behavior and norms, HIV-related research—as conducted in both the biomedical and social sciences—has produced a wealth of information about STD-related sexual behaviors, particularly regarding efficacy and determinants of condom use. The research spawned by the HIV epidemic has allowed sexual behaviors to be studied at a far greater magnitude than has been possible previously. The number of studies on sexual behavior and sexuality has increased substantially, with many providing important information about the range of sexual behaviors and patterns that exist within populations (Catania et al., 1992; Sonenstein et al., 1991; Leigh et al., 1993; Laumann, Gagnon, et al., 1994). Another significant development is that a new level of sexual discourse is developing, characterized by an increased willingness to talk publicly and explicitly about sexuality topics.

Despite the recent surge of research activity regarding sexual behaviors, the knowledge base is still limited, and many epidemiological studies of human sexuality are outdated (Laumann, Gagnon, et al., 1994). While some government funding has been provided, there has been little major or consistent support from either the government or the private sector for behavioral and social science research on human sexuality since the work of Kinsey and his colleagues (di Mauro, 1995). Comprehensive data on contemporary sexual behaviors, attitudes, and practices are limited, and it is not understood how these factors are shaped by different societal, cultural, and familial contexts (Laumann, Gagnon, et al., 1994; di Mauro, 1995).

Societal ambivalence regarding sexuality poses substantial obstacles to research regarding sexual behavior. For example, in 1991, there was unprecedented political interference with scientific research when federal administration officials, under pressure by congressional critics, blocked funding for studies of adolescent and adult sexual behavior after these studies had been approved for funding by a scientific peer-review process at the National Institutes of Health (Suplee, 1991; Laumann, Michael, et al., 1994). Congressional critics alleged that sexual behavior surveys were intended to solely "legitimize homosexual lifestyles" (Laumann, Michael, et al., 1994). The survey was eventually privately funded and became the National Health and Social Life Survey, which is the most comprehensive survey of sexual behavior in the United States in many years (Laumann, Gagnon, et al., 1994).

Researchers in human sexuality come from diverse disciplines such as anthropology, education, history, medicine, psychology, and sociology. Few researchers, however, have had specific training in designing, conducting, and evaluating research in sexuality (di Mauro, 1995). It has been generally, and incorrectly, assumed that conducting sexuality research requires no specific preparation or training other than the ability to integrate questions about sexual behavior into research design. While the inadequacy of sexuality training is well documented for health care professionals and educators (Lief and Karlen, 1976;

Nathan, 1986; Lewis and Freeman, 1987), there has been no review of the extent to which social scientists studying sexuality lack such preparation.

Trends in Sexual Activity

Although the discomfort and secrecy surrounding sexuality in America have limited scientific knowledge and prevented many parents and others from recognizing that adolescents as well as adults are sexually active, there are some scientific data regarding sexual activity. These data suggest that adolescents and young adults are not only sexually active but have very high rates of high-risk sexual behavior.

In the United States, nearly 70 percent of students in the twelfth grade have had sexual intercourse (Figure 3-3), and 27 percent of twelfth-grade students

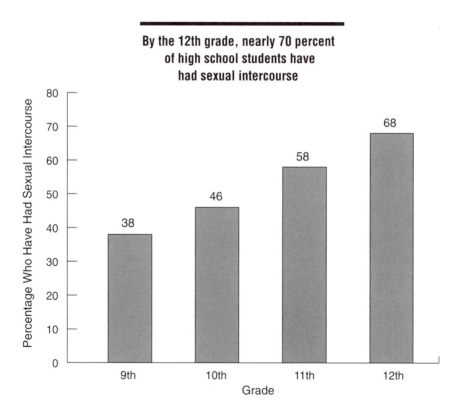

By the 12th grade, nearly 70 percent of high school students have had sexual intercourse

FIGURE 3-3 Percentage of U.S. high school students who reported ever having sexual intercourse, by grade level, 1993. SOURCE: CDC (Centers for Disease Control and Prevention). Youth risk behavior surveillance—United States, 1993. CDC Surveillance Summaries, MMWR 1995;44(No. SS-1).

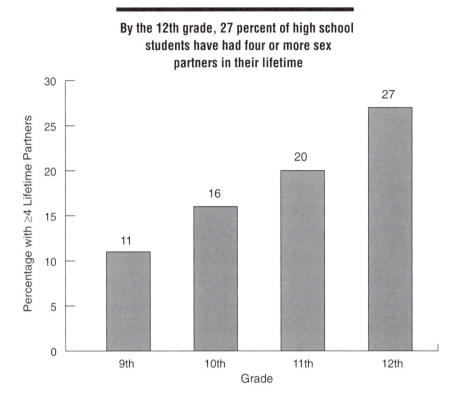

By the 12th grade, 27 percent of high school students have had four or more sex partners in their lifetime

FIGURE 3-4 Percentage of U.S. high school students reporting four or more lifetime sex partners, by grade level, 1993. SOURCE: CDC (Centers for Disease Control and Prevention). Youth risk behavior surveillance—United States, 1993. CDC Surveillance Summaries, MMWR 1995;44(No. SS-1).

have had sex with four or more partners (Figure 3-4). Intercourse among American adolescents has increased dramatically in the last few decades (Hofferth et al., 1987; CDC, 1992c; Kost and Forrest, 1992). Data from the General Social Survey and the 1988 National Survey of Family Growth show that from 1971 to 1988, the proportion of sexually active adolescents and young women ages 15 to 19 years who have had more than one lifetime sex partner increased nearly 60 percent (Kost and Forrest, 1992). In 1971, approximately 39 percent of adolescents and women surveyed had had more than one partner, compared to 62 percent of those surveyed in 1988 (Figure 3-5). Changes in the past few years have not been as great. Data from CDC's Youth Risk Behavior Surveillance System shows that from 1990 through 1993, the proportion of high school students who reported being sexually experienced, ever having sexual intercourse

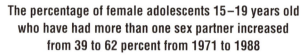

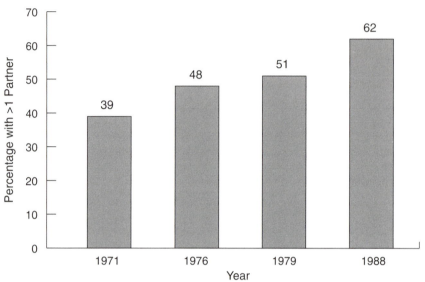

FIGURE 3-5   Prevalence of multiple sex partners among sexually active U.S. female adolescents, 15-19 years old, by year, 1971–1988. SOURCE: Kost K, Forrest JD. American women's sexual behavior and exposure to risk of sexually transmitted diseases. Fam Plann Perspect 1992;24:244-254.

with four or more partners, being sexually active (intercourse during the three months prior to the survey), or having used alcohol or drugs before last sexual intercourse remained constant (CDC, 1995). These data suggest that HIV and other STD prevention activities targeted towards adolescents beginning in the mid- to late 1980s in response to the HIV epidemic may have had a positive effect on some aspects of adolescent sexual activity.

Sexual activity among adolescents is sometimes initiated before the teenage years. A 1992 survey of 2,248 students in grades 6, 8, and 10 from an urban public school district found that 28 percent of sixth-graders and one-half of eighth-graders reported ever having had sexual intercourse (Barone et al., 1996). In an effort to examine the determinants of early onset of sexual intercourse among high-risk adolescents, Mott and colleagues (1996) analyzed a series of data collected through the National Longitudinal Survey of Youth from 1988 through 1992. They found that children were more likely to have early onset of intercourse if their mother had sex at an early age and if she worked extensively.

In addition, African American heritage and early alcohol use among boys and cigarette smoking among girls were associated with early onset of intercourse. Children who attended church and had friends who attended the same church were less likely to initiate sexual intercourse early.

Studies among college and university students give insight on the extent of sexual activity among young adults. A 1991 survey at in a large Midwestern university showed that 80 percent of male and 73 percent of female students had experienced sexual intercourse and that men reported an average of eight lifetime partners and women had an average of six lifetime partners (Reinisch et al., 1995). A survey of a Hawaiian university population found that a history of an STD was reported by 21 percent of women and 16 percent of men (Hale et al., 1993).

The prevalence of high-risk sexual practices among college students remains high. For example, a major study of female college students who sought gynecological care at a student health center during 1975, 1986, and 1989 examined trends in sexual behavior and practices during this time period (DeBuono et al., 1990). Among sexually active women, the percentage who reported that their partner "always or almost always" used a condom increased significantly, from 12 percent in 1975, to 21 percent in 1986, to 41 percent in 1989. However, despite the recognition of HIV infection and other STDs during this period, with the exception of increased condom use, there were no significant changes in sexual practices such as number of partners and other high-risk sexual practices among the students surveyed from 1975 through 1989. A follow-up study, however, showed that almost three-quarters of college women reported "always or almost always" using condoms in 1995 (Peipert et al., 1996). Although condom use has increased substantially, absolute rates are still low in many groups.

During the past several decades, the age of entry into marriage has dramatically increased in the United States. For example, approximately 80 percent of men born during the interval 1933–1942 had married by age 27 compared to only 50 percent of men born during the interval 1953–1962 (Laumann, Gagnon et al., 1994). Coupled with the decreasing age at first intercourse during the last several decades, this means that the length of time between first intercourse and marriage has increased greatly. This phenomenon has increased the potential for spread of STDs because single persons tend to have more sex partners than married persons.

Knowledge and Awareness of STDs

Knowledge and awareness of STDs among Americans is poor. In a 1993 national survey of one thousand women from 18 through 60 years of age, almost two-thirds knew nothing or very little about STDs other than HIV/AIDS, and only 11 percent were aware that STDs can be more harmful to women than to men (EDK Associates, 1994). The lack of knowledge among women in high-risk

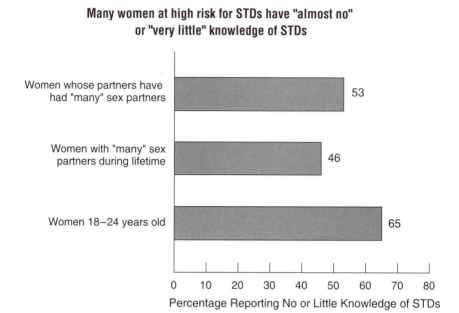

Many women at high risk for STDs have "almost no" or "very little" knowledge of STDs

FIGURE 3-6   Self-reported knowledge of STDs among women by risk groups, 1993. Survey participants were asked to identify number of sex partners as "none," "one," "a few," or "many." SOURCE: EDK Associates, Inc. Women and sexually transmitted diseases: the dangers of denial. New York: American Medical Women's Association, 1994.

groups was dramatic: 65 percent of young women reported "almost none" or "very little" knowledge regarding STDs (Figure 3-6). Survey data suggested that women with greater knowledge and awareness of STDs are more likely to practice protective behaviors such as negotiating for condom use and seeking help from a health care professional.

A recent survey confirmed that many Americans lack sufficient knowledge of STDs (ASHA, 1995). Thirty-two percent of respondents could not name an STD other than HIV/AIDS. Of those who did identify another STD, 44 percent of respondents named syphilis; 37 percent named gonorrhea; few named any other STD. More than half of respondents believed that "all STDs except HIV/AIDS are curable," and they vastly underestimated the prevalence of STDs. Both of those beliefs (that all STDs can be cured and that STD prevalence is not high) are likely to reduce motivation to protect oneself against STDs.

It is interesting to note that adolescents surveyed had greater knowledge of some aspects of STDs than adults (ASHA, 1996). When asked about the prevalence of STDs in the population, 12 percent of the adolescent respondents versus 4 percent of adult respondents correctly stated that the number was one in five people. Although few adolescents could name an STD other than HIV/AIDS, they were more likely than adults to answer correctly that some STDs (in addition to HIV/AIDS) are incurable and that some STDs are asymptomatic.

STDs are far more common than is generally perceived by the general population or health care professionals. For example, while there is widespread awareness of genital herpes infections, there also are many misperceptions about them. Perhaps the single largest misperception concerns the prevalence of herpes infection. In a recent national survey of sexual behavior (Laumann, Gagnon, et al., 1994), 2 percent of survey respondents age 18–59 reported having had genital herpes. In contrast, population-based studies suggest that the prevalence of antibodies to herpes simplex virus type 2, which causes about 85 percent of initial episodes of genital herpes, was 21.7 percent in 1990 (Johnson et al., 1993). The reason for the substantial differences between the low prevalence of self-reported genital herpes infections and the far higher true prevalence of the disease may be misperceptions regarding the clinical manifestations of genital herpes infections. Herpes is most often described as an episodic illness, typically presenting as a painful genital eruption and recurring with similarly painful lesions of shorter duration. In fact, a quite different clinical spectrum of infection exists. Herpes infection may manifest as mild initial episodes and asymptomatic shedding of the virus (Koutsky et al., 1992). Other studies indicate that most genital herpes infections are spread by asymptomatic individuals who often are unaware of their infections (Mertz et al., 1992).

CONCLUSIONS

Biological and social factors contribute to the hidden nature of the STD epidemic. Biological factors, including the lack of signs and symptoms in infected persons, the long lag time from initial infection until signs of severe complications, and the propensity for STDs to more easily infect women than men, contribute to the general lack of awareness of STDs among health professionals and the public. A number of social factors contribute to the risk of STDs and place a disproportionate burden on certain populations in the United States. Poverty and inadequate access to health care, substance use, and sexual abuse all increase an individual's risk for STDs. Lack of health insurance is particularly acute among the age and ethnic groups at greatest risk of STDs. Even for the insured, access to comprehensive STD-related services may be difficult. Sex workers, persons in detention facilities, the homeless, migrant workers, and other disenfranchised persons represent "core" transmitters of STDs in the population. Efforts to prevent STDs in the entire community are not likely to be successful unless these groups receive appropriate STD-related services.

Many Americans are reluctant or unwilling to discuss sexuality and STD-related issues openly or refuse to have the issue appear in the public arena. Such reluctance has devastating consequences for STD prevention efforts. Open and frank communication and the sharing of information regarding sexuality and STDs are essential to preventing high-risk sexual behavior. In order to change behavior, Americans have to feel comfortable discussing sexual health issues; open communication between parents and children, between sexual partners, between teachers and students, and between health care providers and patients is essential. The secrecy surrounding sexuality impedes sexuality education programs for adolescents, open discussion between parents and their children and between sex partners, balanced messages from mass media, education and counseling activities of health care professionals, and community activism regarding STDs. Opponents of sexuality education programs for adolescents are likely to deny the possibility that their children are sexually active. Unfortunately, denial often eliminates the possibility that parents will communicate with their children regarding STDs, and this encourages high-risk behaviors. Children in these families are likely to get their information, which is often inaccurate, from other sources. Lack of comfort with open discussions of sexuality also makes open communication regarding sexual history and negotiating safer sex difficult. In addition, this discomfort has also resulted in a mass media that has not been involved in promoting healthy sexual behaviors. This industry commonly acquiesces to the public's fascination with sex, yet is generally not willing to incorporate and promote factual information regarding STDs and protective behaviors. Furthermore, discomfort and secrecy among health care providers adversely affects the delivery of health services. As a result, many clinicians do not identify potential problems or are ineffective in counseling their patients regarding healthy sexual behavior. Finally, secrecy hinders community activism for STDs. An effective STD prevention program should focus on overcoming all barriers to open communication.

Despite or because of the secrecy surrounding sexuality, adolescents and young adults are becoming increasingly sexually active. Better research is needed to track the problem of STDs and identify possible solutions; much of the data available in this area are seriously outdated or incomplete. There is a compelling need for further training of clinicians, educators, and researchers in the area of human sexuality. The poor understanding of STDs among Americans strongly supports a coordinated campaign to improve knowledge and awareness.

REFERENCES

AAP (American Academy of Pediatrics), Committee on Child Abuse and Neglect. Guidelines for the evaluation of sexual abuse of children. Pediatrics 1991;87:254-60.

AMA (American Medical Association), Council on Scientific Affairs. Health care needs of homeless and runaway youths. JAMA 1989;262:1358-61.

AMA, Council on Scientific Affairs. Health care needs of gay men and lesbians in the United States. JAMA 1996;275:1354-9.

Amaro H. Considerations for prevention of HIV infection among Hispanic women. Psychol Women Q 1988;12:429-43.

Anderson JE, Dahlberg LL. High-risk sexual behavior in the general population: results from a national survey, 1988-1990. Sex Transm Dis 1992;17:320-5.

Aral SO, Holmes KK. Epidemiology of sexual behavior and sexually transmitted diseases. In: Holmes KK, Mårdh PA, Sparling PF, Weisner PJ, Cates W Jr, Lemon SM, et al., eds. Sexually transmitted diseases. 2nd ed. New York: McGraw-Hill, Inc., 1990:19-36.

ARHP, ANPRH (Association of Reproductive Health Professionals and Association of Nurse Practitioners in Reproductive Health). STD counseling practices and needs survey. Silver Spring, MD: Schulman, Ronca, and Bucuvalas, Inc., January 1995.

ASHA (American Social Health Association). International survey reveals lack of knowledge about STDs. STD News. A quarterly newsletter of the American Social Health Association. Fall 1995;3:1,10.

ASHA. Teenagers know more than adults about STDs, but knowledge among both groups is low. STD News. A quarterly newsletter of the American Social Health Association. Winter 1996;3:1, 5.

Barone C, Ickovics JR, Ayers TS, Katz SM, Voyce CK, Weissberg RP. High-risk sexual behavior among young urban students. Fam Plann Perspect 1996:28;69-74.

Bechtel GA, Shepherd MA, Rogers PW. Family, culture, and health practices among migrant farmworkers. J Community Health Nurs 1995;12:15-22.

Bell TA, Farrow JA, Stamm WE, Critchlow CW, Holmes KK. Sexually transmitted diseases in females in a juvenile detention center. Sex Transm Dis 1985;12:140-4.

Bickell NA, Vermund SH, Holmes M, Safyer S, Burk RD. Human papillomavirus, gonorrhea, syphilis, and cervical dysplasia in jailed women. Am J Public Health 1991;81:1318-20.

Blank S, Rubin S, Brome-Bunting M, Masterson M, McDonnell D, Fatt DL, et al. Improving syphilis treatment rates among women inmates in New York City. Proceedings of the twenty-seventh meeting, Society for Epidemiologic Research, June 15-18, 1994, Miami, FL. Salt Lake City: Society for Epidemiologic Research, 1994.

Brandt AM. No magic bullet: a social history of venereal disease in the United States since 1880. New York: Oxford University Press, Inc., 1985.

Brandt AM. AIDS in historical perspective: four lessons from the history of sexually transmitted diseases. Am J Public Health 1988;78:367-71.

Breakey WR, Fischer PJ, Kramer M, Nestadt G, Romanovski AJ, Ross A, et al. Health problems of homeless men and women in Baltimore. JAMA 1989;262:1352-7.

Brown JD, Newcomer SF. Television viewing and adolescents' sexual behavior. J Homosexuality 1991;21:77-91.

Brown JD, Steele JR. Sex and the mass media. Report prepared for The Henry J. Kaiser Family Foundation and presented at "Sex and Hollywood: should there be a government role?" American Enterprise Institute, June 21, 1995, Washington, D.C.

Brown JD, Steele JR. Sexuality and the mass media: an overview. In: SIECUS Report. Sexuality in the media: Part 1. New York: Information and Education Council of the United States, 1996:24:3-9.

Brunham RC, Nagelkerke JN, Plummer FA, Moses S. Estimating the basic reproductive rates of *Neisseria gonorrhoeae* and *Chlamydia trachomatis*: the implications of acquired immunity [see comments]. Sex Transm Dis 1994;21:353-6.

Buchta RM. Attitudes of adolescents and parents of adolescents concerning condom advertisements on television. J Adolesc Health Care 1989;10:220-3.

Buerkel-Rothfuss NL, Strouse JS. Media exposure and perceptions of sexual behaviors: the cultivation hypothesis moves to the bedroom. In: Greenberg BS, Brown JD, Buerkel-Rothfuss NL, eds. Media, sex and the adolescent. Cresskill, NJ: Hampton Press, Inc., 1993:225-47.

Caetano R, Hines AM. Alcohol, sexual practices, and risk of AIDS among blacks, hispanics, and whites. J Acquir Immune Defic Syndr 1995;10:554-61.

Cameron DW, Simonsen JN, D'Costa LJ, Ronald AR, Maitha GM, Gakinya MN, et al. Female to male transmission of human immunodeficiency virus type 1: risk factors for seroconversion in men. Lancet 1989; 2:403-7.

Catania JA, Coates TJ, Stall R, Turner H, Peterson J, Hearst N, et al. Prevalences of AIDS-related risk factors and condom use the United States. Science 1992;258:1101-6.

Cates W Jr. Epidemiology and control of sexually transmitted diseases in adolescents. In: Schydlower M, Shafer MA, eds. AIDS and other sexually transmitted diseases. Philadelphia: Hanly & Belfus, Inc., 1990:409-27.

Cates W Jr. Contraception, contraceptive technology and STD. In: Holmes KK, Sparling PF, Mårdh PA, Lemon SM, Stamm WE, Piot P, Wasserheit JN, eds. Sexually transmitted diseases. 3rd ed. New York: McGraw-Hill, Inc., in press.

CDC (Centers for Disease Control and Prevention). Current trends: heterosexual behaviors and factors that influence condom use among patients attending a sexually transmitted disease clinic—San Francisco. MMWR 1990;39:685-9.

CDC. HIV infection, syphilis, and tuberculosis screening among migrant farm workers—Florida, 1992. MMWR 1992a;41:723-5.

CDC. HIV prevention in the U.S. correctional system, 1991. MMWR 1992b;41:389-91, 397.

CDC. Premarital sexual experience among adolescent women—United States, 1970-1988. MMWR 1992c;39:929-32.

CDC. 1993 Sexually transmitted diseases treatment guidelines. MMWR 1993;42(No. RR-14):56-66.

CDC. Trends in sexual risk behavior among high school students—United States, 1990, 1991, and 1993. MMWR 1995;44:124-5, 131-2.

CDC. Community-level prevention of human immunodeficiency virus infection among high-risk populations: the AIDS Community Demonstration Projects. MMWR 1996a;45(RR-6).

CDC. HIV/AIDS education and prevention programs for adults in prisons and jails and juveniles in confinement facilities—United States, 1994. MMWR 1996b;45:268-71.

Celum CL, Hook EW, Bolan GA, Spauding CD, Leone P, Henry KW, et al. Where would clients seek care for STD services under health care reform? Results of a STD client survey from five clinics. Eleventh Meeting of the International Society for STD Research, August 27-30, 1995, New Orleans, LA [abstract no. 101].

Chilman CS. Adolescent sexuality in a changing American society. Washington, D.C.: U.S. Government Printing Office, 1978 (017-046-00050-1).

Cohen D, Scribner R, Clark J, Cory D. The potential role of custody facilities in controlling sexually transmitted diseases [published erratum appears in Am J Public Health 1992;82:684]. Am J Public Health 1992;82:552-6.

Critchlow CW, Wolner-Hanssen P, Eschenbach DA, Kiviat NB, Koutsky LA, Stevens CE, et al. Determinants of cervical ectopia and of cervicitis: age, oral contraception, specific cervical infection, smoking, and douching. Am J Obstet Gynecol 1995;173:534-43.

Cutler JC, Arnold RC. Venereal disease control by health departments in the past: lessons for the present. Am J Public Health 1988;78:372-6.

Darrow WW. Assessing targeted AIDS prevention in male and female prostitutes and their clients. In: Paccaud F, Vader JP, Gutzwiller F, eds. Assessing AIDS prevention. Basel, Switzerland: Birkhäuser Verlag, 1992:215-31.

David HP, Morgall JM, Osler M, Rasmussen NK, Jensen B. United States and Denmark: different approaches to health care and family planning. Stud Fam Plann 1990;21:1-19.

DeBuono BA, Zinner SH, Daamen M, McCormack WM. Sexual behavior of college women in 1975, 1986, and 1989. N Engl J Med 1990;322:821-5.

Decker MD, Vaughn WK, Brodie JS, Hutcheson RH Jr, Schaffner W. Seroepidemiology of hepatitis B in Tennessee prisoners. J Infect Dis 1984;150:450-9.

DiClemente RJ, Lanier MM, Horan PF, Lodico M. Comparison of AIDS knowledge, attitudes, and behaviors among incarcerated adolescents and a public school sample in San Francisco. Am J Public Health 1991;81:628-30.

Dietz WH, Strasburger VC. Children, adolescents and television. Curr Probl Pediatr 1991;21:8-32.

di Mauro D. Executive summary of sexuality research in the United States: an assessment of the social and behavioral sciences. New York: Social Science Research Council, 1995.

Dolan K, Wodak A, Penny R. AIDS behind bars: preventing HIV spread among incarcerated drug injectors. AIDS 1995;9:825-32.

Doll DC. Tattooing in prison and HIV infection [letter]. Lancet 1988;1:66-7.

Donelan K, Blendon RJ, Hill CA, Hoffman C, Rowland D, Frankel M, et al. Whatever happened to the health insurance crisis in the United States? Voices from a national survey. JAMA 1996;276:1346-50.

Donovan P. Taking family planning services to hard-to-reach populations. Fam Plann Perspect 1996;28:120-6.

Dougherty S. 1996 National Farmworker Health Conference. J Int Assoc Physicians AIDS Care 1996;2:12-16,19.

EBRI (Employee Benefits Research Institute). Children without health insurance. Washington, D.C.: EBRI, Notes, Vol. 16(5), May 1995a.

EBRI. Sources of health insurance and characteristics of the uninsured: analysis of the March 1994 Current Population Survey. Washington, D.C.: EBRI, Special Issue Brief Number 158, February 1995b.

EDK Associates. Women & sexually transmitted diseases: the dangers of denial. New York: EDK Associates, 1994.

EDK Associates. The ABCs of STDs. New York: EDK Associates, 1995.

Edlin BR, Irwin KL, Faruque S, McCoy CB, Word C, Serrano Y, et al. Intersecting epidemics—crack cocaine use and HIV infection among inner-city young adults. The Multicenter Crack Cocaine and HIV Infection Study Team. N Engl J Med 1994;31:1422-7.

Elias CJ, Heise LL. Challenges for the development of female-controlled vaginal microbicides. AIDS 1994;8:1-9.

Elliot S. The sponsor is the surprise in Fox's first condom ad. New York Times, November 19, 1991; Sect. D: 19(col. 1).

Ericksen KP, Trocki KF. Behavioral risk factors for sexually transmitted diseases in American households. Soc Sci Med 1992;34:843-53.

Finelli L, Budd J, Spitalny KC. Early syphilis. Relationship to sex, drugs, and changes in high-risk behavior from 1987-1990. Sex Transm Dis 1993;20:89-95.

Finkelhor D and Associates. A sourcebook on child sexual abuse. Beverly Hills, CA: Sage Publications, 1986.

Fish AN, Fairweather DV, Oriel JD, Ridgeway GL. Chlamydia trachomatis infection in a gynaecology clinic population: identification of high-risk groups and the value of contact tracing. Eur J Obstet Gynecol Reprod Biol 1989;31:67-74.

Flora JA, Maibach EW, Holtgrave D. Communication campaigns for HIV prevention: Using mass media in the next decade. In: IOM. Assessing the social and behavioral science base for HIV/AIDS prevention and intervention [workshop summary, background papers]. Washington, D.C.: National Academy Press, 1995:129-54.

Forrest KA, Washington AE, Daling JR, Sweet RL. Vaginal douching as a possible risk factor for pelvic inflammatory disease. J Natl Med Assoc 1989;81:159-65.

Forst ML. Sexual risk profiles of delinquent and homeless youths. J Community Health 1994;19:101-14.

Freeman HE, Blendon RJ, Aiken LH, Sudman S, Mullix CF, Covey CR. Americans report on their access to health care. Health Aff Millwood 1987;6:6-18.

Freeman HE, Corey CR. Insurance status and access to health services among poor persons. Health Serv Res 1993;28:531-41.

Furstenberg R, Moore K, Peterson J. Sex education and sexual experience among adolescents. Am J Public Health 1985;75:1331-2.

Gerbner G. Women and minorities on television: a study in casting and fate. Report presented to the Screen Actors Guild and the American Federation of Radio and Television Artists, Annenberg School for Communications, Philadelphia, June 1993.

Gerrard M. Sex, sex guilt and contraceptive use. J Pers Soc Psychol 1982;42:153-8.

Gerrard M. Sex, sex guilt and contraceptive use revisited: the 1980's. J Pers Soc Psychol 1987;52:975.

Glaser JB, Greifinger RB. Correctional health care: a public health opportunity. Ann Intern Med 1993;118:139-45.

Greenberg BS, Brown JD, Buerkel-Rothfuss NL, eds. Media, sex and the adolescent. Cresskill, NJ: Hampton Press, 1993.

Greenberg BS, Busselle RW. Soap operas and sexual activity. Report submitted to The Henry J. Kaiser Family Foundation, October 1994.

Greenberg BS, Smith S, Ah Yun J, Busselle R, Rampoldi Hnilo L, Mitchell M, et al. The content of television talk shows: topics, guest and interactions. Departments of Communication and Tele-communication, Michigan State University. Report prepared for The Henry J. Kaiser Family Foundation, November 1995.

Greenberg J, Schnell D, Conlon R. Behaviors of crack cocaine users and their impact on early syphilis intervention. Sex Transm Dis 1992;19:346-50.

Greenberg MSZ, Singh T, Htoo M, Schultz S. The association between congenital syphilis and cocaine/crack use in New York City: a case-control study. Am J Public Health 1991;81:1316-8.

Guidry HM. Childhood sexual abuse: role of the family physician. Am Fam Physician 1995;51:407-14.

Gutman LT, St. Claire K, Herman Giddens ME. Prevalence of sexual abuse in children with genital warts [letter; comment]. Pediatr Infect Dis J 1991;10:342-3.

Hale RW, Char DF, Nagy K, Stockert N. Seventeen-year review of sexual and contraceptive behavior on a college campus. Am J Obstet Gynecol 1993;168 (6 Pt 1):1833-7; discussion 1837-8.

Hall J. The networks' condom cover-up. Raleigh News and Observer, January 31, 1994, C10.

Hammett TM, Widom R, Epstein J, Gross M, Sifre S, Enos T. 1994 Update: HIV/AIDS and STDs in correctional facilities. Washington, D.C.: U.S. Department of Justice, Office of Justice Programs, National Institute of Justice/U.S. Department of Health and Human Services, Public Health Service, CDC, December 1995.

Harris L and Associates. Attitudes about television, sex and contraception. A survey of a cross-section of adult Americans. Conducted for Planned Parenthood Federation of America. February 1987.

Harris L and Associates. Sexual material on American network television during the 1987-88 season. New York: Planned Parenthood Federation of America, 1988.

Hein K, Cohen MI, Marks A, Schonberg SK, Meyer M, McBride A. Age at first intercourse among homeless adolescent females. J Pediatr 1978;93:147-8.

Herold ES, Goodwin MS, Lero DS. Self-esteem, locus of control, and adolescent contraception. J Psych 1979;101:83-8.

Hingson RW, Strunin L, Berlin BM, Hereen T. Beliefs about AIDS, use of alcohol and drugs, and unprotected sex among Massachusetts adolescents. Am J Public Health 1990;80:295-9.

Hofferth SL, Kahn JR, Baldwin W. Premarital sexual activity among U.S. teenage women over the past three decades. Fam Plann Perspect 1987;19:46-53.

Hogan H. Human sexuality, a nursing perspective. Norwalk, CT: Appleton-Century-Crofts Co., 1980.

Holmes MD, Safyer SM, Bickell NA, Vermund SH, Hanff PA, Phillips RS. Chlamydial cervical infection in jailed women. Am J Public Health 1993; 83:551-5.

Horsburgh CR, Jarvis JQ, McArthur T, Ignacio T, Stock P. Seroconversion to human immunodeficiency virus in prison inmates. Am J Public Health 1990;80:209-10.

Hudgins R, McCusker J, Stoddard A. Cocaine use and risky injection and sexual behaviors. Drug Alcohol Depend 1995;37:7-14.

Hyde S. Understanding human sexuality. 5th ed. New York: McGraw Hill, Inc., 1994.

IOM (Institute of Medicine). Understanding the determinants of HIV risk behavior. In: Auerbach JD, Wypijewska C, Brodie HKH, eds. AIDS and behavior. Washington, D.C.: National Academy Press, 1994:78-123.

IOM. Best intentions: unintended pregnancy and the well-being of children and families. Brown SS, Eisenberg L, eds. Washington, D.C.: National Academy Press, 1995.

Jemmott LS, Jemmott JB. Family structure, parental strictness, and sexual behavior among inner-city black male adolescents. J Adolesc Res 1992a;7:192-207.

Jemmott LS, Jemmott JB. Increasing condom-use intentions among sexually active black adolescent women. Nurs Res 1992b;41:273-9.

Jemmott JB, Jemmott LS, Fong GT. Reductions in HIV risk-associated sexual behaviors among black male adolescents: Effects of an AIDS prevention intervention. Am J Public Health 1992; 82:372-7.

Johnson R, Lee F, Hadgu A, McQuillan G, Aral S, Keesling S, et al. U.S. genital herpes trends during the first decade of AIDS—prevalences increased in young whites and elevated in blacks. In: Proceedings of the Tenth Meeting of the International Society for STD Research, August 23-September 1, 1993, Helsinki, Finland [abstract No. 22].

Johnstone H, Tornabene M, Marcinak J. Incidence of sexually transmitted diseases and Pap smear results in female homeless clients from the Chicago Health Outreach Project. Health Care Women Int 1993;14:293-9.

Jones JL, Rion P, Hollis S, Longshore S, Leverette WB, Ziff L. HIV-related characteristics of migrant workers in rural South Carolina. South Med J 1991;84:1088-90.

Judson FN. Gonorrhea. Med Clin North Am 1990;74:1353-67.

Kalichman SC, Kelly JA, Johnson JR, Bulto M. Factors associated with risk for HIV infection among chronic mentally ill adults. Am J Psychiatry 1994;151:221-7.

Keim J, Woodard MP, Anderson MK. Screening for *Chlamydia trachomatis* in college women on routine gynecological exams. J Am Coll Health 1992;41:17-9, 22-3.

Kennedy CA, Skurnick J, Wan JY, Quattronc G, Sheffet A, Quinones M, et al. Psychological distress, drug and alcohol use as correlates of condom use in HIV-serodiscordant heterosexual couples. AIDS 1993;7:1493-9.

Kilborne J. Killing us softly: gender roles in advertising. Adolesc Med: State of the Art Rev 1993;4:635-49.

Kimani J, Maclean IW, Bwayo JJ, MacDonald K, Oyugi J, Maitha GM, et al., Risk factors for *Chlamydia trachomatis* pelvic inflammatory disease among sex workers in Nairobi, Kenya. J Infect Dis 1996;173:1437-44.

Kirby D, Short L, Collins J, Rugg D, Kolbe L, Howard M, et al. School-based programs to reduce sexual risk behaviors: a review of effectiveness. Public Health Rep 1994;109:339-60.

Klassen AD, Williams CI, Levitt EE. Sex and morality in the U.S. Middletown, CT: Wesleyan University Press, 1989.

Klein JD, Brown JD, Childers KW, Oliveri J, Porter C, Dykers C. Adolescents' risky behavior and mass media use. Pediatrics 1993; 92:24-31.

Koelle DM, Benedetti J, Langenberg A, Corey L. Asymptomatic reactivation of herpes simplex virus in women after the first episode of genital herpes. Ann Intern Med 1992;116:433-7.

Koopman C, Rosario M, Rotheram-Borus MJ. Alcohol and drug use and sexual behaviors placing runaways at risk for HIV infection. Addict Behav 1994;19:95-103.

Kosovich DR. Sexuality throughout the centuries. Psychiatr Opin 1978;15:15-9.

Kost K, Forrest JD. American women's sexual behavior and exposure to risk of sexually transmitted diseases. Fam Plann Perspect 1992;24:244-54.

Koutsky LA, Stevens CE, Holmes KK, Ashley RL, Kliviat NB, Critchlow CW, et al. Underdiagnosis of genital herpes by current clinical and viral-isolation procedures. N Engl J Med 1992; 326:1533-9.

Kreiss JK, Hopkins SG. The association between circumcision status and human immunodeficiency virus infection among homosexual men. J Infect Dis 1993;168:1404-8.

Laumann EO, Gagnon JH, Michael RT, Michaels S. The social organization of sexuality: sexual practices in the United States. Chicago, IL: University of Chicago Press, 1994.

Laumann EO, Michael RT, Gagnon JH. A political history of the National Sex Survey of Adults. Fam Plann Perspect 1994;26:34-8.

Lear D. Sexual communication in the age of AIDS: the construction of risk and trust among young adults. Soc Sci Med 1995;41:1311-23.

Lebow MA. Contraceptive advertising in the United States. Women's Health Issues 1994;4:196-208.

Leigh BC, Stall R. Substance use and risky sexual behavior for exposure to HIV. Issues in methodology, interpretation, prevention. Am Psychol 1993;48:1035-45.

Leigh, BC, Temple MT, Trocki KF. The sexual behavior of U.S. adults: results from a national survey. Am J Public Health 1993;83:1400-8.

Leigh BC, Temple MT, Trocki KF. The relationship of alcohol use to sexual activity in a U.S. national sample. Social Science Med 1994;39:1527-35.

Lewis CE, Freeman HE. The sexual history-taking and counseling practices of primary care physicians. West J Med 1987;147:165-7.

Lewis CE, Montgomery K. The AIDS-related experience and practices of primary care physicians in Los Angeles: 1984-89. Am J Public Health 1990;80:1511-3.

Lichter SR, Lichter LS, Rothman S. Prime time. How TV portrays American culture. Washington, D.C.: Regnery Publishing, Inc., 1994.

Lief H, Karlen A. Sex education in medicine. New York: Spectrum Publications, 1976.

Lowry DT, Schidler JA. Prime time TV portrayals of sex, "safe sex" and AIDS: a longitudinal analysis. Journalism Q 1993;70:628-37.

Lowry DT, Towles DE. Soap opera portrayals of sex, contraception, and sexually transmitted diseases. J Communications 1989;39:76-83.

Lowry R, Holtzman D, Truman BI, Kann L, Collins JL, Kolbe LJ. Substance use and HIV-related sexual behaviors among US high school students: are they related? Am J Public Health 1994;84:1116-20.

Mahon N. New York inmates' HIV risk behaviors: the implications for prevention policy and programs. Am J Public Health 1996;86:1211-5.

Manov A, Lowther L. A health care approach for hard-to-reach adolescent runaways. Nurs Clin North Am 1983;18:333-42.

Martensen RL. Syphilis, contagion, and the place of sexuality in late 19th-century America. JAMA 1994;272:69.

Martin HL, Hyange PM, Richardson BA, Chohan B, Hillier SL, Mandaliya K, et al. Association between presence of vaginal lactobacilli and acquisition of HIV and STDs. Eleventh International Conference on AIDS, July 7-12, 1996, Vancouver [abstract no. Tu.C.2692].

Marx R, Aral SO, Rolfs RT, Sterk CE, Kahn JG. Crack, sex, and STD. Sex Transm Dis 1991;18:92-101.

Marx PA, Spira AI, Gettie A, Dailey PJ, Veazey RS, Lackner AA, et al. Progesterone implants enhance SIV vaginal transmission and early virus load. Nature Med 1996;2:1084-9.

Matthews WC, Booth MW, Turner JD, Kessler L. Physicians' attitudes toward homosexuality—survey of California County Medical Society. West J Med 1986;144:106-10.

May RM, Anderson RM. Transmission dynamics of HIV infection. Nature 1987;326:137-42.

Mayden B. Sexuality education for youths in care. A state-by-state survey. Washington, D.C.: Child Welfare League of America Press, 1996.

Mays VM, Cochran SD. Issues in the perception of AIDS risk and risk reduction activities by black and Hispanic/Latina women. Am Psychol 1988;43:949-57.

McCoy HV, Inciardi JA. Women and AIDS: social determinants of sex-related activities. Women Health 1993;20:69-86.

Merrill JM, Laux LF, Thornby JI. Why doctors have difficulty with sex histories. Southern Med J 1990;83:613-17.

Mertz GJ, Benedetti J, Ashley R, Selke SA, Corey L. Risk factors for the transmission of genital herpes. Ann Intern Med 1992;116:197-202.

Miller BC, Monson BH, Norton MC. The effects of forced sexual intercourse on white female adolescents. Child Abuse Negl 1995;19:1289-301.

Moran JS, Peterman T. Sexually transmitted diseases in prisons and jails. Prison J 1989;64:1-6.

Moses S, Plummer FA, Bradley JE, Ndinya-Achola JO, Nagelkerke NJ, Ronald AR. The association between lack of male circumcision and risk for HIV infection: a review of the epidemiological data. Sex Transm Dis 1994;21:201-10.

Moss GB, Clemetson D, D'Costa L, Plummer FA, Ndinya-Achola JO, Reilly M, et al. Association of cervical ectopy with heterosexual transmission of human immunodeficiency virus: results of a study of couples in Nairobi, Kenya. J Infect Dis 1991;164:588-91.

Mostad S, Welch M, Chohan B, Reilly M, Overbaugh J, Mandalya K, et al. Cervical and vaginal HIV-1 DNA shedding in female STD clinic attenders. Eleventh International Conference on AIDS, July 7-12, 1996, Vancouver [abstract no. WeC 333].

Mott FL, Fondell MM, Hu PN, Kowaleski-Jones L, Menaghan EG. The determinants of first sex by age 14 in a high-risk adolescent population. Fam Plann Perspect 1996;28:13-8.

Mutter RC, Grimes RM, Labarthe D. Evidence of intraprison spread of HIV infection. Arch Intern Med 1994;154:793-5.

Nathan SG. Are clinical psychology graduate students being taught enough about sexuality? A survey of doctoral programs. J Sex Res 1986;22:520-4.

NCCHC (National Commission on Correctional Health Care). Standards for health services in jails. Chicago: National Commission on Correctional Health Care, 1992.

NCCHC. Administrative management of HIV in corrections. Position statement. Chicago: National Commission on Correctional Health Care, September 25, 1994.

Oh MK, Cloud GA, Wallace LS, Reynolds J, Strudevant M, Feinstein RA. Sexual behavior and sexually transmitted diseases among male adolescents in detention. Sex Transm Dis 1994;21:127-32.

O'Leary A, Jemmott LS. Future directions. In: O'Leary A, Jemmott, LS, eds. Women at risk: issues in the primary prevention of AIDS. New York: Plenum Press, 1995:257-9.

Olson B. Sex and the soaps: a comparative content analysis of health issues. Journalism Q 1994;71:840-50.

Orbovich C. Case studies of collaboration between family planning agencies and managed care organizations. West J Med 1995;163(3 Suppl):39-44.

Peipert JF, Domagalski L, Boardman L, Daamen M, Zinner SH. College women and condom use, 1975-1995. New Engl J Med 1996;335:211.

Piot P, Islam MQ. Sexually transmitted diseases in the 1990s. Global epidemiology and challenges for control. Sex Transm Dis 1994;21(2 Suppl):S7-S13.

Plichta SB, Abraham C. Violence and gynecological health in women < 50 years old. Am J Obstet Gynecol 1996;174:903-7.

Plummer FA, Ngugi EN. Prostitutes and their clients in the epidemiology and control of sexually transmitted diseases. In: Holmes KK, March P-A, Sparling, PF, Wiesner PJ, Cates W Jr, Lemon SM, et al., eds. Sexually transmitted diseases. 2nd ed. New York: McGraw-Hill, Inc., 1990:71-6.

Plummer FA, Simonsen JN, Chubb H, Slaney L, Kimata J, Bosire M, et al. Epidemiologic evidence for the development of serovar immunity after gonococcal infection. J Clin Invest 1989;83:1472-6.

Poorman S, Albrecht L. Human sexuality and the nursing process. Norwalk, CT: Appleton & Lange Publishing Co., 1987.

Ramos R, Shain, RN, Johnson L. "Men I mess with don't have anything to do with AIDS": Using ethno-theory to understand sexual risk perception. Sociol Q 1995;36:483-504.

Reinisch JM, Hill CA, Sanders S, Ziemba-Davis M. High-risk sexual behavior at a Midwestern university: a confirmatory study. Fam Plann Perspect 1995;27:79-82.

Rickman RL, Lodico M, DiClemente RJ, Morris R, Baker C, Huscroft S. Sexual communication is associated with condom use by sexually active incarcerated adolescents. J Adolesc Health 1994;15:383-8.

Risen CB. A guide to taking a sexual history. Clin Sex 1995;18:39-53.

Rosenbaum S, Shin P, Mauskopf A, Fund K, Stern G, Zuvekas A. Beyond the freedom to choose. Medicaid, managed care, and family planning. West J Med 1995;163(3 Suppl): S33-S38.

Rosenberg MJ, Gollub EL. Commentary: methods women can use that may prevent sexually transmitted diseases, including HIV [see comments]. Am J Public Health 1992;82:1473-8.

Rosenblum L, Darrow W, Witte J, Cohen J, French J, Gill PS, et al. Sexual practices in the transmission of hepatitis B virus and prevalence of hepatitis delta virus infection in female prostitutes in the United States. JAMA 1992;267:2477-81.

SAMHSA (Substance Abuse and Mental Health Services Administration). National Household Survey on Drug Abuse: population estimates 1994. Rockville, MD: Substance Abuse and Mental Health Services Administration, DHHS Publication No. (SMA) 95-3063, September 1995.

Scholes D, Daling JR, Stergachis A, Weiss NS, Wang SP, Grayston JT. Vaginal douching as a risk factor for acute pelvic inflammatory disease. Obstet Gynecol 1993;81:601-6.

Schulte JM, Ramsey HA, Paffel JM, Roberts MA, Williams RL, Blass CM, et al. Outbreaks of syphilis in rural Texas towns, 1991-1992. South Med J 1994;87:493-6.

Schwartz A, Colby DC, Reisinger AL. Variation in Medicaid physician fees. Health Aff Millwood 1991;10:131-9.

Seidman SN, Sterk-Elifson C, Aral SO. High-risk sexual behavior among drug-using men. Sex Transm Dis 1994;21:173-80.

Shafer MA. Sexual behavior and sexually transmitted diseases among male adolescents in detention. Sex Transm Dis 1994;21:181-2.

Shafer MA, Hilton JF, Ekstrand M, Keogh J, Gee L, DiGiorgio-Haag L, et al. Relationship between drug use and sexual behaviors and the occurrence of sexually transmitted diseases among high-risk male youth. Sex Transm Dis 1993;20:307-13.

Sherman BL, Dominick JR. Violence and sex in music videos: TV and rock 'n' roll. J Communication 1986;36:79-93.

Sherman DJ. The neglected health care needs of street youth. Public Health Rep 1992;107:433-40.

Siegel K, Mesango FP, Chen J, Christ G. Factors distinguishing homosexual males practicing risky and safer sex. Soc Sci Med 1989;28:561-9.

Smith LS. Ethnic differences in knowledge of sexually transmitted diseases in North American black and Mexican-American migrant farmworkers. Res Nurs Health 1988;11:51-8.

Smith L, Lanthrop L. AIDS and human sexuality. Can J Public Health 1993;84(1 Suppl):S14-S18.

Sokolow JA. Eros and modernization: Sylvester Graham, health reform, and the origins of Victorian sexuality in America. Cranbury, NJ: Associated University Presses, Inc., 1983.

Sonenstein FL, Ku L, Schulte MM. Reproductive health care delivery. Patterns in a changing market. West J Med 1995;163(3 Suppl):7-14.

Sonenstein FL, Pleck JH, Ku LC. Levels of sexual activity among adolescent males in the United States [published erratum appears in Fam Plann Perspect 1991;23:225]. Fam Plann Perspect 1991;23:162-7.

Stall R, McKusick L, Wiley J, Coates TJ, Ostro DG. Alcohol and drug use during sexual activities and compliance with safe sex guidelines for AIDS. Health Education Q 1986;13:359-71.

Stamm WE, Holmes KK. Chlamydia trachomatis infections in the adult. In: Holmes KK, Mårdh P-A, Sparling PF, Weisner PJ, Cates W Jr, Lemon SM, et al., eds. Sexually transmitted diseases. 2nd ed. New York: McGraw-Hill, Inc., 1990:181-93.

STD Communications Roundtable. STDTALK: spreading the word about sexually transmitted diseases. Washington, D.C.: Ogilvy Adams & Rinehart, 1996.

Strasburger VC. Adolescent sexuality and the media. Pediatr Clin North Am 1989;36:747-73.

Strasburger VC. Television and adolescents: Sex, drugs, and rock 'n' roll. Adoles Med: State of the Art Rev 1990;1:161-94.

Strasburger VC. Adolescent sexuality and the media. Curr Opin Pediatr 1992;4:5948.

Strasburger VC. Adolescents and the media. Medical and psychological impact. Thousand Oaks, CA: Sage Publications, Developmental Clinical Psychology and Psychiatry Series, Vol. 33, 1995.

Strouse JS, Buerkel-Rothfuss N. Media exposure and sexual attitudes and behaviors of college students. In: Greenberg BS, Brown JD, Buerkel-Rothfuss, eds. Media, sex and the adolescent. Cresskill, NJ: Hampton Press, Inc., 1993:277-92.

Stuntzner-Gibson D. Women and HIV disease: an emerging social crisis. Social Work 1991;36:22-7.

Sugerman ST, Hergenroeder AC, Chacko MR, Parcel GS. Acquired immunodeficiency syndrome and adolescents. Knowledge, attitudes, and behaviors of runaway and homeless youths. Am J Dis Child 1991;145:431-6.

Suplee C. Apprehensive NIH defers sex survey; political concerns cited for decision. Washington Post, September 25, 1991, A1.

Thomas JC, Tucker MJ. The development and use of the concept of a sexually transmitted disease core. J Infect Dis 1996;174(Suppl 2):S134-43.

U.S. Department of Justice. Selected findings: violence between intimates, Bureau of Justice Statistics, NCJ-149259. Washington, D.C.: U.S. Department of Justice, 1994.

U.S. Department of Justice. Prisoners at mid-year 1995. Bureau of Justice Statistics, National Prisoner Statistics Series. Washington D.C.: U.S. Department of Justice, December 3, 1995.

Warner DL, Rochat RW, Fichtner RR, Toomey KE, Nathan L, Stoll B, et al. Untreated syphilis in pregnant women: identifying gaps in prenatal care. 123rd Annual American Public Health Association Meeting, October 29-November 2, 1995, San Diego, CA [session 4030].

Wasserheit JN. Effect of changes in human ecology and behavior on patterns of sexually transmitted diseases, including human immunodeficiency virus infection. Proc Natl Acad Sci 1994;91:2430-5.

Webber MP, Lambert G, Bateman DA, Hauser WA. Maternal risk factors for congenital syphilis: a case-control study. Am J Epidemiol 1993;137:415-22.

Weber FT, Gearing J, Davis A, Conlon A. Prepubertal initiation of sexual experiences and older first partner predict promiscuous sexual behavior of delinquent adolescent males—unrecognized child abuse? J Adolesc Health 1992;13:600-5.

Widom R, Hammett TM. Research in brief: HIV/AIDS and STDs in juvenile facilities. Washington, D.C.: U.S. Department of Justice, Office of Justice Programs, National Institute of Justice, April 1996.

Wolner-Hanssen P, Eschenbach DA, Paavonen J, Kiviat N, Stevens C, Critchlow C, et al. Decreased risk of symptomatic chlamydial pelvic inflammatory disease associated with oral contraceptive use. JAMA 1990;263:54-9.

Wolner-Hanssen P, Eschenbach DA, Paavonen J, Stevens CE, Kiviat NB, Critchlow C, et al. Association between vaginal douching and acute pelvic inflammatory disease. JAMA 1990;263:1936-41.

Woods H. Human sexuality in health and illness. St. Louis: C.V. Mosby Co., 1979.

WREI (Women's Research and Education Institute). Women's health care costs and experiences. Washington, D.C.: Women's Research and Education Institute, 1994.

Zelnick M, Kim Y. Sex education and its association with teenage sexual activity, pregnancy, and contraceptive use. Fam Plann Perspect 1982;16:117-26.

4

Prevention of STDs

Highlights

• Americans seriously underestimate their risk for STDs; 77 percent of women and 72 percent of men at high risk for STDs surveyed were not concerned about acquiring an STD.

• There are many individual- and community-based interventions and tools that are effective and can be used immediately to prevent STDs.

ISSUES IN PREVENTION

Americans have not done well in confronting issues associated with sexual behavior in general and with STDs in particular. Partially as a result of our failure to deal with these public health problems in a straightforward and effective manner, the prevalence of STDs is high, and the economic and health impact of STDs is enormous. Contrary to the misperceptions of some, use of available information and interventions could have a rapid and dramatic impact on the incidence and prevalence of STDs in the United States. Many effective and efficient behavioral and biomedical interventions are available. While there have not been rigorous assessments of the impact of many interventions on health outcomes, there is reason to believe that they could have a substantial impact on the risk of acquiring and spreading STDs if there were the resources and national will to implement some of these programs more widely (Hillis, Black, et al., 1995).

A Mathematical Model for Prevention

The rate of spread of communicable diseases in a population is determined by three factors: (1) the rate of exposure of susceptible persons to infected individuals; (2) the probability that an exposed, susceptible person will acquire the infection (i.e., the "efficiency of transmission"); and (3) the length of time that newly infected persons remain infected and are able to spread the infection to others. A simple transmission cycle for STDs is illustrated in Figure 4-1.

The transmission of STDs in a population can also be represented by the

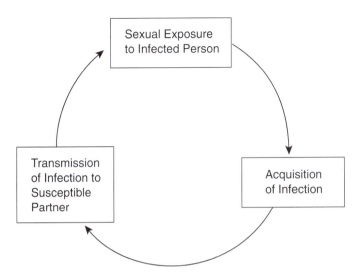

FIGURE 4-1 Basic transmission cycle for STDs.

mathematical model, $R_0 = \beta cD$ (May and Anderson, 1987; Anderson, 1991). In this model, R_0, the reproductive rate of infection, represents the average number of secondary cases of STDs that arise from a new case; c is the mean rate of sexual partner change within the population; β is the mean probability of transmission per exposure; and D is the mean duration of infectiousness of newly infected persons. Thus, interventions can prevent the spread of an STD within a population by reducing the rate of exposure to an STD; lowering the rate of partner change; reducing the efficiency of transmission; or shortening the duration of infectiousness for that STD. An extremely important conclusion from this model is that, for communicable diseases such as STDs, if R_0 remains less than 1, the infection eventually disappears from the population. A sustained prevention program can drive the infection to extinction in the entire population, even when these interventions are provided only to individuals and social networks with the highest rates of transmission (Anderson, 1991).

Anderson and May (1991) have highlighted differences in the epidemiology of communicable and noncommunicable diseases that have important implications for prevention of STDs. First, rates of partner change within the population and patterns of partner mixing greatly influence the spread of STDs. In essence, individuals with the highest rates of partner change, referred to as "core" groups or transmitters, disproportionately increase the rate of spread. Furthermore, mathematical models show that patterns of sex partner mixing and the characteristics of sexual networks are important determinants of the rate of spread of STDs. For example, if individuals with many partners tend to have sex with others who have many partners ("assortative mixing"), infection spreads rapidly at first; and it spreads fastest within "dense" sexual networks with many sexual links over a short period of time (Morris, 1993). Thus, interventions should have the greatest impact if they reach, and are effective among, individuals who have many partners and in "dense" networks with "assortative mixing."

Primary Versus Secondary Prevention

For many infectious diseases, vaccines are a major method of prevention. It is important to recognize that early detection and curative treatment of individuals with communicable diseases provide not only *secondary prevention at the individual level*, but also *primary prevention at the population level* by preventing further transmission. Reduction in the duration of infectivity, particularly among those most likely to transmit the infection to others, lowers the reproductive rate of infection (R_0). Thus, public health efforts to prevent the spread of communicable diseases need to include not only immunization programs but also early detection and curative treatment of communicable diseases, especially those for which vaccines are not available. For these diseases, behavioral interventions are also important.

Behavioral Versus Biomedical Approaches

Historically, STD programs have been based on a biomedical model that focused on the treatment of infected individuals and the development of biological and biomechanical interventions such as drugs, diagnostic tests, and barrier methods. Services have centered on the medical screening and treatment of individuals, coupled in some cases with partner notification. The system for delivering services typically has been composed of health professionals practicing in fixed clinical settings. Traditionally, STD prevention activities have involved episodic therapy driven by symptoms of disease and have provided limited clinical counseling or education to promote behavior change. In recent years, the approach to STD prevention has begun to change as a result of critiques by both affected communities and social and behavioral scientists (Fee and Krieger, 1993). Both biomedical and behavioral health disciplines have made important contributions to the knowledge base for STD prevention (Sparling and Aral, 1991). Because both behavioral and biomedical approaches to STD prevention are necessary, distinguishing between them is unimportant. Federal agencies recently have recognized the need to incorporate both behavioral and biomedical approaches in a more holistic approach.

Wasserheit (1994) examined six changes in patterns of STDs and described how physical and social environmental changes drive these disease patterns. She called for the development of STD prevention programs based on "an appreciation of the role of risk behaviors and macroenvironmental forces" using companion clinic-based and community-based services. In another holistic approach to prevention, Stryker and colleagues (1994) identified several fundamental precedents that need to exist before effective HIV prevention is possible. These factors are: (a) sound policies that promote HIV risk reduction; (b) access to health and social services, including condoms, needles, syringes, and information; (c) interventions shown to motivate behavior change; (d) community-based organizations capable of reaching persons at risk; and (e) development and diffusion of technologies to interrupt HIV transmission. Similar conditions are probably necessary for the prevention of other STDs.

In terms of the mathematical model previously described, current technology can reduce β, the mean probability of transmission per exposure, and D, the mean duration of infectiousness, to zero. This means that we have the technology and resources to interrupt transmission and greatly reduce many STDs in the United States. In this chapter, the committee describes the complex behavioral problems involved in reducing β and c ("the effective mean rate of partner change") and in ensuring that individuals have access to, and make use of, the technologies that can reduce the efficiency of transmission and duration of infectiousness. The committee also evaluates the ability to effectively and efficiently screen for and treat STDs and describes available effective methods for preventing STDs. It should be noted that most of the behavioral interventions discussed in this chapter focus more on reducing efficiency of transmission than on reducing the rate of partner change. This is because many studies of behavioral interventions use consistent condom use as the primary behavioral outcome. In actuality, many behavioral interventions have multiple objectives that include reducing the rate of partner change. Examples of this are school-based interventions that seek to delay the onset of sexual intercourse and also promote condom use. Nevertheless, research on behavioral interventions to reduce the rate of partner change have been underemphasized. It should be noted that reducing the rate of partner change or the patterns of partner selection may affect the dynamics of how groups at differing risk for STDs subsequently interact in populations (Morris, 1996).

The question implicit in the subsequent sections is a perplexing and disturbing one: Why has the United States been unsuccessful in significantly reducing or eliminating a group of diseases that costs thousands of lives and billions of dollars annually in health care costs, despite the fact that effective tools are available?

Figure 4-2 depicts the levels of potential breakdown in steps required to prevent STDs. In regard to the third level (from the top of Figure 4-2), there is currently no way to influence the development of symptoms of STDs. All the other levels, however, represent a point for preventive interventions. Individual- and population-level interventions are needed to (a) reduce individual risk behaviors and high population prevalence of STDs, both of which increase exposure to STDs; (b) promote safe practices and protective methods, such as condom use, necessary to reduce acquisition of an STD by those exposed; (c) educate the

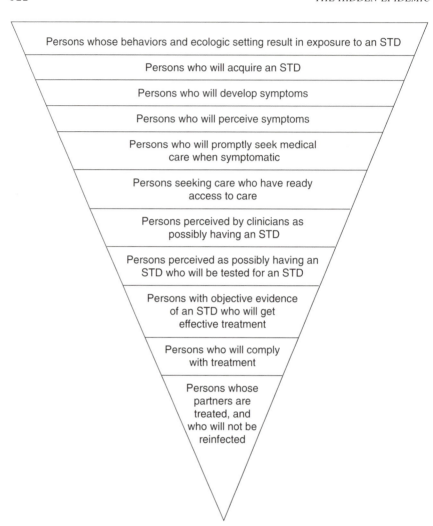

FIGURE 4-2 Schematic representation of the levels of potential breakdown in the steps required for preventing STDs. Each level, except for the third from the top, represents an important point for public health or clinical intervention. ADAPTED FROM: Waller HT, Piot MA. The use of an epidemiological model for estimating the effectiveness of tuberculosis control measures. Bull World Health Organ 1969;41:75-93. Waller HT, Piot MA. Use of an epidemiological model for estimating the effectiveness of tuberculosis control measures. Bull World Health Organ 1970;43:1-16. The model was also described in "Resource allocation model for public health planning—a case study of tuberculosis control," supplement to Vol. 84 of the Bull World Health Organ, 1973.

public, especially adolescents and young adults, to be aware of and recognize symptoms of STDs; (d) motivate prompt health-care-seeking behaviors for symptoms of STDs; (e) ensure access to health care for STDs; (f) train clinicians in risk assessment and diagnosis of STDs; (g) provide access to, and laboratory capabilities for, STD testing; (h) train clinicians how to treat STDs, including use of syndromic treatment when laboratory tests are unavailable or results are pending; (i) make single-dose therapies available for clinicians to dispense directly to patients to ensure compliance; and (j) ensure treatment of sex partners exposed to STDs. The following discussion describes interventions at each of the steps designed to reduce exposure to STDs, reduce transmission to those exposed, and reduce duration of infection.

REDUCING EXPOSURE AND TRANSMISSION

STDs result from exposure to infectious organisms through sexual contact with an infected individual. Risk factors for exposure include the frequency and type of one's sexual behaviors, use or nonuse of contraceptive methods that provide protection against transmission of STDs, and the likelihood that one's partner is infected. The same behavior (e.g., unprotected intercourse with a new partner) will carry very different levels of risk of transmission, depending on the likelihood of STDs in the social network from which one's partner is chosen. For example, individuals may engage in apparently high-risk behaviors but avoid an STD if their sex partners are not infected.

An important strategy for reducing the rate of spread of STDs is to identify and treat infected individuals and their partners. However, it is necessary to supplement this approach with an understanding of how individual behaviors contribute to both exposure and transmission. This is especially important in the case of STDs for several reasons. First, medical treatment will not prevent transmission of some asymptomatic and incurable STDs, such as HIV infection and other viral STDs. For these diseases, initial exposure must be avoided to prevent infection. Second, reduction of STDs will be facilitated not only by secondary prevention through treatment of infected individuals but also by preventing initial infections. Therefore, prevention of most STDs requires modification of the behaviors that place individuals at risk.

In this section, the committee summarizes how individual factors influence exposure to and transmission of STDs. The committee then illustrates how individual factors affect condom use and summarizes behavioral and clinical methods for preventing exposure and reducing transmission of STDs.

Individual Factors

Many factors influence an individual's sexual behavior and risk for STDs. These factors include sexual and other behaviors, perception of risk, and personal skills. There are also costs and obstacles associated with adopting behaviors that reduce individual risk of STDs. In this section, immediate factors that influence individual risk of STDs are summarized. It is important to note that these factors are influenced by the social, contextual factors described in Chapter 3, such as poverty and substance use.

Sexual and Other Behaviors

Aral (1994) recently reviewed the sexual and other behaviors that place individuals at greater risk of exposure to STDs. These behaviors are:

1. *Initiation of sexual intercourse at an early age.* Persons who initiate intercourse at an early age may be at greater risk of STDs because of the longer time they are sexually active and the greater likelihood of risk factors for STDs such as nonvoluntary intercourse, greater number of partners, and less consistent use of condoms. In addition, adolescents are biologically more susceptible to STDs than adults.

2. *Greater number of partners.* The greater the number of partners an individual has, the greater is the risk of exposure. This association may be due to the increased risk of exposure to an infected partner with increasing number of partners and the fact that having multiple partners may be associated with other risk factors such as high-risk partners and less consistent use of condoms.

3. *High-risk partners.* Having sex with a partner who is likely to have had many partners increases the risk of an STD.

4. *Increased frequency of intercourse and certain sexual practices.* The greater is the frequency of intercourse with an infected partner, the greater are the chances of transmission. Risk of HIV infection, hepatitis B virus infection, and other STDs is greater with anal intercourse than with vaginal or oral intercourse.

5. *Lack of circumcision of male partner.* As discussed in Chapter 3, men who are not circumcised appear to have a greater risk of acquiring and transmitting certain STDs, such as HIV infection and chancroid, compared to men who are circumcised. Women with male partners who are circumcised are at reduced risk of exposure compared to those with uncircumcised partners.

6. *Use of vaginal douching.* Women who douche are at higher risk for later complications of STDs, such as pelvic inflammatory disease, as discussed in Chapter 3.

7. *Lack of barrier contraceptive use.* Consistent use of condoms and barrier contraceptives reduces the risk of STDs. As mentioned in Chapter 3 and Table 4-1, hormonal contraceptives may also affect risk of STDs.

Perception of Risk

Americans commonly underestimate their risk for STDs. In a 1993 survey mentioned previously (EDK Associates, 1994), 84 percent of women surveyed were not concerned about acquiring an STD, including 72 percent of women from 18 through 24 years of age, and 78 percent of women reported having had "many" sexual partners during their lifetime. Mays and Cochran (1988) reported on a study of African American college students who believed that African Americans were less likely to get AIDS than European Americans, even though the reverse is true. Of the sexually active women in the sample, almost a third had taken no actions to avoid STDs. Another nationwide survey of 1,000 persons in 1994 found that Americans underestimated their risk of STDs and were therefore not taking appropriate protective measures (EDK Associates, 1995). This survey found that 62 percent of men and 50 percent of women were at moderate to high risk for STDs (see Figure 4-3 for definitions of risk). Single and divorced men and women were most likely to be at high or moderate risk for STDs compared to married persons (Figure 4-3). Among those at high risk for STDs, 77 percent of women and 72 percent of men stated that they were not worried about getting an STD.

Perceived susceptibility has played a central role in most theories of health behavior (e.g., Wallston and Wallston, 1984; Weinstein, 1988). Perceiving one's personal susceptibility as low may arise from the experience of remaining STD- or HIV-free in the face of behavior that is known to be associated with a high risk of acquiring infection, such as engaging in anonymous unprotected sex with multiple partners over a prolonged period of time. Such perceptions may be reinforced by periodic negative testing. With consistent reinforcement of negative results in light of high-risk behavior, beliefs congruent with "genetic immunity" or "super invulnerability" may develop, leading to reduced motivation to adopt protective behaviors.

Knowledge is necessary but not sufficient to motivate action. Without knowledge, individuals may be unaware of risk or not know what actions to take to protect themselves against STDs. However, among those who do have sufficient knowledge, other factors will affect whether they take action. Thus, among populations with sufficient knowledge, knowledge itself is not related to the behavior (Morrison et al., 1994). Morrison and others (1994) studied adolescents who were incarcerated in the juvenile justice system. These adolescents, who reported engaging in high-risk sexual behaviors, had a good deal of knowledge regarding STDs and condoms, but this knowledge was not related to more positive attitudes toward use of condoms. Similarly, Wulfert and Wan (1993) found that college students with better knowledge about the HIV virus and how it is transmitted were no more likely to use condoms compared to those with less knowledge.

In virtually all behavioral theories regarding the reasons individuals either adopt or fail to adopt risk-avoidance strategies, reducing risk is viewed as a principal motivation of behavior (Cleary et al., 1986). Perceived risk is a critical component in the Health Belief Model (Becker and Maiman, 1975) and the Theory of Reasoned Action (Ajzen and Fishbein, 1980) and is reflected in out-

TABLE 4-1 Effects of Contraceptives on STDs and Pregnancy

Contraceptive Method	STDs		Pregnancy
	Bacterial	Viral (including HIV/AIDS)	
Condoms	Protective (if used for STD/HIV prophylaxis)	Protective (if used for STD/HIV prophylaxis)	Protective
Sterilization	Not protective (except against salpingitis)	Not protective	Highly protective
Spermicides with nonoxynol-9	Protective against cervical gonorrhea and chlamydial infection; associated with increased risk of urinary tract infections and altered vaginal flora[a]	No proven protection in vivo	Protective
Diaphragms	Protective against cervical infection; associated with increased risk of altered vaginal flora[b]	Insufficient data	Protective
Oral contraceptives	Associated with increased cervical chlamydial infection; protective against symptomatic pelvic inflammatory disease	Not protective; some studies suggest increased risk for acquisition of HIV;[c] others show no effect[d]	Highly protective
Implantable/injectable contraceptives	Not protective	Not protective; some studies suggest increase risk for acquisition of HIV infection[d,e]	Highly protective
IUDs	Associated with pelvic inflammatory disease in first month after insertion	Not protective	Protective
Rhythm method	Not protective	Not protective	Protective

[a]Hooten TM, Fennell CL, Clark AM, Stamm WE. Nonoxonol-9: differential antibacterial activity and enhancement of bacterial adherence to vaginal epithelial cells. J Infect Dis 1991;164:1216-9.

[b]Hooten TM, Roberts PL, Stamm WE. Effects of recent sexual activity and use of a diaphragm on the vaginal microflora. Clin Infect Dis 1994;19:274-8.

[c]Plummer FA, Simonsen JN, Cameron DW, Ndinya-Achola JO, Kreiss JK, Gakinya MN, et al. Co-factors in male-female transmission of human immunodeficiency virus type 1. J Infect Dis 1991;163:233-9.

Nyange P, Martin H, Mandaliya K, Jackson D, Ndinya-Achola JO, Ngugi E, et al. Cofactors for heterosexual transmission of HIV to prostitutes in Mombasa Kenya. Proceedings of the 9th International Conference on AIDS and STD in Africa. 1994 December 10-14; Kampala, Uganda.

Mostad S, Welch M, Chohan B, Reilly M, Overbaugh J, Mandalya K, et al. Cervical and vaginal HIV-1 DNA shedding in female STD clinic attenders. Eleventh International Conference on AIDS, July 7-12, 1996, Vancouver [abstract no. WeC 333].

Cates W Jr. Contraception, contraceptive technology and STD. In: Holmes KK, Sparling PF, Mårdh PA, Lemon SM, Stamm WE, Piot P, Wasserheit JN, eds. Sexually transmitted diseases. 3rd ed. New York: McGraw-Hill, Inc., in press.

[d]Cates W Jr., et al., in press. (see above)

[e]Marx PA, Spira AI, Gettie A, Dailey PJ, Veazey RS, Lackner AA, et al. Progesterone implants enhance SIV vaginal transmission and early virus load. Nature Med 1996;2:1084-9.

Mostad et al., 1996. (see above)

Spira AI, Marx PA, Patterson BK, Mahoney J, Koup RA, Wolinsky SM, et al. Cellular targets of infection and route of viral dissemination following intravaginal inoculation of SIV into rhesus macaques. J Exp Med 1996;183:215-25.

OTHER SOURCES: CDC. Update: barrier protection against HIV infection and other sexually transmitted diseases. MMWR 1993;42:589-97; Cates W Jr, Stone. Family planning, sexually transmitted diseases, and contraceptive choice: a literature update. Fam Plann Perspect 1992;24:75-84; Ehrhardt AA, Wasserheit JN. Age, gender, and sexual risk behaviors for sexually transmitted diseases in the United States. In: Research issues in human behavior and sexually transmitted disease in the AIDS era. Wasserheit JN, Aral SO, Holmes KK, Hitchcock PJ, eds. Washington, DC: American Society for Microbiology, 1991; Hatcher RA, Trussell J, Stewart F, et al. Contraceptive technology, 16th revised ed. New York, NY: Irvington Publishers, Inc.; 1994: Table 4-2.; IOM. Contraceptive research and development: looking to the future. Harrison PF, Rosenfield A, editors. Washington, D.C.: National Academy Press, 1996.

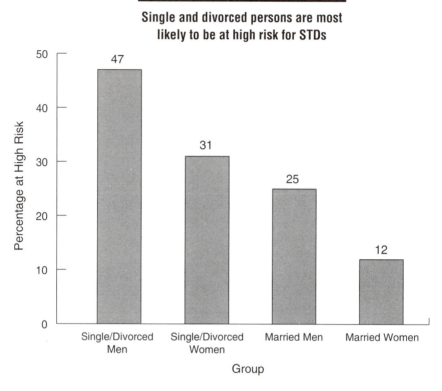

FIGURE 4-3 Proportion of persons at high risk for STDs by marital status and gender, 1994. High risk was defined as having at least two of the following: (a) six or more sex partners in lifetime, (b) partners who have had sex with six or more people or have no knowledge of their partners' sexual history, or (c) more than one sex partner in the past year. Moderate risk was defined as having one of these characteristics. SOURCE: EDK Associates, Inc. The ABCs of STDs. New York: EDK Associates, 1995.

come expectancies in social learning theory (Bandura, 1977). All of these models predict that behavior change will be greater when individuals perceive that they are at risk of infection and that the behavior being recommended will reduce that risk. In addition to the reasons mentioned previously for why individuals fail to adopt protective behaviors, there are other explanations for why the association between perceived risk and protective behaviors is weak.

Link Between Perceived Risk and Protective Behaviors

Given the centrality of perceived risk to the theoretical models as well as to many intervention programs, it is surprising that the empirical evidence linking perceived risk and health-protective behavior is weak. Confirming that risk perceptions directly lead to adoption of protective behavior is very difficult (Baldwin and Baldwin, 1988). Some studies have demonstrated a relationship between perceived risk of STDs and preventive behaviors (Janz and Becker, 1984; Joseph et al., 1987; Hingson et al., 1990; Weisman et al., 1991; Pendergrast et al., 1992; Stiffman et al., 1992) and number of sex partners (Catania et al., 1989), but others have failed to find such an association (Kegeles et al., 1989; Weisman et al., 1989; Shafer and Boyer, 1990; Cleary et al., 1991, 1995; Orr and Langefeld, 1993; Wulfert and Wan, 1993).

There are several possible explanations for why perception of risk has not been systematically linked to behaviors that reduce the risk of STDs. One is the difficulty of assessing risk adequately in such studies. Perceptions of risk involve perceptions of both the severity of the outcome, such as getting an STD, and the likelihood of its occurrence (Yates and Stone, 1992). Individuals are likely to differ in the extent to which they feel vulnerable to acquiring different STDs and in their views of the gravity of different STDs. Perceived risk usually has been assessed globally, but individuals are likely to have partner-specific perceptions of risk (Weisman et al., 1991; Pilkington et al., 1994; Ellen et al., 1996) and partner-specific patterns of condom use (Magura et al., 1994; Morris et al., 1995).

A second methodological reason why perceived risk has not been consistently linked with behavior may be that the temporal ordering of variables is hard to assess in cross-sectional studies. Individuals who perceive themselves at higher risk should be more likely to take protective action. However, if individuals are engaging in health-protective actions, their perception of risk may drop, and perceived risk would be negatively related to behavior. Longitudinal studies are needed to determine the temporal ordering of risk perceptions and change in risk behaviors.

Finally, there are substantive reasons why perceived risk may not be closely linked to behavior. Perceived risk of STDs may be necessary to motivate health-protective behavior or behavior change but may not be sufficient. There are other powerful factors that influence these behaviors. In addition to having knowledge, individuals need to be motivated to reduce risk behaviors. Behaviors that reduce the risk of STDs, such as reducing the number of sex partners and using a condom consistently, have substantial personal costs associated with them. Unless these costs are offset by a strong motivation to reduce risk or by other reasons to engage in these behaviors, it is unlikely that the person will take these actions.

Individuals may show different degrees of motivation based on their risk perception. For example, persons at relatively low risk for acquiring STDs or HIV infection may be easily stimulated to adopt behaviors that are self-protective, while high-risk individuals may be less able to control sexual impulses that lead to diminished self-protective strategies (Joseph et al., 1987) or such individuals perceive little actual benefit in changing behavior given other pressing life concerns.

An example of a barrier to protective behavior was seen early in the HIV epidemic, when men who were targeted for HIV risk-reduction behavior were asked to engage in behaviors, such as condom use, for which they had never been socialized. Using condoms was a new behavior for most men who had sex with men during the 1980s. The committee hypothesizes that a related barrier to adoption of condom use and reduction of unsafe sexual practices (e.g., anonymous partners) was the association of sexual behavior with self-identity. As the gay movement matured during the 1970s in the United States, a growing number of gay men equated their sexual practices with their own identity. Thus, admonitions to alter sexual behaviors were in direct conflict with the self-identities of gay men, and this conflict frustrated well-meaning attempts to alter behavior. However, this barrier is now diminishing with new generations of young Americans who have become socialized in the AIDS era.

Finally, most sexual risk-reduction efforts for STDs require mutual consent of at least two people. This requires communication about expectations, agreement on the value of engaging in protective strategies, and an understanding of sexual pleasure for each person. Communication regarding sexual behavior is problematic in the best of situations. Experience in the conduct of HIV prevention trials suggests that sexual negotiation and empowerment strategies may be perceived as meaning either that one's partner does not trust one or that there is a "hidden" reason why condom use is being added to an ongoing relationship. Neither of these perceptions builds trust or mutual respect, and these strategies may be extremely difficult to introduce into a stable relationship.

Personal Skills

An individual needs motivation, personal skills, and interpersonal resources to implement complicated behavior changes in the face of the types of barriers discussed above. These include interpersonal communication and negotiation skills and a sense of self-efficacy regarding accomplishment of the relevant behaviors (Bandura, 1990; Wulfert and Wan, 1993). For example, individuals who are able to communicate more readily about sex appear to be more effective in their use of condoms (Brien et al., 1994; Rickman et al., 1994; Shoop and Davidson, 1994).

The best evidence that having specific skills enhances STD-reducing behavior comes from evaluations of programs that provide training in specific behavioral skills. St. Lawrence and colleagues (1995) conducted a randomized trial of an educational program versus education with behavioral skills training. The latter intervention included problem-solving skills, assertion and refusal skills, and training in proper use of condoms. African American adolescents who were sexually active and who received the latter intervention increased condom use and had a lower frequency of unprotected intercourse compared to those who received only the educational program. In addition, adolescents who had not begun sexual activity and who received the skills intervention were less likely to become sexually active in the next year compared to those who received only the educational program.

In addition to having specific skills, individuals having a greater sense of self-efficacy regarding their ability to enact the behaviors will be more likely to be effective (Bandura, 1990). Self-efficacy beliefs are important because they affect motivation to initiate behavior and to persevere if obstacles are encountered. Thus, men who feel that they can use condoms each time they have intercourse and women who feel that they will be able to get their partners to use a condom consistently should be more likely to implement the behaviors needed to achieve this goal (e.g., obtaining condoms, having them accessible at the time of intercourse, using them). Several studies have shown that greater self-efficacy and confidence in one's ability to use condoms predicts both a stronger intention to use condoms and more effective use of condoms (Marin et al., 1993; Schaalma et al., 1993; Wulfert and Wan, 1993; Mahoney et al., 1995; Rotheram-Borus et al., 1995).

An important determinant of self-efficacy is one's comfort level and acceptance of individual sexuality. Persons who have developed negative emotions regarding premarital sex, such as guilt and denial, are less likely to practice protective behaviors, such as use of contraceptives, compared to those who do not have such emotions (Herold and McNamee, 1982; Gerrard, 1987; Morrison and Shaklee, 1990; Gerrard et al., 1993). In addition, persons who are embarrassed about their sexual activity are less likely to use condoms consistently (Hingson et al., 1990; Koniak-Griffin et al., 1994).

Behavioral Methods

Behavioral interventions represent promising approaches to preventing STDs. While there are many reports of behavioral interventions to prevent STDs including HIV infection, most studies have not been conducted in a methodologically sound manner to determine their effectiveness in improving health outcomes (Oakley et al., 1995; Oakley, Fullerton, Holland, et al., 1995). Many studies, however, show that behavioral interventions can have a positive effect on self-reported sexual health behaviors. A meta-analysis of 12 controlled studies of risk-reduction interventions for HIV infection found that the mean weighted effect of such behavioral interventions on self-reported sexual behaviors was positive and statistically significant (Kalichman et al., 1996). In addition, two recent studies have demonstrated that certain feasible behavioral interventions are effective in reducing the risk of STDs (Kamb et al., 1996; Shain et al., 1996) and support a strong role for such interventions as part of a comprehensive approach to preventing STDs. An advantage of behavioral interventions is that they can be effective in preventing all STDs, in contrast to some biomedical interventions that are specific for only certain STDs.

A variety of strategies can lead to sustained behavior changes that reduce the risk of STDs. These intervention strategies include individually focused interventions relying heavily on one-on-one counseling that occurs independent of, or jointly with, STD testing; group- or community-based interventions (Kelly, 1994); and structural or "macro" level legislative solutions. A review of federally funded HIV prevention studies that evaluated the impact of individual- and community-based behavioral interventions found that most interventions had positive effects on knowledge of AIDS and sexual behavior such as increased rates of condom use (IOM, 1994). The intent of STD preventive interventions is to reduce the incidence of new STDs by assisting individuals in changing behaviors in ways that decrease risk of contracting STDs. Altering precursors of sexual decision making and actual sexual practices, such as increasing rates of condom use, reducing number of partners, or decreasing rates of unprotected sex, will ultimately reduce the number of new cases of STDs.

While reduced STD incidence and sexual behavior change are the primary endpoints in STD risk-reduction interventions, other endpoints also have merit. For example, several important studies in STD prevention have utilized changes in risk behavior intentions, condom use attitudes, and perceived vulnerability as principal outcome measures. Community-level interventions based on "stages of change" theoretical models (Prochaska and DiClemente, 1983) have defined success on the basis of shifting community attitudes towards greater readiness to enact a specific behavior change, stronger change intentions, or future resolve to engage in protective behavior. "Social marketing" approaches to condom promotion have included condom sales in the community as an indicator of programmatic success. Success needs to be judged independently for specific target populations and for desired behavioral and disease outcomes.

Among adolescents, delaying sexual intercourse or intermittent avoidance of sexual activity is effective in STD risk reduction (Kirby, 1980). Furthermore, it has been well documented (Gold et al., 1994; Ku et al., 1994) that it is easier to encourage consistent condom use in sexual relationships with nonprimary partners than in primary relationships. Thus, the context of behavioral change strategies needs to be specified.

The literature on the effectiveness of HIV prevention programs contains some findings applicable for developing other effective STD prevention programs. Holtgrave and others (1995) found that successful prevention programs that were able to avert, reduce, or modify HIV-risk-related behaviors or their determinants had the following characteristics:

1. basis in real specific needs and community planning;
2. culturally competent messages;
3. clearly defined audience, objectives, and interventions;
4. basis in behavioral and social science theory and research;
5. quality monitoring and adherence to plans;

6. use of evaluation findings and midcourse corrections; and
7. sufficient resources.

The study's authors also concluded that some behaviorally based prevention programs are cost saving, and others are likely to be cost-effective relative to other health programs.

Theoretical Approaches to STD and HIV Risk Reduction

A number of theoretical approaches drawn from the social and behavioral sciences have been employed in developing STD prevention interventions (Cleary et al., 1986, 1995). These models were derived from efforts to promote change in nonsexual health-risk behaviors, such as smoking cessation, cardiovascular risk reduction, and cancer prevention. The dominant model guiding most STD prevention interventions has been social learning theory (also referred to as social cognitive or cognitive-behavioral theory), originally proposed by Bandura (1977). This approach postulates that specific skills are needed to alter risk behaviors. These skills can be imparted through modeling, rehearsal, or practice opportunities. Behavior change interventions have heavily focused on training participants in condom use skills, sexual assertiveness, safer sex negotiations and communication strategies, and self-management skills to deal with situations that might trigger vulnerability to high-risk sexual behavior (Kelly, 1994). Other theoretical approaches that are appropriately focused on the individual-level determinants of high-risk behavior and behavior change include the Theory of Reasoned Action (Ajzen and Fishbein, 1980) and the Precaution-Adoption Process (Weinstein, 1988).

At the community level, one approach that has been very popular over the past decade in STD prevention has been the "stages of change" formulation mentioned previously (Prochaska and DiClemente, 1983). This approach was originally developed to explain the process of changing health habits, primarily smoking, and postulates that people are at varying levels of readiness for change. Understanding the different levels of readiness for each person allows tailoring interventions that can successfully move the individual further along the continuum of change—towards action and then behavioral maintenance. While this approach has been widely discussed in the literature (Catania et al., 1990; O'Reilly and Higgins, 1991), there have been few empirical demonstrations of its utility in influencing behavior change at the community level.

Community-norm-change models that focus on influencing social or peer group norms regarding sexual behavior have proven particularly appropriate in studies of sexual risk practices of adolescents, heterosexual adults, and gay men. One approach for producing normative change at the community level is the "diffusion of innovation" model (Rogers, 1983) in which normative change attributable to advocacy by key, popular "opinion leaders" leads to accepted new behavioral norms in the population. This strategy has been viewed as extremely successful in interventions focused on gay men. A second approach, "social marketing" (Andreasen, 1995), uses media campaigns to change attitudes towards condoms and improve their availability.

Individual-Focused Interventions

Intensive small-group risk-reduction interventions, largely guided by cognitive-behavioral theory, have been shown to be very effective in promoting self-protective behavior change (Kelly, 1994; Cleary et al., 1995). These studies have included randomized trials with gay men (Kelly et al., 1991), homeless and runaway adolescents (Rotheram-Borus et al., 1991), adolescents at risk for STDs (Jemmott et al., 1992; St. Lawrence et al., 1995), low-income and adult women of certain ethnic groups (Hobfoll et al., 1994; DiClemente and Wingood, 1995) and at-risk mentally ill men and women (Kalichman et al., 1994). These interventions have been delivered in small-group programs with 6 to 18 hours of contact time, allowing time to practice risk-reduction skills and review successes and problems encountered in enacting these behaviors. These interventions produced evidence of change in self-reported sexual risk behavior, usually on the order of 30 to 70 percent reduction in the frequency of unprotected sex from pre-intervention levels. While none of these studies incorporated STD incidence as a primary outcome measure, each study did utilize some method to validate self-reported behavioral changes. A limitation to these studies is that long-term maintenance of behavior change effects has not been examined.

Brief interventions focused on influencing knowledge and attitudes have been successful (Kalichman et al., 1994) but have had little impact on sexual behavior practices. Other strategies have focused on counseling and HIV testing as a method of increasing perceptions of vulnerability and promoting self-protection from STDs. Analyses of these strategies suggest that while these approaches have merit, the counseling, as practiced in field conditions, leaves much to be desired in meeting minimal criteria for being "successful" (Giesecke et al., 1991; Higgins et al., 1991).

Preliminary results of a major randomized, controlled trial evaluating the impact of enhanced prevention counseling for HIV and STD risk reduction strongly support individual-focused counseling (Kamb et al., 1996). Among public STD clinic patients, those who received a series of counseling sessions based on the Health Belief Model or the Theory of Reasoned Action were significantly more likely to adopt certain protective behaviors and less likely to acquire new STDs at six months of follow-up compared to those who received only educational messages.

In its latest report, the U.S. Preventive Services Task Force concluded that the ability of primary care clinicians to influence high-risk sexual behavior is limited, but that there is consistent evidence that Americans have changed their behavior in response to information regarding STDs, including HIV infection, provided through a variety of clinical and other settings. Although the task force determined that the effectiveness of clinician counseling in the primary care setting is unproven, the group recommended that primary care clinicians counsel their adolescent and adult patients regarding measures to prevent STDs, and that such counseling should be tailored to the risk factors, needs, and abilities of each patient (U.S. Preventive Services Task Force, 1996). The CDC and several physician organizations have also recommended that primary care clinicians counsel their adolescent and adult patients regarding measures to prevent STDs (ACOG, 1992; AMA, 1993; CDC, 1993a; AAP, Committee on Adolescence, 1994; AAFP, 1994). Clinician counseling does not work in isolation and is a necessary component of appropriate clinical management of STDs. This is because clinician counseling takes advantage of opportunities to educate patients when they are most receptive to health messages and effectively reinforces messages from other sources (Bigelow et al., 1986).

Couple-based interventions to prevent high-risk sexual behaviors are also promising approaches to prevention. In this approach, both members in a relationship are the focus of an intervention. Perhaps the best evidence to support the effectiveness of such an approach is from HIV counseling studies among discordant couples.[1] In one study, after multiple HIV testing and counseling sessions, condom use among discordant couples increased from 4 percent to 57 percent after one year of follow-up (Allen et al., 1992).

Community-Based Interventions

Community-based interventions to promote behavior change include interventions that target specific high-risk groups, such as female sex workers and adolescents, as well as interventions that attempt to change community norms, most commonly through mass media messages. A number of intervention trials involving high-risk groups such as gay men (Kelly et al., 1991, 1992), injection drug users and their sex partners, female sex workers, and youth in high-risk situations have been successful in improving knowledge and promoting behavior change (O'Reilly and Higgins, 1991; IOM, 1994). Some interventions have been modeled after the Diffusion of Innovation Theory and have successfully utilized peer opinion leaders and educators to change norms in a community by endorsing condoms and educating regarding their use (Kelly et al., 1991, 1992). For example, a multicity trial that recruited popular gay men to educate other gay men who frequented bars resulted in a dramatic decline in the frequency of unprotected intercourse after several months (Kelly et al., 1992). Studies in Tanzania show that community-based interventions to improve syndromic management of

---

[1]A couple where one partner is infected and the other is not.

STDs and health-care-seeking behavior significantly reduce HIV transmission and population incidence of urethritis and syphilis (Grosskurth et al., 1995a, b; Mwijarubi et al., 1996).

One major community-based intervention for disenfranchised groups that may be directly applicable to community-based STD prevention is the AIDS Community Demonstration Projects initiative (CDC, 1996a). These programs were initiated in 1989 to target populations at high risk of HIV infection in five cities, such as intravenous drug users and their sex partners, female sex workers, men who have sex with men, and youths in high-risk situations. The goal of these programs was to determine the efficacy of a specific community-based intervention among hard-to-reach populations, and one of the two main objectives was to increase consistent condom use among these populations.[2] The intervention included distribution of printed materials that described "role models" who successfully changed their behaviors and provided basic HIV and condom information. Peers and other community network members were used extensively to distribute materials. Preliminary data indicate that high rates of exposure to the intervention can be achieved within two years of the initiation of the program. In addition, for the three sexual behaviors examined, the mean stages of change-continuum value among persons who reported exposure to the intervention was greater than that among persons who did not report exposure to the intervention.[3] Replications of successful interventions among high-risk groups are being undertaken in the United States and abroad, and the results will shed light on the long-term impact and applicability of these approaches to other communities at risk.

In January 1994, the CDC implemented its Prevention Marketing initiative for HIV and STD prevention (U.S. Conference of Mayors, 1994). This initiative was motivated by research on community interventions showing that they were most effective when designed and managed by the communities themselves. As part of this program, the CDC is contributing funds for pilot prevention-marketing interventions and is providing technical assistance to state and local health departments, community coalitions, and other partners. The initiative uses commercial marketing techniques, including mass media messages, and community involvement to promote healthy sexual behaviors. The social marketing approach adapted by the CDC includes the concepts of the right product, the right price, the right place, and the right promotion (DeJong, 1989).

Public health workers recognize that, in order for behavior change to occur, the community environment should not be a barrier but should be supportive of

---

[2]The other main objective was to increase the use of bleach by intravenous drug users to clean injecting drug equipment.

[3]The stages of change continuum represents a series of steps on a behavior change continuum from precontemplation to adoption and maintenance of the behavior change. The higher the stages of change-continuum value, the greater is the progression of the individual from the precontemplation stage to the maintenance stage of behavior change.

such changes. In response to this issue, "enabling approaches" to prevention have recently gained attention (Tawil et al., 1995; O'Reilly and Piot, 1996). These interventions are intended to either remove barriers to adoption of protective behaviors or to erect barriers to risky behaviors. An example of how structural or environmental changes can significantly reduce risky sexual behaviors is the "100% Condom Program" that was implemented nationwide in Thailand by the Thai HIV/AIDS Prevention and Control Program in 1992, along with a mass media condom-promotion campaign and wide distribution of condoms to prevent the spread of HIV among sex workers (Rojanapithayakorn and Hanenberg, 1996). The program enforced universal use of condoms among sex workers through the use of sanctions against sex establishments where condoms were not being consistently used. This intervention was effective apparently because it supported desired behavior change and did not reduce the income of sex workers. An extensive evaluation of the program among Thai army male conscripts showed that the proportion of men who had sex with sex workers fell, the proportion who used condoms with sex workers increased, and the seroprevalence of HIV and the proportion with a history of an STD declined significantly after program implementation (Nelson et al., 1996). These data indicate that environmental interventions that adequately address structural or other barriers to behavior change are necessary for the adoption of healthy sexual behaviors.

School-Based Interventions

School is an obvious venue for providing information regarding STDs and for preventing the initiation of high-risk sexual behaviors among adolescents. More than half of teenagers surveyed in 1995 indicated that the school was their primary source of information (ASHA, 1996). As of mid-1994, 45 states and approximately 91 percent of school districts required schools to offer health education (Collins et al., 1995). Five states required a separate course devoted almost entirely to health topics in all elementary schools, 14 required such courses at the middle/junior high school level, and 28 required such courses in senior high school. A 1994 survey of state education agencies and teachers by the CDC showed that 28 of 43 states and the District of Columbia and 81 percent of school districts required teaching STD prevention in a required course (CDC, 1996b). In addition, 39 states plus the District of Columbia required HIV prevention education. As of September 1995, 22 states and the District of Columbia had legal mandates that required schools to provide both sexuality and STD/HIV education; an additional 15 states require schools to provide only STD/HIV education; and 13 states did not require schools to provide sexuality or STD/HIV education (NARAL Foundation, 1995). Many of the states that require education in STD/HIV mention education only for HIV/AIDS, not other STDs, in their laws. Although many states require schools to provide instruction in HIV or STD prevention, these legal mandates are often underfunded and restrictive in the content of the instruction (NARAL Foundation, 1995). For example, in Louisiana, schools are required to teach that abstinence is the expected norm for students, but the law makes no mention of instruction regarding STD prevention. In addition, 19 states prohibit or restrict school health and education programs from making contraceptives, or in some cases information regarding contraceptives, available to students. The number of restrictive laws enacted or considered by states increased in 1995 (NARAL Foundation, 1995). Another important limitation of current school-based education is the lack of consistent STD-related education at lower grade levels.

The majority of health education teachers recently surveyed reported that they taught about sexual abstinence (76 percent); how to prevent STDs (75 percent); signs and symptoms of STDs (70 percent); and other topics related to risk factors for STDs (Collins et al., 1995). In the CDC survey mentioned previously, among teachers who taught in health education classes, 78 percent taught about sexual behaviors that transmit HIV (and other STDs), but only 37 percent taught about correct use of condoms (CDC, 1996b). The preparation of teachers who provide instruction on these topics is inconsistent. For example, while 86 percent of states and 33 percent of school districts that required instruction in STDs reported providing training on the topic (CDC, 1996b), only 16 percent of teachers surveyed reported receiving training on teaching STD prevention during the two years prior to the survey.

A 1989 survey of more than 4,200 seventh- through twelfth-grade teachers in specialties most likely to be responsible for sex education found that most teachers believed that information regarding HIV infection, other STDs, and pregnancy should be covered by the seventh and eighth grades at the latest (Forrest and Silverman, 1989). There was a gap between what the teachers think should be taught and what actually occurs. For example, almost all teachers believed that sex education information for students should include sexual decision-making and abstinence and birth control methods, but only 82 to 84 percent of teachers reported being in schools that provided instruction in these areas. Teachers cited (a) pressure from parents, the community, and school administration; (b) lack of appropriate teaching materials; and (c) lack of student interest as potential barriers to teaching sex education.

An IOM committee[4] that is preparing a report on the role of comprehensive school health programs in the United States has come to the conclusion that health education does not commence at a sufficiently early age; the period prior to high school appears to be the most crucial for shaping attitudes and behaviors. By the time students reach high school, many are already engaging in risky behaviors or at least have formed accepting attitudes toward these behaviors. For

---

[4]IOM Committee on Comprehensive School Health Programs in Grades K-12.

this reason, the committee believes that sequential, age-appropriate health education before high school is essential.

In many communities, there is considerable controversy regarding the role of "abstinence-based" (i.e., delaying intercourse until marriage) versus harm-reduction approaches (i.e., promoting use of condoms) to school-based education curriculum design. Some communities and school boards, in spite of predominant scientific evidence to the contrary, believe that harm-reduction approaches such as condom promotion encourage sexual intercourse among adolescents. Because of the controversial nature of school-based STD education programs, it has been strongly suggested that health departments and private organizations that desire to implement such programs work closely with school administrators, health educators, teachers, parents, and students throughout the planning and implementation process (Molbert et al., 1993).

It should be noted that although school-based programs will reach the overwhelming number of adolescents in the United States, as discussed in Chapter 3, a sizable number of adolescents are homeless, in detention facilities, or otherwise not attending school. These youths, who are at high risk for STDs because they are likely to be sexually active, have a history of being sexually abused, and use drugs and alcohol, present many challenges to prevention efforts. Information regarding the effectiveness of interventions to prevent STDs among youths who are not in school settings are limited (Rotheram-Borus et al., 1991).

Effectiveness of School-Based Programs. The quality of studies that have evaluated the effectiveness of school-based programs to reduce risky sexual behaviors varies greatly. Many studies that have evaluated the effectiveness of school-based programs in reducing risky sexual behaviors have used some type of experimental design, commonly randomization of students or schools to intervention and control groups to measure program effectiveness. Other evaluation methodologies include the use of data from national surveys of adolescent sexual behavior to relate past participation in health education programs to subsequent sexual health behaviors. Limitations of many of these studies include lack of appropriate control or comparison groups, insufficient sample size of students and resulting inadequate statistical power, variability of the time frame chosen for postintervention follow-up, and difficulty in accurately measuring health outcomes. For example, studies based on national surveys of adolescent sexual behavior are problematic because they rely on the recall of the respondent's past participation in health education activities. In addition, many specifics regarding the scope and quality of health education programs are not captured, thereby essentially grouping together programs of varying quality and scope. Because of ethical concerns and other problems associated with assessment of rates of STDs among students, it is not feasible to evaluate the direct impact of such programs on rates of STDs in most situations. Therefore, most studies evaluate effectiveness on the basis of changes in self-reported risky sexual behaviors such as frequency of unprotected sexual intercourse.

The overwhelming proportion of peer-reviewed evaluations of the effectiveness of sex and AIDS and STD education programs have reported positive changes or no effect of programs on sexual health behaviors such as condom use and onset of sexual intercourse (Kirby et al., 1994). In a few studies based on national survey data, mixed outcomes (positive, negative, or no effect) have also been documented (Dawson, 1986; Marsiglio and Mott, 1986; Ku et al., 1993). Kirby and colleagues recently completed a comprehensive review of 23 studies of school-based sex and AIDS and STD education programs that were published in peer-reviewed journals and evaluated their impact on sexual behavior (Kirby et al., 1994) The authors found that some but not all programs were effective and that programs having the following six characteristics had a clear impact on behavior:

1. narrowly focused on reducing sexual risk-taking behaviors that lead to HIV or other STDs or unintentional pregnancy;
2. utilized social learning theories as a foundation for development;
3. provided basic, accurate information about the risks of unprotected intercourse and methods of avoiding unprotected intercourse through experiential activities designed to personalize this information;
4. included activities that address social or media influences on sexual behaviors;
5. reinforced clear and appropriate values to strengthen individual values and group norms against unprotected sex; and
6. provided modeling and practice in communication and negotiating skills.

The authors concluded that, contrary to the concerns of some individuals and groups, such educational programs do not increase sexual activity among students. Studies of specific programs found that programs that included instruction on contraception either delayed the onset of sexual intercourse or had no effect on onset. In addition, a previous IOM committee (IOM, 1995:233) evaluated 23 local programs, including school-based programs, related to unintended pregnancy and concluded that:

> Sexuality education programs that provide information on both abstinence and contraceptive use neither encourage the onset of sexual intercourse nor increase the frequency of intercourse among adolescents. In fact, programs that provide both messages appear to be effective in delaying the onset of sexual intercourse and encouraging contraceptive use once sexual activity has begun, especially among younger adolescents.

A recent nationwide survey revealed that respondents wanted information on STDs from multiple sources and rated health care professionals and school-based programs most frequently as being "very effective" sources of information on STDs (EDK Associates, 1995). Factors affecting the acceptance and effectiveness of school-based programs include community norms related to the appropriateness of the inclusion of certain topics in school curricula and the knowledge of teachers about, and attitudes towards, issues related to STDs. It is important to recognize that there is substantial heterogeneity in teacher and community attitudes towards how health curricula should deal with these topics. Competing demands on time and resources, political and religious attitudes, and beliefs about the effects of the teaching of such topics on children's attitudes and behavior vary tremendously. It is important to be aware of, and address when feasible, such factors that might inhibit the implementation of effective programs.

A significant barrier to implementation of effective school-based interventions is inadequate support for dissemination of such programs. To address this issue, the "Research to Classroom Project," sponsored by the Division of Adolescent and School Health, CDC, is the largest federal program to disseminate school-based curricula for reducing sexual risk behaviors. Under this program, the CDC identifies curricula that have been evaluated and shown to be effective in reducing specific risky behaviors and meet other selection criteria, and then provides resources, including training and technical assistance, to ensure that such curricula are disseminated on a national level.

Condom Availability in Schools. To address barriers to adolescent condom usage, approximately 431 schools in 50 school districts in 21 states have condom availability programs as part of HIV and STD prevention efforts, primarily in large urban public high schools (Kirby and Brown, 1996). Ninety-two percent of schools that made condoms available are high schools; these high schools represent only 2.2 percent of all public high schools in the United States (Kirby and Brown, 1996). The 50 school districts with condom availability programs represent only 0.3 percent of all U.S. high school districts. In 1994, there were a total of 9,573 middle schools, 20,059 high schools, and 14,881 school districts in the United States (U.S. Department of Education, National Center for Education Statistics, 1995). Massachusetts, New York State, and the District of Columbia are the only states or jurisdictions to recommend that their schools consider condom availability for students as part of a comprehensive HIV prevention program (NARAL Foundation, 1995). In addition, Los Angeles, New York City, and other cities have mandated condom availability in high schools as part of a comprehensive effort to prevent HIV infection (Kirby and Brown, 1996). In 1992, a survey of superintendents or their designees of 299 middle and high school districts found that only 8 percent of middle and high school students are in districts that have approved condom distribution programs (Leitman et al., 1993). Of schools with condom distribution programs in place, students were not given access to condoms before grade 9. Most districts with approved programs were located in the East and West and in areas with a large proportion of students of lower socioeconomic status. Most schools with condom availability programs are located in Los Angeles and New York City because of these cities' mandates on condom availability. Condom availability programs have used a variety of mechanisms for distributing condoms in schools (Stryker et al., 1994; Advocates for Youth, 1995; Kirby and Brown, 1996). Many schools provide condoms through school health professionals, teachers, principals, or counselors. In only a small percentage of cases are condoms provided in bowls and baskets (5 percent) or through vending machines (3 percent) (Kirby and Brown, 1996). In 81 percent of schools with programs, some type of parental consent (active or passive) is required for student participation. Approximately half of schools that make condoms available require education and counseling before condoms are provided; students are commonly informed regarding use of condoms and that not having sex is the best protection against STDs. An analysis of utilization of condom availability programs showed that students in alternative schools, smaller schools, schools that made condoms available through bowls and baskets, and schools with health clinics obtained more condoms per person per year than did students in other schools (Kirby and Brown, 1996).

There are only limited data on the effectiveness of condom availability programs in schools to increase protective sexual behaviors and decrease STD rates, since these programs are relatively few and newly established (Kirby, 1993; Stryker et al., 1994). In addition, many condom availability programs were not designed to measure program effectiveness (Stryker et al., 1994). One study, however, estimated that an additional 6 to 13 percent of students would have had sexual intercourse without protection if their school had not provided contraceptives (Kirby et al., 1991). Preliminary data from the evaluation of the New York City program indicate that girls considered embarrassment and confidentiality concerns as main barriers to using the program (Guttmacher et al., 1995a). After implementation of condom availability programs in New York City high schools, 69 percent of parents surveyed supported condom availability for their children in school; 85 percent believed that providing condoms to students would either have no effect on, or would decrease the frequency of, sexual activity among the students; and 75 percent believed that providing condoms would result in students practicing safer sex (Guttmacher et al., 1995b).

There seems to be wide public support for school condom availability programs. A 1991 survey showed that 74 percent of adults surveyed favored condom availability in high school and 47 percent favored availability in junior high schools (The Roper Organization, 1991). Among Denver high school students, 85 percent believed that condoms should be provided in their school and 76 percent believed that having access to condoms would not affect the frequency of sexual activity among students (Fanburg et al., 1995). In New York City public high schools where passive parental permission is required for participation, fewer than 2 percent of parents have submitted written denials of participation for their children (Guttmacher et al., 1995b). Health care provider groups have strongly endorsed condom availability for adolescents through schools (AAP, Committee on Adolescence, 1995; AMA, 1996).

Condom availability in schools is an emotionally and politically charged issue. Some of the other the major issues associated with condom availability programs are related to parental consent, funding of condom purchases, staffing and counseling, and legal liability. Opponents of condom availability in schools believe that providing or promoting condoms to adolescents hastens the onset of sexual intercourse, increases sexual activity, and violates parental autonomy in this area. There is no evidence, however, that condom availability or promotion programs increase sexual activity (Kirby, 1994). A study of three school-based clinics that provided contraceptives showed that students in these schools did not initiate sexual intercourse earlier or have intercourse more frequently compared to students in schools without such programs (Kirby et al., 1991). Another study of a high school condom availability program found that the benefit of the program in protecting a sexually active student against STDs and pregnancy was more than three times greater than the risk of encouraging a nonsexually active student to have intercourse (Wolk and Rosenbaum, 1995). In addition, a study of a community-based condom promotion and distribution program among Latino adolescents compared rates of sexual activity in the intervention city with a comparable city without such an intervention (Sellers et al., 1994). Researchers found that, compared to their counterparts in the control city, male adolescents in the intervention city were significantly less likely to initiate sexual intercourse, and female adolescents in the intervention city were significantly less likely to have multiple partners. There were no significant differences in the onset of sexual activity for female adolescents, multiple partnership among male adolescents, or the frequency of sex for male or female adolescents in the two cities.

The funding of condom availability programs can be as contentious as the programs themselves. Schools and local health departments are increasingly under budgetary constraints, and there are several concerns regarding the use of federal funds for these programs (Brindis, 1993). An examination of major condom availability programs in several cities demonstrates that a mix of funding sources, including public and private funds, is necessary to sustain these programs (Brindis, 1993; Stryker et al., 1994). A series of focus group discussions with school superintendents and board members in 1992 revealed that, although they may be supportive of condom availability programs under certain conditions, school officials were unlikely to be leaders in initiating condom availability programs (Greene, 1993).

School condom availability programs in Falmouth (Massachusetts), New York City, and Philadelphia have been challenged in the courts (Mahler, 1996). Program opponents have generally argued that such programs violate parental and religious rights. In January 1996, however, the U.S. Supreme Court declined to review *Curtis v. School Committee of Falmouth*. In this case, the Massachusetts Supreme Judicial Court upheld the school district's program that allowed students in grades 7–12 access to condoms on request without a procedure for parents to refuse participation on behalf of their children (Mahler, 1996).

Mass Media Interventions

An important community-based approach to reducing STDs is to use mass media to disseminate information and promote specific behavior changes. There is compelling evidence that properly designed mass media campaigns can have beneficial effects on health behaviors. Flay (1987) reviewed 40 mass media programs focused on smoking and concluded that information and motivation programs generally produced positive changes in awareness, knowledge, and attitudes. Extensive national campaigns also produced meaningful behavior change. In many ways, changing knowledge and attitudes regarding smoking is less difficult than for STDs. Yet, because there is widespread lack of awareness and information regarding STDs, it is possible that national campaigns would have a greater impact on STDs compared to well-recognized issues such as smoking.

A recent review of HIV prevention mass media campaigns (Flora et al., 1995) concluded that, with the exception of campaigns in Australia and Britain, most of the campaigns that were intended to increase knowledge were successful (Appendix E). The results were mixed with respect to attitude change. Programs designed to change behaviors were largely successful. One prominent example is a Swiss multimedia campaign to promote condom use among adolescents and young adults that has significantly increased condom use among these groups (Wasserfallen et al., 1993). In addition, this campaign, which incorporated explicit messages regarding sexuality, did not result in increased sexual activity among young people. Authors of studies in Italy and Zaire have attributed reductions in HIV infection rates to mass media campaigns (Flora et al., 1995). As mentioned previously, perceived risk is an essential element in almost all models of behavioral risk reduction. The only studies to examine the impact of media campaigns on perceived risk were done in Brazil, France, and the Philippines, and the campaigns were deemed successful (Flora et al., 1995).

Other Methods

Effective interventions are available to prevent exposure to and reduce transmission of STDs. Biomedical methods, such as vaccines and antibiotic therapy, require education of, access to, and compliance among individuals. Similarly, condom use requires behavioral modification to utilize the intervention appropriately. Partner notification and treatment clearly has both behavioral and technical components. Thus, the technical expertise provides methods for intervening in the transmission of STDs, but utilizing the technology requires applying clinical and behavioral interventions concurrently.

Prophylaxis

An important method of preventing acquisition of an STD is to protect persons who have been exposed. Antimicrobial therapy is frequently administered to individuals exposed to bacterial infections. Currently, the only effective vaccine available for prevention of an STD is hepatitis B vaccine. Vaccines for herpes simplex virus are in clinical trials, and vaccines for other STDs are in various stages of development (NIH, 1996).

Although an effective vaccine against hepatitis B virus infection has been available for over a decade, the vaccine's impact has been small because the initial vaccination strategy of selective vaccination of persons with identifiable risk factors was not successful (CDC, 1991b). The Advisory Committee on Immunization Practice (ACIP) recommended in 1991 that hepatitis B vaccine become a routine childhood immunization to protect against later exposures in adolescence or adulthood (CDC, 1991b). Immunization of certain adults, including men who have sex with men and heterosexual persons at high risk for STDs, was also recommended. In 1994, the advisory committee further recommended vaccination of all 11–12-year-old children who had not been previously vaccinated as part of a routine adolescent immunization visit (CDC, 1995b). Current data on hepatitis B vaccination coverage of persons in high-risk groups, including sexually active adolescents and men who have sex with men, are limited, but vaccination coverage is considered to be low (CDC, 1996c; Frank Mahoney, CDC, Hepatitis Branch, personal communication, July 1996). In a recent study, only 3 percent of young men who have sex with men in the San Francisco area were adequately vaccinated against hepatitis B virus (CDC, 1996c). Reasons for inadequate vaccination of adolescents and men who have sex with men include lack of awareness among clinicians of groups at high risk for hepatitis B virus infection and lack of clinical opportunities to provide immunization, especially for adolescents (CDC, 1991b).

Hepatitis B vaccination of adolescents has been successfully implemented in school-based clinics, primary care clinics, and other clinical settings (CDC, 1994b; Kollar et al., 1994). Initiatives to administer hepatitis B vaccine to STD clinic patients show that such programs are feasible, although completion of all three vaccine doses is sometimes problematic (Moran et al., 1992; Lafferty et al., 1995). Since 1994, hepatitis B vaccine has been accessible free of charge under the Vaccines for Children program for children less than 19 years of age at high risk for hepatitis B virus infection, including adolescents seen in STD clinics and correctional facilities (CDC, 1994a). To be eligible for the program, children must be enrolled in Medicaid, have no health insurance, be an American Indian/ Alaska Native, or have health insurance that does not cover hepatitis B immunization. Outside of limited federal demonstration projects, there are no major programs or public funds to increase vaccination of adults at high risk for sexually transmitted hepatitis B virus infection. Frequency of coverage for adult hepatitis B immunization among private health plans is unclear but is considered to be low (Eric Mast, CDC, Hepatitis Branch, personal communication, October 1996). A recent economic analysis of various immunization strategies to prevent hepatitis B showed that perinatal prevention (screening of pregnant women and prophylaxis of infants) and routine infant immunization would reduce the 4.8 percent lifetime risk of hepatitis B virus infection by at least 68 percent, compared with a 45 percent reduction of lifetime risk for adolescent vaccination (Margolis et al., 1995). The authors concluded that adolescent vaccination of those who were not currently immunized should be considered part of a national strategy against hepatitis B virus infection.

Condoms

With the exception of not having sexual intercourse with an infected partner, using a new latex condom during every act of sexual intercourse is currently the most effective method of preventing exposure to STDs (CDC, 1993b). When used correctly and consistently (during every act of intercourse), condoms are highly effectively against bacterial and viral STDs including HIV infection (Cates and Stone, 1992; Roper et al., 1993; Weller, 1993). Several studies that have followed "discordant" partners show that consistent condom use significantly reduces the transmission of STDs including HIV infection (Laurian et al., 1989; European Study Group on Heterosexual Transmission of HIV, 1992).

Failure to use a condom correctly and consistently, rather than potential defects of the condom itself, is considered to be the major barrier to condom effectiveness (Cates and Stone, 1992; CDC, 1993b). Many incidents of condom breakage and leakage are associated with improper handling or inappropriate use of lubricants.

Data show that condom use has increased in the United States in the last few decades (DeBuono et al., 1990; Pleck et al., 1993; Peterson, 1995). Data from the National Survey of Family Growth show that, among women who had their first intercourse premaritally at 15–19 years of age, the proportion who used a condom at first intercourse rose from 28 percent during 1980–1982 to 55 percent during June 1988–November 1990 (Peterson, 1995). In addition, data from the CDC's Youth Risk Behavior Surveillance System show that, from 1990 through 1993, the proportion of high school students who reported using condoms at last sexual intercourse increased significantly from 46.2 percent to 52.8 percent (CDC, 1995a). Among unmarried sexually experienced women of reproductive age, approximately 30 percent reported using a condom for disease prevention every time or most times that they have intercourse (Anderson et al., 1996).

Although the first female condom was introduced in the 1920s, the polyurethane female condom has only recently been approved for use in the United States and represents an important alternative to the male condom (CDC, 1993b; IOM, 1996). A major advantage of the female condom is the greater control that women have over its use compared to the male condom. Other advantages include insertion before intercourse, it protects a greater area of the vagina, and it is less likely to break than the male condom (Gollub and Stein, 1993). The female condom is an effective mechanical barrier to viruses including HIV (CDC, 1993b). The Food and Drug Administration has recently approved labeling for the female condom to reflect annual pregnancy protection failure rates of 21 percent for "typical use" (the product is used inconsistently or incorrectly) and 5 percent for "perfect use" (the product is used consistently and correctly every time).[5] These data are consistent with results of a multisite study that found a six-month 2.6 percent unintended pregnancy rate (and no STDs) for U.S. women who used the female polyurethane condom consistently and correctly (Farr et al., 1994). Although a percentage of women in this study reported liking the female condom, there is insufficient experience with the female condom to determine its long-term acceptability (IOM, 1996). Potential disadvantages of the female condom include its relatively high cost, its appearance, and its acceptance by women (Gollub and Stein, 1993). The female condom represents one of the few female-controlled contraceptive methods that are effective against STDs. Many factors may influence individual behavior related to condom use. Understanding the impact of these individual factors is important in effectively promoting condom use as a measure to prevent STDs. Although studies on condom use behavior have increased in the last decade, many of the determinants of correct and consistent condom use have not been adequately examined (Roper et al., 1993).

Adolescence. Behavioral factors that influence condom use among adolescents include sufficient knowledge and skills, perceptions of condoms, ability to communicate with partners, and perception of condom use by peers (Brown et al., 1992; Orr and Langefeld, 1993; AAP, Committee on Adolescence, 1995). Other major factors that influence whether condoms are used by adolescents include access, availability, confidentiality, and cost (Kirby et al., 1994; AAP, Committee on Adolescence, 1995). Magura and others (1994) found that male adolescents of certain ethnic groups in the juvenile justice system were more likely to report using condoms if condoms were accessible. A sample of college males reported that not having condoms available was a major factor in their lack of condom use (Franzini and Sideman, 1994). The importance of ready access to condoms was underscored by another study that found that adolescents who carry condoms are almost three times more likely to use a condom during sexual

---

[5] These failure rates may differ from those cited in package inserts of some earlier lots of female condoms. The original labeling indicated an annual pregnancy protection failure rate of 26 percent for "typical use" (a range of 21 to 26 percent is also cited) and did not give an estimate for "perfect use." The newer estimates reflect the Food and Drug Administration's approval for the manufacturer to cite the lower estimated failure rate under "typical use" and the rate under conditions of "perfect use."

intercourse compared to other adolescents (Hingson et al., 1990). Embarrassment in obtaining and using condoms is also an important factor that may discourage their use (Hingson et al., 1990). In a sample of female adolescents who were pregnant or who already had a child, Koniak-Griffin and colleagues (1994) found that poor condom use was associated with greater embarrassment.

Age. Condom use among men declines with age. For example, data show that the rate of reported condom use at last intercourse steadily declined with increasing age from 39 percent of men 20–25 years old to 17 percent of men 35–39 years old in 1991 (Pleck et al., 1993). In 1992, 28 percent of adults 18–24 years of age surveyed reported using a condom at last intercourse compared to 19 percent of adults 30–34 years of age and 12 percent of adults 40–44 years of age (Laumann et al., 1994). These data may reflect the tendency to rely on contraceptive methods other than condoms as men grow older, establish long-term relationships, and depend more on female-controlled contraceptives such as oral contraceptives and sterilization (Landry and Camelo, 1994). Age also seems to be associated with the comfort level of persons in negotiating condom use with partners. For example, a national survey revealed that 69 percent of women 18–24 felt "very comfortable" in asking a new partner to use a condom compared to 55 percent of women 25–34 and 40 percent of women 35–44 years (EDK Associates, 1994).

Educational Level, Race, and Gender. Men with higher levels of education report higher rates of condom use compared to less educated men (Tanfer et al., 1993), but studies have failed to show that socioeconomic status is independently associated with condom use (Pleck et al., 1991; Ku et al., 1992). African American women are almost twice as likely to use condoms compared to women of other races (Anderson et al., 1996). In addition, African American men are more likely to have used condoms during their last episode of intercourse compared to either European American or Hispanic men (Laumann et al., 1994). The rate of condom use at first intercourse for African Americans, however, is lower than that for European American men independent of age at initial intercourse (Ku et al., 1993). Women generally report slightly lower rates of condom use at last intercourse compared to men. In 1992, 18 percent of men and 15 percent of women reported such use (Laumann et al., 1994).

Ability to Negotiate Use. Even if the individual has a condom, negotiating its use with one's partner may be difficult. Condom use may be particularly difficult in a romantic relationship. For a woman, asking a partner to use a condom (or for a man, using one himself) may convey a lack of trust in the partner. Women may fear that their partner will react angrily to the suggestion. Marin and colleagues (1993) found that Hispanic women's fear of an angry response by their partners to a request to use condoms predicted their reported use of condoms. In some cultures, suggestions about condom use may prompt male partners to view the woman as "loose" (Mays and Cochran, 1988). Sexual communication between partners has been found to be an important determinant of condom use (Catania et al., 1992). In addition, studies have found that college students tended to use condoms in casual relationships, but when they became more committed and developed trust in the relationship, they stopped using them (Pilkington et al., 1994; Lear, 1995).

Perceptions of Condoms. Several studies show that persons who believe that condoms require interrupting the act of intercourse and that they reduce sexual pleasure are less likely to use condoms compared to those who did not have such beliefs (Wulfert and Wan, 1993; Norris and Ford, 1994; Ramos et al., 1995). In one study, adolescents who believed that condoms did not reduce sexual pleasure were more than three times as likely to use condoms compared to other adolescents (Hingson et al., 1990). In another study, men who felt that condoms would be uncomfortable or painful to use were less likely to intend to use them (Kegeles et al., 1989) Among unmarried women, favorable perceptions of the effectiveness of condoms strongly predict condom use (Anderson et al., 1996).

Competing Concerns. Concerns that compete with protective behaviors are important determinants of condom use. Disenfranchised and poor persons in particular may have more immediate survival concerns, such as obtaining money for food and shelter, that may hinder the implementation of protective health behaviors (Mays and Cochran, 1988; Donovan, 1996). In addition, if one or both partners wish to conceive, the desire for pregnancy may undermine conscientious use of condoms (Adler and Tschann, 1993). The impact of other contraceptive use on condom use is discussed in the following section.

Other Contraceptives and Dual Protection

Among sexually active women 15–44 years of age at risk of unintended pregnancy, 12 percent do not use a method of contraception (Peterson, 1995). As reflected in the high rates of unintended pregnancy in the United States, it is clear that many persons are not using contraceptives consistently or correctly (IOM, 1995). Among women who use contraception, the most common methods are female sterilization, oral contraceptives, and the condom. Barriers to contraceptive access include the cost of contraceptives, inadequate coverage of contraceptives by health insurance plans, and inadequate training and skills of some health care professionals in providing contraceptive services (IOM, 1995). These problems are particularly difficult for adolescents.

Women who rely on sterilization, oral contraceptives, or another method for protecting against pregnancy are less likely to use condoms compared to other women. For example, studies show that women who have been surgically sterilized are less likely to report condom use (CDC, 1992a, b). Women who used oral contraceptives, had been pregnant, were surgically sterilized, wanted future births, or were older were less likely to use condoms for disease prevention than other women (Anderson et al., 1996; Santelli et al., 1996).

The effectiveness of various contraceptives against STDs (including HIV infection) and pregnancy is summarized in Table 4-1. Of the methods listed, condoms are the most protective method against STDs, including HIV infection, but are not the most effective pregnancy-prevention method. In contrast, surgical sterilization is most effective against pregnancy but confers no protection against STDs. Spermicides, such as nonoxynol-9, are effective against most STDs in vitro (Cates and Stone, 1992) and have been found to be partially effective against gonorrhea and chlamydial infection in clinical trials (Louv et al., 1988). Epidemiological and biological studies, however, have indicated that excessive use of nonoxynol-9 may irritate the vaginal lining, thus potentially facilitating HIV infection (Cates et al., 1992). There has been some debate about how women should be counseled regarding the relative effectiveness of condoms, diaphragms, and spermicides. Some believe that women should be counseled that both condoms and spermicides are effective against STDs (Rosenberg and Gollub, 1992; Stein, 1992). However, most believe that the effectiveness of spermicides against STDs other than gonorrhea and chlamydial infection is uncertain and that condoms should remain the primary recommended strategy for STDs including HIV infection (Cates et al., 1992). Hormonal contraceptives may actually increase the risk for cervical infections, but their effects on STD transmission and sequelae remain unclear (Cates and Stone, 1992). The IUD seems to increase the risk for STDs, especially around the time of insertion (Cates and Stone, 1992).

No single method of preventing STDs or pregnancy confers the maximum level of protection for both conditions (Cates and Stone, 1992). Use of dual protection—that is, one to protect against STDs and another to protect against pregnancy—is especially important for women. Women who use a contraceptive other than a condom are not fully protected against STDs. To obtain maximum protection against STDs and pregnancy, a condom (male or female) should be used with another effective contraceptive. There seems to be public interest in simultaneous protection against STDs and pregnancy, and dual use of contraceptives has increased (IOM, 1995). However, it is not clear how well the public understands the need for dual protection against STDs and pregnancy.

As mentioned in Chapters 2 and 3, women are more vulnerable to STDs than men. Additional contraceptive methods that are female-controlled and effective against all STDs need to be developed (Cates et al., 1992; Rosenberg and Gollub, 1992; Stein, 1992). In particular, topical microbicides that are effective against HIV and other STDs but do not impair a woman's ability to become pregnant would be an important female-controlled method for STD prevention (Elias and Heise, 1994). Another IOM committee has identified the development of chemical or physical barriers to conception and to transmission of STDs as a major priority in a research agenda focused on women (IOM, 1996). Currently, researchers are attempting to develop methods of protection that are not harmful to beneficial microbes and the lining of the lower reproductive tract (unlike nonoxynol-9) but are active against pathogenic organisms (IOM, 1996).

Partner Notification and Treatment

Partner notification has been a component of STD programs in the United States for many years (Rothenberg and Potterat, 1990). Championed by Surgeon General Thomas Parran at the first National Conference on Venereal Disease Control in 1936, it became an integral component of efforts against syphilis in this country after penicillin became widely available in the 1940s (Brandt, 1985). STD patient interviews followed by partner notification were considered to be the cornerstones of the early federal efforts against syphilis implemented by the Venereal Disease Branch at the National Communicable Disease Center, now known as the CDC. Partner notification has continued to be supported through current federally funded STD programs.

Because the incubation period for early syphilis is long (an average of three weeks, but anywhere from 10 to 90 days from exposure to onset of symptoms), partner notification could break the "chain of transmission" not only by identifying "source" cases of illness and partners with clinical or serologic evidence of disease, but also by identifying and treating partners exposed to syphilis. By providing treatment to exposed but asymptomatic partners, a potential case could be prevented by treatment of "incubating" syphilis.

When the syphilis model was expanded to include the referral of partners exposed to gonorrhea (Potterat et al., 1989; Alary et al., 1991; CDC, DSTD/HIVP, 1992) and chlamydial infection (Katz et al., 1988; Alary et al., 1991), the rationale for partner notification had to be modified, since the incubation periods are shorter for gonorrhea (usually a week or less) and chlamydial infection (one to two weeks). Therefore, therapy of partners with incubating infections was not possible; instead, emphasis was placed on locating asymptomatic infected female partners of symptomatic men and on providing early treatment to prevent complications (CDC, DSTD/HIVP, 1992).

Identification of partners exposed to treatable bacterial STDs makes intuitive sense as an STD prevention strategy. "Source" cases—those exposing others to an STD—require treatment to break the chain of transmission. Partners who have been exposed to an already infected and infectious individual are at greatest risk for developing STD infection themselves. Treatment of infected or exposed partners will not only cure or prevent the infection (as in the case of incubating syphilis) but will both prevent STD transmission to future partners and directly benefit the exposed individual by preventing complications of untreated infection. Partner notification followed by partner treatment, therefore, is considered to be a strategy that benefits the individual index patient, his or her partner, and the community as a whole.

Evaluation of STDs in men generally requires less time and less equipment and is easier to perform (a pelvic examination is not required) than in women. Nonetheless, for a number of reasons, clinicians, especially those who primarily treat women, often do not routinely examine and treat male sex partners of women found to have STDs. In some instances, clinicians do not counsel women regarding the importance of partner treatment. In other instances, women with STDs are given medications to give to their partners. This latter practice, although widespread, is of unproven benefit and is the subject of a recently initiated multicenter study conducted by the CDC. When utilized, this approach has several disadvantages for preventing STDs including the small but real risk of adverse drug reactions in unseen "patients," the inability to screen the partner for other STDs, and the lack of opportunity to examine and counsel the partner.

Techniques in Partner Notification. The method and intensity of partner outreach activities traditionally have varied according to the clinical setting. In dedicated public STD clinics, emphasis has been placed on the activities of trained program staff, commonly called "disease intervention specialists," to interview STD patients and identify names and the whereabouts of partners.[6] The role of these "disease intervention specialists" will be discussed in detail in Chapter 5. Originally called "contact tracing" and now referred to as "provider referral," this method of partner notification relies on intensive interviews with patients about their sexual histories and partners, followed by active outreach by public health staff to identify and locate partners to ensure that they are examined and treated. Although labor intensive and costly, provider referral is still carried out within most public health programs for syphilis and selected other STDs (Rothenberg and Potterat, in press).

Any efforts by patients to notify their own partners about STD exposure without assistance from public health staff is called "patient referral." STD programs and staff have emphasized provider referral as the notification method of choice, especially for syphilis and to a lesser extent for other bacterial STDs identified in STD clinics, since the benefits of ensuring that partners receive preventive treatment have been thought to outweigh the substantial costs in staff time. Few efforts have been made to identify partners of individuals with other viral STDs such as herpes simplex or hepatitis B virus (Munday et al., 1983). The

---

[6]The term "disease intervention specialist" is commonly used to refer to a nonphysician health professional who is involved with educating and counseling persons with STDs and has responsibility for partner notification activities. A "disease intervention specialist" may be a federal, state, or local government employee. Sometimes this term is confused with the term "public health advisor" which comes from a CDC job series title. A "public health advisor" is a nonphysician CDC staff member assigned to state or local health departments in STD prevention and other areas. This person may function as a "disease intervention specialist" or may have management or supervisory responsibilities.

cost of carrying out provider referral is significantly higher than that for patient referral (Oxman et al., 1994).

Partner notification performed for patients seen outside of the STD clinic setting has never been well developed or documented. Although disease intervention specialists make intensive efforts to identify partners of syphilis patients seen in public STD clinics and in private practice and to follow up on positive tests reported by laboratories, little effort is generally made to support partner notification for patients treated for gonorrhea or chlamydial infection in private health care settings such as physician offices and hospital emergency rooms (Toomey, 1990). Little is known about the practices of private providers regarding partner follow-up, and no systematic national efforts have been made to educate private sector providers regarding the importance of partner treatment as an essential component of STD-related care.

When the provider referral model was applied to HIV prevention and AIDS, other concerns about partner notification emerged (Potterat et al., 1989; Toomey and Cates, 1989; Giesecke et al., 1991; Bayer and Toomey, 1992; Rothenberg and Potterat, in press). The long asymptomatic incubation period for HIV infection makes partner follow-up difficult (Rutherford et al., 1991), and curative therapies are not available. Exposed partners who are identified and not yet infected can benefit substantially from risk-reduction counseling to change behavior, thereby potentially preventing future HIV infection among at-risk partners. HIV-infected persons benefit from early intervention since retroviral therapy and prophylaxis against opportunistic infections are beneficial when utilized appropriately.

Although confidentiality has been ensured with provider referral for STDs, concern about the scope and limits of confidentiality—as well as doubt about the relevance and potential efficacy of partner notification in preventing any STD—have emerged. As the debate regarding partner notification intensified, some public health leaders questioned the value of any provider referral activities (Bayer and Toomey, 1992).

Effectiveness of Partner Notification. Temporal trends suggest that partner notification contributed to the reduction of syphilis and congenital syphilis after the program was widely implemented in the 1950s (Baumgartner et al., 1962). In addition, published reports have documented the effectiveness of partner notification strategies in controlling focal outbreaks of gonorrhea and chancroid (Handsfield et al., 1982, 1989; Blackmore et al., 1985; Zenilman et al., 1988) and in targeting intervention for specific high-risk populations (Yorke et al., 1978; Phillips et al., 1980). In some countries, such as Sweden, partner notification for gonorrhea, syphilis, and chlamydial infection has been highly effective (Ramstedt et al., 1991). The effectiveness of partner notification strategies for STD prevention, however, has not been rigorously evaluated in terms of STD incidence or prevalence in the population at large or rates of reinfection among index patients.

Instead, STD programs emphasize "yields" from interviews and volume of activity as indirect programmatic indicators of efficacy (CDC, DSTD/HIVP, 1992; Rothenberg and Potterat, in press). Recent studies suggest that provider referral for STDs, as it is currently performed by disease intervention specialists, is not working effectively. In many programs, fewer than one partner can be found per index patient, although index patients often report having many partners during the interview period (Gunn et al., 1995). A number of factors may contribute to the diminishing utility of provider referral as traditionally carried out in public STD clinics. Concerns about the safety of the interviewers working in high-crime communities, as well as concerns about the cultural sensitivity of the STD interviewers, continue to be raised by both supporters and critics of the process.

Crack cocaine use and the exchange of sex for drugs have emerged as major risk factors in recent epidemics of syphilis (Marx et al., 1991), other STDs (Schwarcz et al., 1992), and HIV infection (Edlin et al., 1994). The large number of often anonymous partners involved in sex-for-drug activities have reduced the efficacy of traditional patient interviewing to identify partners, to the point that many have questioned the continued utility of provider referral in these populations (Andrus et al., 1990; Oxman and Doyle, 1996). Implementing alternative case-finding methods (CDC, 1991a; Engelgau et al., 1995) and refocusing partner outreach toward communities and social networks (Klovdahl et al., 1994; Trotter et al., 1995; Gunn et al., 1995; Rothenberg and Narramore, 1996), rather than traditional partner identification, have been suggested as more effective strategies for reaching high-risk individuals for intervention and prevention activities (Rothenberg and Potterat, in press).

Research evidence concerning the effectiveness of partner notification is sparse at best. Oxman and others (1994) recently reviewed published studies in this area and found the following:

1. simple forms of assistance for improving patient referral, such as telephone calls, can be effective;

2. provider referral results in more partners being notified than does patient referral for HIV infection;

3. evidence supporting provider referral as being more effective than patient referral for syphilis is weak;

4. evidence is inconsistent regarding the effectiveness of health care professional referral compared with patient referral for gonorrhea and chlamydial infection; and

5. there is only weak evidence to support the notion that trained interviewers are more effective than regular health care professionals at identifying partners, and there is no evidence that this slightly increased effectiveness has any practical importance for STD prevention.

Screening

Screening programs for many STDs are cost-effective and, sometimes, cost-saving (Handsfield et al., 1986; Arevalo and Washington, 1988; Trachtenberg et al., 1988; Randolph and Washington, 1990; Britton et al., 1992; Hillis, Nakashima, et al., 1995; Scholes et al., 1996). For example, using a decision model, Trachtenberg and colleagues (1988) estimated net savings of more than $60 million (in 1986 dollars) over the first five years of a California statewide chlamydia-screening program for asymptomatic women in family planning clinics. The CDC estimates that approximately $12 in costs associated with the complications of chlamydial and gonococcal infection could be saved for every $1 spent on early detection and treatment (CDC, DSTD/HIVP, 1995).

There are many examples of successful comprehensive screening programs. The Wisconsin chlamydia prevention program is a comprehensive program supported by state funding that includes public-private collaborations, screening in family planning and STD clinics, low-cost laboratory services, integrated information systems, and evaluation of program effectiveness (Addiss et al., 1994; Hillis, Nakashima, et al., 1995). In Wisconsin, substantial declines in the prevalence and incidence of chlamydial infections were observed statewide after the implementation of selective chlamydia screening in family planning clinics and universal screening in large STD clinics, in conjunction with other statewide interventions. Rates of positive laboratory tests for chlamydia, hospitalization for pelvic inflammatory disease, and ectopic pregnancy also declined. In addition, an Indianapolis chlamydia program that included screening demonstrated a 63 percent decrease in chlamydial infections among adolescent girls attending adolescent health clinics for the first time during the 8.75 years of the program (Katz et al., 1996).

The success of a CDC and Office of Population Affairs initiative begun in 1988 in Public Health Service Region X to reduce chlamydia rates led to the Preventive Health Amendments of 1992 that authorized federal funding for expansion of activities to prevent infertility associated with chlamydial and gonococcal infections. Appropriated funds of $12.2 million in fiscal year 1995 have allowed the CDC to screen and treat at least half of at-risk women and their sex partners using family planning and STD clinics in 4 of 10 regions; to initiate screening and treatment services in the other 6 regions; and to implement research and evaluation activities at 5 sites (CDC, Division of STD Prevention, unpublished data, 1996). The CDC estimates that $175 million per year, including $90 million in public funding, is needed to fully implement a national chlamydia prevention program to screen and treat all female adolescents and women between 15 and 34 years of age (CDC, DSTD/HIVP, 1995).

In the primary care setting, screening and treating women at increased risk for asymptomatic chlamydial infection significantly reduces the rate of subsequent pelvic inflammatory disease (Scholes et al., 1996). The U.S. Preventive

Services Task Force (1996) recently recommended a group of screening activities for primary care clinicians based on the age of the patient and risk category. A summary of the task force's recommendations related to STD screening and counseling is presented in Appendix F. These clinical guidelines were developed after an extensive review of data, studies, and expert opinions. It is important to note that the task force recommendations were based on evidence of prevention effectiveness rather than on cost-effectiveness or other considerations. Recognizing the limited amount of time available to primary care clinicians during patient visits, the task force only recommended interventions that were shown to be effective by peer-reviewed studies. The intent is that clinicians would choose from the specific recommended interventions and tailor them to the health needs of the individual patient. The task force evaluated and made specific recommendations for the following diseases and conditions related to sexual intercourse: hepatitis B virus infection, syphilis, gonorrhea, HIV infection, chlamydial infection, genital herpes, cervical cancer, and unintended pregnancy. Several medical professional societies, other organizations, and government agencies have also published guidelines regarding screening for STDs (U.S. Preventive Services Task Force, 1996). The recommendations of these organizations and agencies are very similar. For example, no major organizations recommend screening of the general population for chlamydial infection, genital herpes simplex virus, hepatitis B virus infection, or syphilis. The recommendations of these groups, however, often vary in the criteria recommended for selecting risk groups for screening.

Not all STD screening programs are cost-effective. State laws requiring premarital and prenatal screening in order to prevent syphilis transmission date back to the 1930s and 1940s (Brandt, 1985). As a result of data showing that only approximately 1 percent of syphilis infections were detected by premarital screening, many states have repealed their premarital testing requirements (Felman, 1981). As of 1996, however, 15 states still require premarital syphilis testing as a requirement for marriage licenses (CDC, Division of STD Prevention, unpublished data, 1996). The number of previously undetected cases of syphilis identified through premarital testing is extremely low (Felman, 1981; Haskell, 1984). In addition, studies show that premarital tests for syphilis or HIV infection are not cost-effective and have little public health impact (Haskell, 1984; Cleary et al., 1987; Peterson and White, 1990). In contrast, screening for syphilis during pregnancy has been shown to be cost-saving; the economic benefits of the national screening program in Norway were almost four times the program cost (Stray-Pederson, 1983).

Inadequate resources and other considerations may preclude implementation of widespread screening protocols or other intervention programs. In such situations, methods for identifying individuals or groups at particularly high risk are helpful in targeting interventions and maximizing effectiveness (Stergachis et al., 1993). For example, a study of public STD clinics in Dade County, Florida, found that it is possible to identify persons at highest risk for STDs using routinely collected clinical data (Richert et al., 1993). Thirty-nine percent of those at highest risk for STDs were reinfected within a year compared to 7 percent of those at the lowest risk.

REDUCING DURATION OF INFECTION

In addition to effective interventions designed to prevent exposure and reduce the efficiency of disease transmission, effective interventions to reduce the duration of infection are currently available. Reducing duration of STDs can be accomplished primarily by ensuring early diagnosis and treatment of infected persons and by reducing barriers to diagnostic and treatment services. Reducing the duration of STDs among infected individuals is an effective method of preventing STDs in the population because reducing duration will reduce the period of time that an individual is infectious and, consequently, reduce the number of partners exposed to infection. In addition, early detection and treatment prevents complications of STDs in infected individuals. This is illustrated by the trials in Tanzania demonstrating that early detection and treatment reduces active syphilis and symptomatic urethritis (Mwijarubi et al., 1996). In this section, the committee reviews the diagnostic tests available for STDs and the barriers to diagnosis and treatment.

Early Diagnosis and Treatment

Early, specific diagnosis and treatment of symptomatic and asymptomatic individuals will prevent further transmission of STDs to their partners. Currently available diagnostic and therapeutic technologies are adequate for containment or eradication of bacterial STDs in the United States. While improved diagnostic tests and more effective therapies would facilitate the task, the fact that countries such as Sweden have, for all practical purposes, eradicated endemic gonorrhea and syphilis indicates that bacterial STDs can be contained with current biomedical technologies. Diagnostic techniques are similarly effective for viral STDs; however, in general, curative therapeutic agents for viral STDs are not currently available.

Diagnostic Tests for STDs

Traditionally, diagnostic tests for STDs are used by clinicians to evaluate either persons who suspect they have an STD or sex partners of infected individuals. Appropriate diagnosis of an STD often requires multiple specific diagnostic tests because of the variety of STDs. Further complicating the diagnosis of STDs is the availability of several different diagnostic tests for each STD. No single test can be relied upon to provide timely (i.e., in less than 30 minutes) and accurate diagnosis of symptomatic individuals while also being utilized for accurate detection of asymptomatic persons in the context of screening. Unfortunately, many clinicians fail to appreciate that no single laboratory test is optimal for use in all settings.

"Syndromic diagnosis," which utilizes the patient's history, results of physical examination, and rapid laboratory tests, can be utilized for the diagnosis of clinical syndromes. This allows appropriate treatment for infected individuals in a single visit. This approach is relatively inexpensive when compared to conducting specific laboratory testing. Unfortunately, syndromic diagnosis is not always specific even though, for many of the syndromes, only one or two STD pathogens are usually the cause. The major curable STD syndromes in adults include urethritis in males; vaginal discharge, cervicitis, and pelvic inflammatory disease in women; and genital ulcers in both men and women. In clinical practice in the United States, it is common to initiate syndromic treatment for urethritis in men and cervicitis and pelvic inflammatory disease in women (while results of laboratory testing are pending), using treatments effective against all of the common bacteria that can cause these syndromes. For genital ulcers and vaginal discharge, it is more common to perform rapid tests before initiating treatment. Since syndromic treatment, by definition, is used only for persons with symptoms or signs of a clinical syndrome, this approach is not useful in detecting mild or asymptomatic infection. It should also be noted that, like any diagnostic test, the predictive value and therefore diagnostic utility of syndromic diagnosis will vary with the prevalence of the disease being tested for in the population. In low-prevalence populations, construing all cervicitis or urethritis to represent an STD may result in a large number of false positive diagnoses, unnecessary treatment, and potential psychological distress.

Laboratory testing for specific causative infectious agents is necessary for the detection of minimally symptomatic and asymptomatic individuals. There are STDs, such as gonorrhea, for which the antimicrobial resistance patterns of the pathogen are important. The isolation of the pathogen permits a determination of sensitivity or resistance to appropriate antibiotics. In addition, laboratory isolation of the pathogen allows specific testing for epidemiological purposes to track the spread of infection in a population. Although analyses of antimicrobial resistance patterns for STDs are seldom used to guide individual treatment, they are essential to develop community-based treatment guidelines. Unfortunately, some specific laboratory tests are often not available at clinical sites other than dedicated STD clinics and, even when available, the test results are often not available during the initial patient visit. In addition, the expense of these tests may limit their availability and utility.

Specific laboratory tests often guide therapeutic decisions. Ideally, the test could distinguish between past and present infection. The adequacy of specimens collected and specimen transport conditions are important modifiers of test performance. For example, there may be nonpathogenic microorganisms present in some of the sites being sampled, and specimens must be managed to preserve the integrity of the more labile organisms. For STDs, specimen collection procedures, such as a pelvic examination or obtaining a urethral swab, may be a disincentive for patients to seek testing or for providers to perform the test. Although diagnostic tests are available for each of the common STDs, they will not be appropriately utilized if the test is too expensive or limited in availability (Hitchcock et al., 1991).

Culturing

Culturing of the pathogen is a common laboratory test for specific diagnosis of many STDs. When available, organism-specific cultures are often the "gold standard" for etiologic diagnosis. However, recently available amplified nucleic acid detection tests, such as polymerase chain reaction (PCR) or ligase chain reaction (LCR), may soon displace culturing as these tests become more available and assessment of these tests is completed (Rumpianesi et al., 1996). The only bacterial STD that is very commonly diagnosed by culturing in North America is gonorrhea. The sensitivity of the culture technique is subject to conditions that affect pathogen viability, including transport time and conditions. The specificity is 100 percent with no false positive results except in cases of laboratory error. The medium for optimal culture diagnosis, however, may not be uniformly available. Currently, in the United States, nonamplified probe tests are probably performed almost as often as culture for the diagnosis of gonorrhea.

Microscopy

Results of microscopy are rapidly available and are of considerable importance in refining syndromic diagnoses. Sensitivity of this technique, however, varies with the pathogen suspected and the expertise of the microscopist. The preferred method for diagnosis of urethritis in men and vaginal discharge syndromes in women is the microscopic examination of materials. Because microscopy requires time, clinicians are discouraged from using it. Different stains and methodology are necessary for diagnosis of different STDs. Microscopic evaluation of Papanicolaou (Pap) stained smears of cervical specimens is a useful test for detection of malignant and premalignant cellular changes related to human papillomavirus infection.

Antibody Detection Tests

Currently, serological tests to detect antibodies against STDs are most often used for the diagnosis of syphilis, HIV infection, and viral hepatitis in North America. One of the advantages of serological testing is that multiple evaluations for different pathogens can be performed on a single serum specimen. The presence of antibody in a single serum, however, may not distinguish between previ-

160 THE HIDDEN EPIDEMIC

ous infection and existing infection. This is of particular importance if the disease has been appropriately treated in the past but the serological test remains positive. Potentially, serological testing can lead to false positive results if antibodies against an infection other than the one tested for produce a positive reaction in the assay. Serological tests are particularly useful for screening because they can be performed in large numbers by automation and by central laboratories that can process entire groups of sera at once.

Antigen Detection Tests

These tests use pathogen-specific antibodies to detect proteins, carbohydrates, or lipid-carbohydrates present on the surface of STD pathogens. They have been extensively used for the diagnosis of STDs such as hepatitis B virus infection, chlamydial infection, and genital herpes and are potentially very useful for syphilis. For example, a fluorescent antibody kit used fluorescein-labeled antichlamydia antibodies to stain specimens collected from the urethra or cervix and then visualize chlamydial organisms under a fluorescent microscope. An alternate approach is solid phase immunoassay and involves a variety of formats that have been widely used in STD diagnostics. These tests can be used to detect organisms than cannot be cultured (grown in the laboratory) or that are difficult to culture. Many have become relatively inexpensive, and some can be used for rapid diagnosis of STDs in the clinic. However, these tests, particularly the rapid tests, are generally less sensitive than culture tests (for the culturable organisms) or genomic detection tests, which are therefore beginning to replace the antigen detection tests and are described below.

Tests Based on Genetic Markers

There are two basic types of genetically based tests available. Nonamplified tests use a nucleic acid probe to detect the extremely small amount of an infectious organism's unique genetic sequence (nucleic acid) present in an infected person. In contrast, amplified tests first make many copies of an organism's genetic sequence, thereby magnifying the "signal" of the organism and enhancing the ease of detection.

Since the late 1980s, the availability of nonamplified nucleic acid detection tests has significantly increased the availability of diagnostic testing for chlamydial infection and gonorrhea in North America. Currently, most specific diagnoses of chlamydial infections are accomplished using these methods. Compared to culture, nucleic acid probe tests are more practical for STD diagnosis in many settings because they are less expensive and because specimens do not need to be handled and transported under ideal conditions. On the other hand, these tests are usually less sensitive than culturing, especially for patients with small infectious burdens, such as asymptomatic patients.

Nucleic acid amplification tests, such as PCR and LCR, are increasingly being utilized for diagnosis of many infections and will likely be considered the standard for diagnosis of STDs in the future. Chlamydia, gonorrhea, and HIV diagnostic tests from one or more manufacturers are currently approved by the Food and Drug Administration. Prototype tests for the diagnosis of syphilis, genital herpes, human papillomavirus, trichomonas, and most other sexually transmitted pathogens are in various stages of development. Because these assays amplify genetic material from infectious organisms, their specificity can approach 100 percent if the proper genetic sequences are selected for the test; their sensitivity is a function of the amplification process. In certain situations, such as when tests are performed soon after therapy, false positive results may be a problem. Nucleic acid amplification tests have been as sensitive as culture for several STDs, and the detection of some pathogens such as chlamydia and herpes virus has been improved by these tests. The causative pathogens of human papillomavirus and syphilis cannot be cultured but can be detected using these sensitive techniques. In addition, the sensitivity of these tests has enabled clinicians to use more easily collected specimens for diagnosis, such as simple urine and vaginal swabs, rather than specimens obtained by more invasive sampling techniques. Lastly, the tests are not dependent on the presence of viable organisms in the specimen; therefore, handling and transport of specimens are relatively easy.

Treatment for STDs

The diagnosis of an STD should lead to either curative and/or preventive therapy for the infected individual. Although ideal therapy does not exist for many infections, highly effective antimicrobial therapy is available for all bacterial STDs as well as those caused by protozoa and ectoparasites (CDC, 1993a). They are administered to eradicate infection and to prevent its complications. In contrast, drugs for viral STDs have largely been limited to alleviating symptoms because they cannot eradicate the organism. However, many viral STDs (e.g., HIV infection, genital herpes, hepatitis B virus infection) are increasingly being viewed as suppressible infections with new therapies. These treatments suppress viral replication and thereby reduce transmission and may be considered to be a viable approach for preventing STDs.

Utilization of antimicrobial drugs is guided by both syndromic and etiologic diagnoses. The STD Treatment Guidelines published by the CDC provide the current standards for therapy of STDs (CDC, 1993a). A significant barrier to appropriate treatment is failure to comply with a full course of medication. To address this problem, effective single-dose therapy for several STDs (e.g., chancroid, gonorrhea, syphilis, trichomoniasis) has been available for some time, and single-dose therapy for chlamydial infection has recently become available. These single-dose regimens have been shown to be as effective as multiple-dose regimens (CDC, 1993a; Thorpe et al., 1996; Zenilman, 1996). Some single-dose therapies, however, are substantially more expensive than standard multiple-dose medications.[7]

Various clinical encounters for potential health problems other than STDs can provide a valuable opportunity for clinicians to evaluate and, if appropriate, treat persons for STDs. In particular, persons seeking health services for unintended pregnancy, contraception, or potential HIV infection are also at high risk for STDs. In addition, such encounters provide "teaching moments" where patients are more likely to be receptive to prevention messages (Bigelow et al., 1986). Thus, examples of underutilized opportunities to both prevent and treat STDs are clinical encounters for family planning services, evaluation of an unintended pregnancy, and encounters for HIV testing and counseling. Newer technologies, such as noninvasive diagnostic tests for STDs, would make the evaluation of patients in the above clinical venues much more practical.

Barriers to Diagnosis and Effective Treatment

Although many useful diagnostic tests and effective drugs for STDs are available, they have not been successfully used on a national basis. Several major barriers prevent early diagnosis and treatment of infected persons. These include inadequate access to health care, lack of health-care-seeking behavior, inadequate training of health care providers, inadequate financial and physical access to laboratory tests, and geographic factors.

Inadequate access to effective health care, as discussed in Chapter 3, is the major impediment to appropriate diagnosis and treatment of STDs, particularly because the young and certain ethnic and racial groups, who have the highest rates of STDs, are the least likely to have health insurance coverage. In the United States, diagnosis and treatment cannot occur without the direct assistance of a licensed health care provider. Factors that prevent persons from seeking health care for potential STDs, including lack of perception of risk, misinformation and lack of knowledge about STDs, and the social stigma of STDs, are mentioned in Chapter 3. Inadequate training of health care providers is a serious barrier to early diagnosis and treatment of STDs because it results in clinicians who are not aware of the scope of STDs and lack the clinical skills necessary for diagnosing and managing an STD. This issue is discussed further in Chapter 5. In addition, although newer laboratory tests hold much promise for improved screening and diagnosis, financial and physical accessibility to these tests presents a barrier to

---

[7]The CDC-negotiated price (only available to public STD clinics and family planning programs) for azithromycin, the single-dose therapy for chlamydial infection, is $9.50 per dose, compared to approximately $2 (average cost to public STD clinics and family planning programs) for multiple-dose doxycycline (Cathleen Walsh, CDC, Division of STD Prevention, personal communication, June 1996).

clinician diagnosis. Expense is especially problematic in publicly sponsored facilities, and accessibility is also difficult in remote areas.

Geographic factors also present challenges to diagnosis and treatment of STDs. Specifically, some regions of the United States and rural areas have to overcome unique obstacles in ensuring access to STD-related services. For example, states along the national borders may have difficulty in identifying and reaching partners because of language and cultural barriers. These regions may also have difficulty in ensuring effective treatment of STDs as people seek care on both sides of the border. In rural areas, low population density makes it difficult to ensure convenient access to STD-related services and to maintain a ready group of health care professionals who are adequately trained and available to provide such services, especially during outbreak situations. In anticipation of sporadic demands for services, some health departments have organized provider networks.

CONCLUSIONS

There are many behavioral interventions that have been shown to change health risk behaviors, including sexual behavior. There also are biomedical interventions that are highly effective. If these interventions could be widely implemented in a comprehensive fashion, they would likely have a substantial impact on the prevention of STDs. The three primary goals of both individual- and population-based interventions are to prevent exposure to an STD, prevent acquisition of infection once exposed, and prevent transmission of the infection to others. Given the variety of factors that influence the risk for STDs, it is clear that a multifaceted approach to prevention that integrates both biomedical and behavioral interventions is needed.

Individual factors that increase risk of STDs, such as high-risk sexual behavior, misperception of risk, and lack of personal skills, need to be targeted on a national basis because of the high prevalence of these factors in the general population. Individual behavior, however, is clearly influenced by social factors such as inadequate access to health care. Many individual- and community-level behavioral interventions have been shown to be effective in changing risk behaviors for STDs. Promotion of condom use, in particular, will continue to be a central strategy for preventing STDs. Given the high rates of sexual activity among adolescents, school-based health programs deserve particular emphasis. Although not all school-based programs to reduce risky sexual behaviors have been effective, there is little evidence of adverse outcomes. Interventions that involve the mass media also can have beneficial effects on knowledge and health behavior, especially for adolescents. Clinical methods that are effective in preventing exposure and reducing transmission include prophylaxis and partner notification and treatment. Although treatment of sex partners of infected persons is critical to STD prevention, the traditional methods for identifying partners need to be reevaluated and redesigned in light of the changing epidemiology and social context of STDs. The duration of sexually transmitted infections and thus the period during which infected individuals are infectious to others can be reduced primarily by ensuring early diagnosis and treatment of infected persons through screening programs and by improving the clinical skills of health care providers. Appropriate use and interpretation of diagnostic tests and access to laboratory services are essential in ensuring accurate diagnosis and treatment. Barriers to early detection and treatment, such as inadequate access to health care and lack of health-care-seeking behavior, need to be addressed.

REFERENCES

AAFP (American Academy of Family Physicians). Age charts for periodic health examination. Kansas City, MO: American Academy of Family Physicians, 1994 (reprint no. 510).

AAP (American Academy of Pediatrics), Committee on Adolescence. Sexually transmitted diseases. Pediatr 1994;94 (Pt. 1):568-72.

AAP, Committee on Adolescence. Condom availability for youth. Pediatr 1995;95:281-5.

ACOG (American College of Obstetricians and Gynecologists). Human immunodeficiency virus infection. Washington, D.C.: American College of Obstetricians and Gynecologists, 1992. [Technical Bulletin No. 169.]

Addiss DG, Vaughn ML, Hillis SD, Ludka D, Amsterdam L, Davis JP. History and features of the Wisconsin *Chlamydia trachomatis* control program. Fam Plann Perspect 1994;26:83-9.

Adler NE, Tschann, JM. Conscious and preconscious motivation of pregnancy among female adolescents. In: Lawson A, Rhode D, eds. The politics of pregnancy: adolescent sexuality and public policy. New Haven, CT: Yale University Press, 1993:144-58.

Advocates for Youth. Condom availability in schools: an integral component to comprehensive school health programs. Washington, D.C., 1995.

Ajzen I, Fishbein M. Understanding attitudes and predicting social behavior. Englewood, NJ: Prentice-Hall, 1980.

Alary M, Joly JR, Poulin C. Gonorrhea and chlamydia infection: comparison of contact tracing performed by physicians or by a specialized service. Can J Public Health 1991;82;132-4.

Allen S, Tice J, Van de Perre P, Serufilira A, Hudes E, Nsengumuremyi F, et al. Effect of serotesting with counselling on condom use and seroconversion among HIV discordant couples in Africa. British Med J 1992;304:1605-9.

AMA (American Medical Association). HIV blood test counseling. Physician guidelines. 2nd ed. Chicago: American Medical Association, 1993.

AMA. Policy compendium on reproductive health issues affecting adolescents. Gans Epner JE, ed. Chicago: American Medical Association, 1996.

ASHA (American Social Health Association). Teenagers know more than adults about STDs, but knowledge among both groups is low. STD News. A quarterly newsletter of the American Social Health Association. Winter 1996;3:1, 5.

Anderson JE, Brackhill R, Mosher WD. Condom use for disease prevention among unmarried U.S. women. Fam Plann Perspect 1996;28:25-8, 39.

Anderson RM. The transmission dynamics of sexually transmitted diseases: the behavioral component. In: Wasserheit JN, Aral SO, Holmes KK, Hitchcock PJ, eds. Research issues in human behavior and sexually transmitted diseases in the AIDS era. Washington, D.C.: American Society for Microbiology, 1991:38-60.

Anderson RM, May RM. Infectious diseases of humans: dynamics and control. Oxford, England: Oxford University Press, Inc., 1991.

Andreasen AR. Marketing social change. San Francisco: Jossey-Bass, 1995.

Andrus JK, Fleming DW, Harger DR, Chin MY, Bennet DV, Horan JM, et al. Partner notification: can it control epidemic syphilis [see comments]? Ann Intern Med 1990;112:539-43.

Aral SO. Sexual behavior in sexually transmitted disease research. An overview. Sex Transm Dis 1994;21(March-April Suppl):S59-S64.

Arevalo JA, Washington AE. Cost-effectiveness of perinatal screening and immunization for hepatitis B virus. JAMA 1988;259:365-9.

Baldwin JD, Baldwin JI. Factors affecting AIDS-related sexual risk-taking behavior among college students. J Sex Res 1988;25:181-96.

Bandura A. Social learning theory. Englewood, NJ:Prentice-Hall, 1977.

Bandura A. Perceived self-efficacy in the exercise of control over AIDS infection. Eval Program Plann 1990;13:9-17.

Baumgartner L, Curtis AC, Gray AL, Kuechle BE, Richman TL. The eradication of syphilis: a task force report. Washington, D.C.: Government Printing Office, 1962. [Public Health Service Publication No. 918.]

Bayer R, Toomey KE. HIV prevention and the two faces of partner notification [see comments]. Am J Public Health 1992;82:1158-64.

Becker MH, Maiman LA. Sociobehavioral determinants of compliance with health and medical care recommendations. Medical Care 1975;13:10-24.

Bigelow GE, Rand CS, Gross J, Burling TA, Gottlieb SH. Smoking cessation and relapse among cardiac patients. In: Tims FM, Leukefeld CG, eds. Relapse and recovery in drug abuse. NIDA Research Monograph No. 72, DHHS Publication No. (ADM) 86-1473. Washington D.C.: Government Printing Office, 1986.

Blackmore CA, Limpakarnjanarat K, Rigan-Perez JG, Albritton WL, Greenwood JR. An outbreak of chancroid in Orange County California: descriptive epidemiology and disease-control measures. J Infect Dis 1985;151:840-4.

Brandt AM. No magic bullet: a social history of venereal disease in the United States since 1880. New York: Oxford University Press, Inc., 1985.

Brien TM, Thombs DL, Mahoney CA, Wallnau L. Dimensions of self-efficacy among three distinct groups of condom users. J Am Coll Health 1994;42:167-74.

Brindis CD. Funding and policy options. In: Samuels SE, Smith MD, eds. Condoms in the schools. Menlo Park, CA: Henry J. Kaiser Family Foundation, 1993:37-61.

Britton TF, DeLisle S, Fine K. STDs and family planning clinics: a regional program for chlamydia control that works. Am J Gynecol Health 1992;6:80-7.

Brown LK, DiClemente RJ, Park T. Predictors of condom use in sexually active adolescents. J Adolesc Health 1992;13:651-7.

Catania JA, Coates TH, Kegeles S, Fullilove MT, Peterson J, Marin B, et al.. Condom use in multi-ethnic neighborhoods of San Francisco: the population-based AMEN (AIDS in Multi-Ethnic Neighborhoods) Study. Am J Public Health 1992;82:284-7.

Catania JA, Dolcini MM, Coates TJ, Kegeles SM, Greenblatt RM, Puckett S, et al. Predictors of condom use and multiple-partnered sex among sexually-active adolescent women: implications for AIDS-related health interventions. J Sex Res 1989;26:514-24.

Catania JA, Kegeles SM, Coates TJ. Towards an understanding of risk behavior. An AIDS risk reduction model (ARRM). Health Educ Q 1990; 17:53-72.

Cates W Jr, Stewart FH, Trussell J. Commentary: the quest for women's prophylactic methods—hopes vs science. Am J Public Health 1992;82:1479-82.

Cates W Jr, Stone KM. Family planning, sexually transmitted diseases, and contraceptive choice: a literature update. Fam Plann Perspect 1992;24:75-84.

CDC (Centers for Disease Control and Prevention). Alternate case-finding methods in a crack-related syphilis epidemic—Philadelphia. MMWR 1991a;40:77-80.

CDC. Hepatitis B virus: a comprehensive strategy for eliminating transmission in the United States through universal childhood vaccination: recommendations of the Immunization Practices Advisory Committee (ACIP). MMWR 1991b;40(RR-13):1-20.

CDC. HIV-risk behaviors of sterilized and nonsterilized women in drug-treatment programs—Philadelphia, 1989-1991. MMWR 1992a;41:149-52.

CDC. Surgical sterilization among women and use of condoms—Baltimore, 1989-1990. MMWR 1992b;41:568-75.

CDC. 1993 Sexually transmitted diseases treatment guidelines. MMWR 1993a;42(No. RR-14):56-66.

CDC. Update: barrier protection against HIV infection and other sexually transmitted diseases. MMWR 1993b;42:589-91, 597.

CDC. ACIP approves additional groups covered under the vaccines for children (VFC) program. [Memorandum to immunization program managers from Director, National Immunization Program, and Chief, Hepatitis Branch.] September 9, 1994a.

CDC. Hepatitis B vaccination of adolescents—California, Louisiana, and Oregon, 1992-1994. MMWR 1994b;43:605-9.

CDC. Trends in sexual risk behavior among high school students—United States, 1990, 1991, and 1993. MMWR 1995a;44:124-5, 131-2.

CDC. Update: recommendations to prevent hepatitis B virus transmission—United States. MMWR 1995b;44:574-5.

CDC. Community-level prevention of human immunodeficiency virus infection among high-risk populations: the AIDS Community Demonstration Projects. MMWR 1996a;45(RR-6).

CDC. School-based HIV-prevention education—United States, 1994. MMWR 1996b;45:760-5.

CDC. Undervaccination for hepatitis B among young men who have sex with men—San Francisco and Berkeley, California, 1992-1993. MMWR 1996c;45:215-7.

CDC, DSTD/HIVP (Division of STD/HIV Prevention). Approaches to partner notification and syphilis; partner notification and gonorrhea. Centers for Disease Control and Prevention. Internal working documents, 1992.

CDC, DSTD/HIVP. Plan for a national partnership to prevent STD-related infertility. Draft internal document, January 10, 1995.

Cleary PD, Barry MJ, Mayer KH, Brandt AM, Gostin L, Fineberg HV. Compulsory premarital screening for the human immunodeficiency virus: technical and public health considerations. JAMA 1987;258:1757-62.

Cleary PD, Rogers TF, Singer E, Avorn J, Van Devanter N, Perry S, et al. Health education about AIDS among seropositive blood donors. Health Educ Q 1986;13:317-29.

Cleary PD, Van Devanter N, Rogers TF, Singer E, Shipton-Levy R, Steilen M, et al. Behavior changes after notification of HIV infection. Am J Public Health 1991;81:1586-90.

Cleary PD,Van Devanter N, Steilen M, Stuart A, Shipton-Levy R, McMullen W, et al. A randomized trial of an education and support program for HIV-infected individuals. AIDS 1995;9:1271-8.

Collins JL, Small ML, Kann L, Collins Pateman B, Gold RS, Kolbe LJ. School health education. J School Health 1995;65:302-11.

Dawson DA. The effects of sex education on adolescent behavior. Fam Plann Perspect 1986;18:162-70.

DeBuono BA, Zinner SH, Daamen M, McCormack WM. Sexual behavior of college women in 1975, 1986, and 1989. N Engl J Med 1990;322:821-5.

DeJong W. Condom promotion: the need for social marketing program in America's inner cities. Am J Health Promot 1989;3:5-10.

DiClemente RJ, Wingood GM. A randomized controlled trial of an HIV sexual risk reduction intervention for young African American women. JAMA 1995;274:1271-6.

Donovan P. Taking family planning services to hard-to-reach populations. Fam Plann Perspect 1996;28:120-6.

EDK Associates. Women & sexually transmitted diseases: the dangers of denial. New York: EDK Associates, 1994.

EDK Associates. The ABCs of STDs. New York: EDK Associates, 1995.

Edlin BR, Irwin KL, Faruque S, McCoy CB, Work C, Serrano Y, et al. Intersecting epidemics—crack cocaine and HIV infection among inner-city young adults. The Multicenter Crack Cocaine and HIV Infection Study Team. N Engl J Med 1994;331:1422-7.

Elias CJ, Heise LL. Challenges for the development of female-controlled vaginal microbicides. AIDS 1994;8:1-9.

Ellen JM, Cahn S, Eyre SL, Boyer CB. Types and attributes of adolescent sexual partnerships and their association with condom use. J Adolesc Health 1996;18:417-21.

Engelgau MM, Woernle CH, Rolfs RT, Greenspan JR, O'Cain M, Gorsky, RD. Control of epidemic early syphilis: the results of an intervention campaign using social networks. Sex Transm Dis 1995;22:203-9.

European Study Group on Heterosexual Transmission of HIV. Comparison of female to male and male to female transmission of HIV in 563 stable couples. Br Med J 1992;304:809-13.

Fanburg JT, Kaplan DW, Naylor KE. Student opinions of condom distribution at a Denver, Colorado, high school. J Sch Health 1995;65:181-5.

Farr G, Gabelnick H, Sturgen K, Dorflinger L. Contraceptive efficacy and acceptability of the female condom. Am J Public Health 1994;84:1960-4.

Fee E, Krieger N. Understanding AIDS: historical interpretations and the limits of biomedical individualism. Am J Public Health 1993;83:1477-86.

Felman Y. Repeal of mandated premarital tests for syphilis: a survey of state health officers. Am J Public Health 1981;71:155-9.

Flay BR. Mass media and smoking cessation: a critical review. Am J Public Health 1987;77:153-60.

Flora JA, Miabach EW, Holtgrave D. Communication campaigns for HIV prevention: using mass media in the next decade. In: IOM. Assessing the social and behavioral science base for HIV/ AIDs prevention and intervention. Background papers. Washington, D.C.: National Academy Press, 1995:129-54.

Forrest JD, Silverman J. What public school teachers teach about preventing pregnancy, AIDS and sexually transmitted diseases [see comments]. Fam Plann Perspect 1989;21:65-72.

Franzini LR, Sideman LM. Personality characteristics of condom users. J Sex Educ Ther 1994;20:110-8.

Gerrard M. Sex, sex guilt and contraceptive use revisited: the 1980s. J Pers Soc Psychol 1987;52:975-80.

Gerrard M, Gibbons FX, McCoy SB. Emotional inhibition of effective contraception. Anxiety, Stress, and Coping 1993;6:73-88.

Giesecke J, Ramstedt K, Granath F, Ripa T, Rado G, Westrell M. Efficacy of partner notification for HIV infection. Lancet 1991;33:1096-100.

Gold RS, Skinner MJ, Ross MW. Unprotected anal intercourse in HIV-infected and non-HIV-infected gay men. J Sex Res 1994; 3159-77.

Gollub EL, Stein ZA. Commentary: the new female condom—item 1 on a women's AIDS prevention agenda. Am J Public Health 1993;83:498-500.

Greene BZ. The view from schools: four focus groups. In: Samuels SE, Smith MD, eds. Condoms in the schools. Menlo Park, CA: Henry J. Kaiser Family Foundation, 1993:25-36.

Grosskurth H, Mosha F, Todd J, Mwijarubi E, Klokke A, Senkoro K, et al. Impact of improved treatment of sexually transmitted diseases on HIV infection in rural Tanzania: randomized controlled trial [see comments]. Lancet 1995a;346:530-6.

Grosskurth H, Mosha F, Todd J, Senkoro K, Newell J, Klokke A, et al. A community trial of the impact of improved STD treatment on the HIV epidemic in rural Tanzania: 2 baseline survey results. AIDS 1995b;9:927-34.

Gunn RA, Montes JM, Toomey KE, Rolfs RT, Greenspan JK, Spitters CE, et al. Syphilis in San Diego County 1983-1992: crack cocaine, prostitution, and the limitations of partner notification. Sex Transm Dis 1995;22:60-6.

Guttmacher S, Lieberman L, Hoi-Chang W, Ward D, Radosh A, Rafferty Y, Freudenberg N. Gender differences in attitudes and use of condom availability programs among sexually active students in New York City public high schools. J Am Med Women's Assoc 1995a;50:99-102.

Guttmacher S, Lieberman L, Ward D, Radosh A, Rafferty Y, Freudenberg N. Parents' attitudes and beliefs about HIV/AIDS prevention with condom availability in New York City public high schools. J Sch Health 1995b;65:101-6.

Handsfield HH, Jasman LL, Roberts PL, Hanson VW, Kothenbeutel RL, Stamm WE. Criteria for selective screening for *Chlamydia trachomatis* infection in women attending family planning clinics. JAMA 1986;255:1730-4.

Handsfield HH, Rice RJ, Roberts MC, Holmes KK. Localized outbreak of penicillinase-producing *Neisseria gonorrhoea*. Paradigm for introduction and spread of gonorrhoea in a community. JAMA 1989;261:2357-61.

Handsfield HH, Sandstrom EG, Knapp JS, Perine PL, Whittington, WL, Sayers DE, et al. Epidemiology of penicillinase-producing *Neisseria gonorrhoea* infections: analysis by auxotyping and serogrouping. N Engl J Med 1982;306:950-4.

Haskell RJ. A cost-benefit analysis of California's mandatory premarital screening program for syphilis. West J Med 1984;141:538-41.

Herold ES, McNamee JE. An explanatory model of contraceptive use among young single women. J Sex Res 1982;18:289-304.

Higgins DL, Galavotti C, O'Reilly KR, Schnell DJ, Moore M, Rugg DL, et al. Evidence for the effects of HIV antibody counseling and testing on risk behaviors. JAMA 1991;266:2419-29.

Hillis S, Black C, Newhall J, Walsh C, Groseclose SL. New opportunities for chlamydia prevention: applications of science to public health practice. Sex Transm Dis 1995;22:197-202.

Hillis SD, Nakashima A, Amsterdam L, Pfister J, Vaughn M, Addiss D, et al. The impact of a comprehensive chlamydia prevention program in Wisconsin. Fam Plann Perspect 1995;27:108-11.

Hingson RW, Strunin L, Berlin BM, Hereen T. Beliefs about AIDS, use of alcohol and drugs, and unprotected sex among Massachusetts adolescents. Am J Public Health 1990;80:295-9.

Hitchcock PJ, Wasserheit JN, Harris JR, Holmes KK. Sexually transmitted diseases in the AIDS era. Development of STD diagnostics for resource-limited settings is a global priority. Sex Transm Dis 1991;18:133-5.

Hobfoll SE, Jackson AP, Lavin J, Britton PJ, Shepherd JB. Reducing inner-city women's AIDS risk activities. Health Psychol 1994;13:397-403.

Holtgrave DR, Qualls NL, Curran JW, Valdiserri RO, Guinan ME, Parra WC. An overview of the effectiveness and efficiency of HIV prevention programs. Public Health Rep 1995;110:134-46.

IOM (Institute of Medicine). Understanding the determinants of HIV risk behavior. In: Auerbach JD, Wypijewska C, Brodie HKH, eds. AIDS and behavior. Washington, D.C.: National Academy Press, 1994:78-123.

IOM. Best intentions: unintended pregnancy and the well-being of children and families. Brown SS, Eisenberg L, eds. Washington, D.C.: National Academy Press, 1995.

IOM. Contraceptive research and development: looking to the future. Harrison PF, Rosenfield A, eds. Washington, D.C.: National Academy Press, 1996.

Janz NK, Becker MH. The health belief model: a decade later. Health Educ Q 1984;11:1-47.

Jemmott JB, Jemmott LS, Fong GT. Reductions in HIV risk-associated sexual behaviors among black male adolescents: effects of an AIDS prevention intervention. Am J Public Health 1992;82:392-77.

Joseph JG, Montgomery SB, Emmons CA, Kirscht JP, Kessler RC, Ostrow DG, et al. Perceived risk of AIDS: assessing the behavioral and psychosocial consequences in a cohort of gay men. J Appl Soc Psychol 1987;17:231-50.

Kalichman SC, Kelly JA, Johnson JR, Bulto M. Factors associated with risk for HIV infection among chronic mentally ill adults. Am J Psychiatry 1994;151:221-7.

Kalichman SC, Carey MP, Johnson BT. Prevention of sexually transmitted HIV infection: a meta-analytic review of the behavioral outcome literature. Ann Behav Change 1996;18:6-15.

Kamb ML, Douglas JM, Rhodes F, Bolan G, Zenilman J, Iatesta M, et al. A multi-center, randomized controlled trial evaluating HIV prevention counseling (Project RESPECT): Preliminary results. Eleventh International Conference on AIDS, July 7-12, 1996, Vancouver [abstract no. Th.C.4380].

Katz BP, Blythe MJ, Van der Pol B, Jones RB. Declining prevalence of chlamydial infection among adolescent girls. Sex Transm Dis 1996;23:226-9.

Katz BP, Danos CS, Quinn TS, Caine V, Jones RB. Efficiency and cost-effectiveness of field follow-up for patients with *Chlamydia trachomatis* infection in a sexually transmitted diseases clinic. Sex Transm Dis 1988;15:11-6.

Kegeles SM, Adler NE, Irwin CD. Adolescents and condoms. Am J Dis Child 1989;143:911-5.

Kelly JA. Sexually transmitted disease prevention approaches that work. Interventions to reduce risk behavior among individuals, groups, and communities. Sex Transm Dis 1994;21[2 Suppl]:S73-S75.

Kelly JA, St. Lawrence JS, Diaz YE, Stevenson LY, Hauth AC, Grasfield TL, et al. HIV risk behaviors reduction following intervention with key opinion leaders of population: an experimental analysis. Am J Public Health 1991;81:168-71.

Kelly JA, St. Lawrence JS, Stevenson LY, Hauth AC, Kalichman SC, Diaz YE, et al. Community AIDS/HIV risk reduction: the effects of endorsements by popular people in three cities. Am J Public Health 1992;82:1483-9.

Kirby D. The effects of school sex education programs: a review of the literature. J Sch Health 1980;50:559-63.

Kirby D. Research and evaluation. In: Samuels SE, Smith MD, eds. Condoms in the schools. Menlo Park, CA: Henry J. Kaiser Family Foundation, 1993:89-109.

Kirby D. Sexuality and HIV education programs in schools. In: Garrison J, Smith MD, Besharov DJ, eds. Sexuality and American social policy: a seminar series. Sex education in the schools. Menlo Park, CA: Henry J. Kaiser Family Foundation, 1994;1-41.

Kirby DM, Brown NL. Condom availability programs in U.S. schools. Fam Plann Perspect 1996;28:196-202.

Kirby D, Short L, Collins J, Rugg D, Kolbe L, Howard M, et al. School-based programs to reduce sexual risk behaviors: a review of effectiveness. Public Health Rep 1994;109:339-60.

Kirby D, Waszak C, Ziegler J. Six school-based clinics: their reproductive health services and impact on sexual behavior. Fam Plann Perspect 1991;23:6-16.

Klovdahl AS, Potterat JJ, Woodhouse DE, Muth JB, Muth SQ, Darrow WW. Social networks and infectious disease: the Colorado Springs study. Soc Sci Med 1994;38:79-88.

Kollar LM, Rosenthal SL, Biro FM. Hepatitis B vaccine series compliance in adolescents. Pediatr Infect Dis J 1994;13:1006-8.

Koniak-Griffin D, Nyamathi A, Vasquez R, Russo AA. Risk-taking behaviors and AIDS knowledge: experiences and beliefs of minority adolescent mothers. Health Educ Res 1994;9:449-63.

Ku L, Sonenstein FL, Pleck JH. The association of AIDS education and sex education with sexual behavior and condom use among teenage men [published erratum appears in Fam Plann Perspect 1993 Jan-Feb;25:36]. Fam Plann Perspect 1992;24:100-6.

Ku L, Sonenstein FL, Pleck JH. Factors influencing first intercourse for young men. Public Health Rep 1993;108:680-94.

Ku L, Sonenstein FL, Pleck JH. The dynamics of young men's condom use during and across relationships. Fam Plann Perspect 1994;26:246-51.

Lafferty W, Ditmer D, Krekeler B, Stoner B, Tyrea T, Sucato G, et al. Feasibility of vaccinating high-risk adolescents for hepatitis B at STD clinic sites. Eleventh Meeting of the International Society for STD Research, New Orleans, August 27-30, 1995 [abstract no. 193].

Landry DJ, Camelo TM. Young unmarried men and women discuss men's role in contraceptive practice. Fam Plann Perspect 1994;26:222-7.

Laumann EO, Gagnon JH, Michael RT, Michaels S. The social organization of sexuality: sexual practices in the United States. Chicago, IL: University of Chicago Press, 1994.

Laurian Y, Peynet J, Verroust F. HIV infection in sexual partners of HIV seropositive patients with hemophilia. N Engl J Med 1989;320:183.

Lear D. Sexual communication in the age of AIDS; the construction of risk and trust among young adults. Soc Sci Med 1995; 41:1311-23.

Leitman R, Kramer E, Taylor H. A survey of condom programs. In: Samuels SE, Smith MD, eds. Condoms in the schools. Menlo Park, CA: Henry J. Kaiser Family Foundation, 1993:1-23.

Louv WC, Austin H, Alexander WJ, Stagno S, Cheeks J. A clinical trial of nonoxynol-9 as a prophylaxis for cervical *Neisseria gonorrhoeae* and *Chlamydia trachomatis* infections. J Infect Dis 1988;158:518-23.

Magura S, Shapiro JL, Kang S-Y. Condom use among criminally-involved adolescents. AIDS Care 1994;6:595-603.

Mahler K. Condom availability in the schools: lessons from the courtroom. Fam Plann Perspect 1996;28:75-7.

Mahoney CA, Thombs KL, Ford OJ. Health belief and self-efficacy models: their utility in explaining college student condom use. AIDS Educ Prev 1995;7:32-49.

Margolis HS, Coleman PJ, Brown RE, Mast EE, Sheingold SH, Arevalo JA. Prevention of hepatitis B virus transmission by immunization. An economic analysis of current recommendations. JAMA 1995;274:1201-8.

Marin BV, Gomez CA, Tschann JM. Condom use among Hispanic men with secondary female sexual partners. Public Health Rep 1993;108:742-50.

Marsiglio W, Mott F. The impact of sex education on sexual activity, contraceptive use and premarital pregnancy among American teenagers. Fam Plann Perspect 1986;18:151-62.

Marx R, Aral SO, Rolfs RT, Sterk CE, Kahn JG. Crack, sex, and STD. Sex Transm Dis 1991;18:92-101.

May RM, Anderson RM. Transmission dynamics of HIV infection. Nature 1987;326:137-42.

Mays VM, Cochran SD. Issues in the perception of AIDS risk and risk reduction activities by black and Hispanic/Latina women. Am Psychol 1988;43:949-57.

Molbert W, Boyer CB, Shafer MA. Implementing a school-based STD/HIV prevention intervention: collaboration between a university medical center and an urban school district. J Sch Health 1993;63:258-61.

Moran JS, Peterman TA, Weinstock HS, Bolan GA, Harden JW, Fleenor ME, et al. Hepatitis B vaccination trials in sexually transmitted disease clinics: implications for program development. Proceedings of the 26th National Immunization Conference, June 1992, St. Louis, MO:107-9.

Morris M. Epidemiology and social networks. Sociological Methods Res 1993;22:99-126.

Morris M, Pramualratana A, Podhisita C, Wawer MJ. The relational determinants of condom use with commercial sex partners in Thailand. AIDS 1995;9:507-15.

Morris M. Behavior change and non-homogeneous mixing. In: Isham V, Medley G, eds. Models for infectious human diseases. Cambridge, England: Cambridge University Press, 1996.

Morrison DM, Baker SA, Gillmore MR. Sexual risk behavior, knowledge, and condom use among adolescents in juvenile detention. J Youth Adolesc 1994;23:271-88.

Morrison DM, Shaklee H. Poor contraceptive use in the teenage years: situational and developmental interpretations. Adv Adolesc Mental Health 1990;4:51-69.

Munday PE, McDonald W, Murray-Sykes KM, Harris JR. Contact tracing in hepatitis B infection. Br J Vener Dis 1983;59:314-6.

Mwijarubi E, Grosskurth H, Mosha F, Mayaud P, Mugey K, Todd J, et al. Improved STD treatment significantly reduces prevalence of syphilis and symptomatic urethritis in rural Tanzania. Eleventh International Conference on AIDS, July 7-12, 1996, Vancouver [abstract LB.C.6062].

NARAL (National Abortion Rights Action League) Foundation. Sexuality education in America: a state-by-state review, 1995. Rev. ed. Washington, D.C., September 1995.

Nelson KE, Celentano DD, Eiumtrakol S, Hoover DR, Beyrer C, Suprasert S, et al. Changes in sexual behavior and a decline in HIV infection among young men in Thailand. New Engl J Med 1996;335:297-303.

NIH (National Institutes of Health). The Jordan report: accelerated development of vaccines 1996. Bethesda, MD: National Institutes of Health, National Institute of Allergy and Infectious Diseases, Division of Microbiology and Infectious Diseases, 1996.

Norris AE, Ford K. Associations between condom experiences and beliefs, intentions, and use in a sample of urban, low-income, African-American and Hispanic youth. AIDS Educ Prev 1994;6:27-39.

Oakley A, Fullerton D, Holland J, Arnold S, France-Dawson M, Kelley P, et al. Sexual health education interventions for young people: a methodological review. Br Med J 1995;310:158-62.

Oakley A, Fullerton D, Holland J. Behavioural interventions for HIV/AID prevention. AIDS 1995;9:479-86.

O'Reilly KR, Higgins DL. AIDS Community Demonstration Projects for HIV prevention among hard-to-reach groups. Public Health Rep 1991;106:714-20.

O'Reilly KR, Piot P. International perspectives on individual and community approaches to the prevention of sexually transmitted disease and human immunodeficiency virus infection. J Infect Dis 1996;174(Suppl 2):S214-S222.

Orr DP, Langefeld CD. Factors associated with condom use by sexually active male adolescents at risk for sexually transmitted disease. Pediatr 1993;91:873-9.

Oxman AD, Scott EA, Sellors JW, Clarke JH, Millson ME, Rasooly I, et al. Partner notification for sexually transmitted diseases: an overview of the evidence. Can J Public Health 1994;85(1 Suppl):S41-7.

Oxman GL, Doyle L. A comparison of the case-finding effectiveness and average costs of screening and partner notification. Sex Transm Dis 1996;23:51-7.

Pendergrast RA, DuRant RH, Gaillard GL. Attitudinal and behavioral correlates of condom use in urban adolescent males. J Adolesc Health 1992;13:133-9.

Peterson LR, White CR. Premarital screening for antibodies to human immunodeficiency virus type 1 in the United States. The Premarital Screening Study Group. Am J Public Health 1990;80:1087-90.

Peterson LS. Contraceptive use in the United States: 1982-90. Advance data, No. 260. Hyattsville, MD: National Center for Health Statistics, February 14, 1995.

Phillips L, Potterat JJ, Rothenberg RB, Pratt C, King RD. Focused interviewing in gonorrhea control. Am J Public Health 1980;70:705-8.

Pilkington CJ, Kern W, Indest D. Is safer sex necessary with a "safe" partner? Condom use and romantic feelings. J Sex Res 1994;31:203-10.

Pleck JH, Sonenstein FL, Ku L. Changes in adolescent males' use of and attitudes toward condoms, 1988-1991. Fam Plann Perspect 1993;25:106-10, 17.

Pleck JH, Sonenstein FL, Ku LC. Adolescent males' condom use: relationships between perceived cost-benefits and consistency. J Marriage Fam 1991;53:733-46.

Potterat JJ, Spencer NE, Woodhouse DE, Muth JB. Partner notification in the control of human immunodeficiency virus infection. Am J Public Health 1989;79:874-6.

Prochaska JD, DiClemente CC. Stages and processes of self-change of smoking: toward an integrative model of change. J Consult Clin Psychol 1983;51:390-5.

Ramos R, Shain, RN, Johnson L. "Men I mess with don't have anything to do with AIDS": Using ethno-theory to understand sexual risk perception. Sociological Q 1995;36:483-504.

Ramstedt K, Giescecke J, Forssman L, Granath L. Choice of sexual partner according to rate of partner change and social class of partners. Int J STD AIDS 1991;2:428-31.

Randolph AG, Washington AE. Screening for *Chlamydia trachomatis* in adolescent males: a cost-based decision analysis. Am J Public Health 1990;80:545-50.

Richert CA, Peterman TA, Zaidi AA, Ransom RL, Wroten JE, Witte JJ. A method for identifying persons at high risk for sexually transmitted infections: opportunity for targeting intervention. Am J Public Health 1993;83:520-4.

Rickman RL, Lodico M, DiClemente RJ, Morris R, Baker C, Huscroft S. Sexual communication is associated with condom use by sexually active incarcerated adolescents. J Adolesc Health 1994;15:383-8.

Rogers EE. Diffusion of innovations. New York: Free Press, 1983.

Rojanapithayakorn W, Hanenberg R. The 100% Condom Program in Thailand. AIDS 1996;10:1-7.

The Roper Organization. AIDS: public attitudes and education needs. 1991. [Poll conducted for Gay Men's Health Crisis, New York.]

Roper WL, Peterson HB, Curran JW. Commentary: condoms and HIV/STD prevention—clarifying the message. Am J Public Health 1993;83:501-3.

Rosenberg MJ, Gollub EL. Commentary: methods women can use that may prevent sexually trans-mitted diseases, including HIV. Am J Public Health 1992;82:1473-8.

Rothenberg R, Narramore J. The relevance of social network concepts to sexually-transmitted dis-ease-control. Sex Transm Dis 1996;23:24-9.

Rothenberg RB, Potterat JJ. Strategies for management of sex partners. In: Holmes KK, Mårdh P-A, Sparling PF, Wiesner PJ, Cates W Jr, Lemon SM, et al., eds. Sexually transmitted diseases. 2nd ed. New York: McGraw Hill, Inc., 1990:1081-6.

Rothenberg RB, Potterat JJ. Partner notification for STD/HIV. In: Holmes KK, Sparling PF, Mårdh P-A, Lemon SM, Stamm WE, Piot P, et al., eds. Sexually transmitted diseases. 3rd ed. New York: McGraw Hill, Inc., in press.

Rotheram-Borus MJ, Koopman C, Haignere C, Davies M. Reducing HIV sexual risk behaviors among runaway adolescents. JAMA 1991;266:1237-41.

Rotheram-Borus MJ, Rosario M, Reid H, Koopman C. Predicting patterns of sexual acts among homosexual and bisexual youths. Am J Psychiatry 1995;152:588-95.

Rumpianesi F, Donati M, Negosanti M, D'Antuono A, La Placa M, Cevenini R. Detection of *Chlamy-dia trachomatis* by a ligase chain reaction amplification method. Sex Transm Dis 1996;23:177-80.

Rutherford GW, Woo JM, Neal DP, Rauch KJ, Geohegan C, McKinney KC, et al. Partner notifica-tion and the control of human immunodeficiency virus infection. Two years of experience in San Francisco. Sex Transm Dis 1991;18:107-10.

Santelli JS, Kouzis AC, Hoover DR, Polacsek M, Burwell LG, Celentano DD. Stage of behavior change for condom use: the influence of partner type, relationship and pregnancy factors. Fam Plann Perspect 1996;28:101-7.

Schaalma H, Kok G, Peters L. Determinants of consistent condom use by adolescents—the impact of experience of sexual intercourse. Health Educ Res 1993;8:255-69.

Scholes D, Stergachis A, Heidrich FE, Andrilla H, Holmes KK, Stamm WE. Prevention of pelvic inflammatory disease by screening for cervical chlamydial infection. New Engl J Med 1996;334:1362-6.

Schwarcz SK, Bolan GA, Fullilove M, McCright J, Fullilove R, Kohn R, et al. Crack cocaine and the exchange of sex for money or drugs. Risk factors for gonorrhea among black adolescents in San Francisco. Sex Transm Dis 1992;19:7-13.

Sellers DE, McGraw SA, McKinlay JB. Does the promotion and distribution of condoms increase teen sexual activity? Evidence from an HIV prevention program for Latino youth. Am J Public Health 1994;84:1952-8.

Shain R, Piper J, Newton E, Perdue S, Ramos R, Dimmitt J, et al. Preventing sexually transmitted disease among minority women: results of a controlled randomized trial at 12 months' follow-up. Eleventh International Conference on AIDS, July 7-12, 1996, Vancouver [abstract no. Mo.D.1773-Mo.D.1779].

Shafer MA, Boyer CB. Psychosocial and behavioral factors associated with risk of sexually transmitted diseases, including human immunodeficiency virus infection, among urban high school students. J Pediatr 1990;119:826-33.

Shoop DM, Davidson PM. AIDS and adolescents: the relation of parent and partner communication to adolescent condom use. J Adolesc 1994;17:137-48.

Sparling PF, Aral SO. The importance of an interdisciplinary approach to prevention of sexually transmitted diseases. In: Wasserheit JN, Aral SO, Holmes KK, Hitchcock PJ, eds. Research issues in human behavior and sexually transmitted diseases in the AIDS era. Washington, D.C.: American Society for Microbiology, 1991:1-8.

Stein ZA. Editorial: the double bind in science policy and the protection of women from HIV infection. Am J Public Health 1992;82:1471-2.

Stergachis A, Scholes D, Heidrich FE, Sherer DM, Holmes KK, Stamm WE. Selective screening for *Chlamydia trachomatis* infection in a primary care population of women. Am J Epidemiol 1993;138:143-53.

Stiffman AR, Earls F, Dore P, Cunningham R. Changes in acquired immunodeficiency syndrome-related risk behavior after adolescence: relationships to knowledge and experience concerning human immunodeficiency virus infection. Pediatr 1992;89:950-6.

St. Lawrence JS, Jefferson KW, Alleyne E, Brasfield TL. Comparison of education versus behavioral skills training interventions in lowering sexual HIV-risk behavior of substance-dependent adolescents. J Consult Clin Psychol 1995;63:154-7.

Stray-Pederson B. Economic evaluation of maternal screening to prevent congenital syphilis. Sex Transm Dis 1983:167-72.

Stryker J, Samuels SE, Smith M. Condom availability in schools: the need for improved program evaluations. Am J Public Health 1994;84:1901-6.

Tanfer K, Grady WR, Klepinger DH, Billy JOG. Condom use among US men, 1991. Fam Plann Perspect 1993;25:61-6.

Tawil O, Verster A, O'Reilly KR. Enabling approaches for HIV/AIDS prevention: can we modify the environment and minimize the risk? AIDS 1995;9:1299-306.

Thorpe EM, Stamm WE, Hook EW III, Gall SA, Jones RB, Henry K, et al. Chlamydial cervicitis and urethritis: single dose treatment compared with doxycycline for seven days in community based practises. Genitourin Med 1996;72:93-7.

Toomey KE. HIV infection: the dilemma of patient confidentiality [editorial]. Am Fam Physician 1990;42:955-6.

Toomey KE, Cates WC Jr. Partner notification for the prevention of HIV infection. AIDS 1989;3(1 Suppl):S57-S62.

Trachtenberg AI, Washington AE, Halldorson A. A cost-based decision analysis for chlamydia screening in California family planning clinics. Obstet Gynecol 1988;71:101-8.

Trotter RT 2d, Rothenberg RB, Coyle S. Drug abuse and HIV prevention research: expanding paradigms and network contributions to risk reduction. Connections 1995;18:29-45.

U.S. Conference of Mayors. CDC's Prevention Marketing initiative: a multi-level approach to HIV prevention. Washington, D.C.: U.S. Conference of Mayors, HIV Capsule Report, Issue 2, July 1994.

U.S. Department of Education, National Center for Education Statistics. Digest of education statistics 1995. Washington, D.C.: U.S. Department of Education, Office of Educational Research and Improvement, NCES 95-029, October 1995.

U.S. Preventive Services Task Force. Guide to clinical preventive services. 2nd ed. Washington, D.C.: U.S. Department of Health and Human Services, 1996.

Wallston BS, Wallston KA. Social psychological models of health behavior: an examination and integration. In: Baum A, Taylor SE, Singer JE, eds. Handbook of psychology and health, Vol. 4. Hillsdale, NJ: Erlbaum, 1984.

Wasserfallen F, Stutz ST, Summermater D, Hausermann M, Duboi-Arber F. Six years of promotion of condom use in the framework of the National Stop AIDS Campaign: experiences and results in Switzerland. Ninth International Conference on AIDS, June 6-11, 1993, Berlin [abstract no. WS-D27-3].

Wasserheit JN. Effect of changes in human ecology and behavior on patterns of sexually transmitted diseases, including human immunodeficiency virus infection. Proc Natl Acad Sci 1994;91:2430-5.

Weinstein ND. The precaution adoption process. Health Psychol 1988;7:355-86.

Weisman CS, Nathanson CA, Ensminger M, Teitelbaum MA, Robinson JC, Plichta S. AIDS knowledge, perceived risk and prevention among adolescent clients of a family planning clinic. Fam Plann Perspect 1989;21:213-7.

Weisman CS, Plichta S, Nathanson CA, Ensminger M, Robinson JC. Consistency of condom use for disease prevention among adolescent users of oral contraceptives. Fam Plann Perspect 1991;23:71-4.

Weller SC. A meta-analysis of condom effectiveness in reducing sexually transmitted HIV. Soc Sci Med 1993;36:1635-44.

Wolk LI, Rosenbaum R. The benefits of school-based condom availability—cross-sectional analysis of a comprehensive high school-based program. J Adolesc Health 1995;17:184-8.

Wulfert E, Wan CK. Condom use: a self-efficacy model. Health Psychology 1993;12:346-53.

Yates JF, Stone ER. The risk construct. In: Yates JF, ed. Risk-taking behavior. Chichester, NY: John Wiley & Sons, 1992:1-25.

Yorke JA, Hethcote HW, Nold A. Dynamics and control of the transmission of gonorrhea. J Am Vener Dis Assoc 1978;5:51-6.

Zenilman JM. Gonococcal susceptibility to antimicrobials in Baltimore, 1988-1994. What was the impact of ciprofloxcin as first-line therapy for gonorrhea? Sex Transm Dis 1996; 23:213-8.

Zenilman JM, Bonner M, Sharp KL, Rabb JA, Alexander ER. Penicillinase-producing *Neisseria gonorrhoeae* in Dade County, Florida: evidence of core-group transmitters and the impact of illicit antibiotics. Sex Transm Dis 1988;15:45-50.

5

Current STD-Related Services

Highlight
* The total annual costs associated with selected STDs are approximately 43 times the total national investment in STD prevention and 94 times the national investment in biomedical and clinical research on STDs every year.

Current STD-related services and activities in the United States comprise several components, including the delivery of clinical services by health care providers, disease surveillance and information systems, training and education of health care professionals, and funding of activities and programs. Most of the components are publicly sponsored programs; but some programs, such as training and education of health professionals, are carried out by both the public and private sectors. Components such as national health surveys are directed and supported by the federal government, while others, such as disease surveillance, involve all levels of government and the private sector. Although the private sector is primarily involved in delivery of clinical services to persons with private health care insurance, this situation is rapidly changing and may have significant implications for the delivery of STD-related services.

CLINICAL SERVICES

Clinical services for STDs—screening, diagnosis and treatment of STDs, patient counseling, and partner notification and treatment—are provided primarily in one of three settings:

* dedicated public STD clinics, operated by local health departments; [1]

---

[1] The committee uses the term "dedicated public STD clinics" to refer to publicly funded clinics whose main purpose is to provide STD-related services. Other clinics that provide STD-related services in the context of other services, such as community health centers, family planning clinics, migrant health centers, and school-based clinics, are not considered to be dedicated public STD clinics. The term "categorical STD clinics" is not used because it invites confusion with "categorical funding."

- community-based health clinics, operated by community-based health professionals or agencies that usually receive public funds; and
- private health care settings, including private physician offices, health-plan-affiliated facilities, private clinics, and private hospital emergency rooms.

The public, community-based, and private settings for STD-related care serve somewhat different, albeit overlapping, population groups, each of which has different needs related to STD prevention.

Health Care Professionals and Prevention Activities

There is a broad range of health care professionals involved in STD-related care. Most clinicians who provide STD-related care in public or private settings emphasize diagnosis and treatment and, to a lesser extent, management of sex partners rather than other approaches to STD prevention (Bowman et al., 1992). Most clinicians do not provide adequate STD risk assessment, prevention counseling, or other STD-related education, despite the fact that they may include some STD screening in their patients' medical evaluation (Lewis and Freeman, 1987; Lewis et al., 1987; Gemson et al., 1991; Bowman et al., 1992; Russell et al., 1992). In a 1986 survey of California internists, only 10 percent reported asking new patients questions that were specific enough to assess their risk of STDs (Lewis and Freeman, 1987). In a more recent national survey of primary care physicians and other health care providers (registered nurses, nurse practitioners, nurse midwives, and physician assistants), only 39 percent of physicians and 49 percent of other primary care providers reported conducting risk assessment for STDs for all or most of their new adult patients (ARHP and NANPRH, 1995). A survey of 961 physicians in the Washington, D.C., area found that only 37 percent of respondents reported regularly asking new adult patients about their sexual practices and that 60 percent did so for new adolescent patients (Boekeloo et al., 1991). Reasons typically cited for these deficits, as mentioned elsewhere in this report, include (a) health professionals' common skepticism of the efficacy of health education and behavioral interventions; (b) pressures to see large numbers of patients in a brief amount of time; (c) personal discomfort regarding taking accurate, nonjudgmental sex and STD histories, attributed to lack of training and other reasons; and (d) a widespread misconception that STDs and issues related to sexuality are too "sensitive" to discuss. The last perception is not correct; one study found that patients who were asked questions about sexual and STD histories at their initial visit to primary health care providers tended to leave those interactions with a greater sense of confidence that their providers would provide high-quality care compared to patients who did not have such histories taken (Lewis and Freeman, 1987). It has been suggested that simulated patients be used to improve clinician skills in risk assessment and counseling (Rabin et al., 1994).

Dedicated Public STD Clinics

The earliest public STD clinics were established in the 1910s, despite substantial resistance by organized medical societies (Brandt, 1985). The concept of dedicated public STD clinics is based on evidence that many persons with STDs prefer anonymous and confidential services, cannot afford to obtain care elsewhere, and are unable to obtain care from private sector health care professionals who are unable or unwilling to provide STD care. These clinics are often seen as the "safety net" for STD-related services. Historically, the stigma associated with having a disease associated with sexual intercourse has discouraged more universal use of public STD clinics and prompt health-seeking behavior for symptoms of STDs in general (Brandt, 1985). Public STD clinics and HIV programs provide the largest proportion of specialized STD-related care in the United States. Various government agencies support STD prevention activities by providing funds, setting standards, or by directly providing care. Public STD clinics usually receive a combination of federal, state, and local funds. The only federal agency that supports dedicated public STD clinics is the CDC, which primarily funds patient education, partner notification, outreach, and other prevention services rather than direct clinical services. State and local health departments also provide financial support for these clinics and programs and are often given responsibility for operating the clinics under federal policies and guidelines.

Persons Served

A recent five-center survey of more than 2,500 patients attending dedicated public STD clinics in the United States showed that users of such clinics are generally young (38 percent under 25 years of age), disproportionately of certain racial or ethnic groups (49 percent African American), and at high risk for multiple STDs (Celum et al., 1995). Approximately 15 to 20 percent of patients attending these clinics are adolescents; the median age of patients attending these clinics is approximately 23 years. The clinics generally provide care for approximately twice as many men as women. Persons who use dedicated public STD clinics tend to have a high prevalence of other health problems, including HIV infection, unintended pregnancy, and drug and alcohol use (Kassler et al., 1994; Zenilman et al., 1994; Weinstock et al., 1995). For example, in one inner-city public STD clinic, 46 percent of women attending the clinic were not using contraception and two-thirds had at least one prior pregnancy (Upchurch et al., 1987).

A significant proportion of dedicated public STD clinic patients have private insurance coverage. In the survey by Celum and others (1995) mentioned above, approximately 31 percent of male and 24 percent of female patients seen in dedicated public STD clinics had private health insurance (Figure 5-1). These data suggest that a large number of privately insured patients use public STD

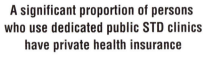

A significant proportion of persons who use dedicated public STD clinics have private health insurance

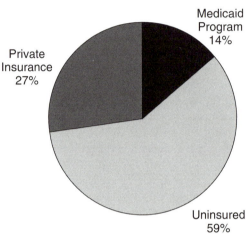

Medicaid
Program
14%

Private
Insurance
27%

Uninsured
59%

FIGURE 5-1 Distribution of health insurance status among persons using public STD clinics, 1995. SOURCE: Celum CL, Hook EW, Bolan GA, Spauding CD, Leone P, Henry KW, et al. Where would clients seek care for STD services under health care reform? Results of a STD client survey from five clinics. Eleventh Meeting of the International Society for STD Research, August 27-30, 1995, New Orleans, LA [abstract no. 101].

clinics without acknowledging their health insurance status. In such situations, the local health department ends up paying the cost of the services (Gary Richwald, Los Angeles County STD Program, personal communication, November 1995).

Patients may be referred to public STD clinics by health care providers who either have made a diagnosis requiring treatment or feel that the STD can be better managed by health care providers in public STD clinics. Reasons cited by clinic patients for seeking medical care included genitourinary symptoms (55–70 percent of individuals); notification of recent sexual contact with a partner diagnosed with an STD (15–20 percent); and perceived risk and desire for STD screening (approximately 20 percent) (Celum et al., 1995).

Services Provided

Publicly funded STD-related services are provided both by dedicated public STD clinics and within the context of primary care by community-based programs. Dedicated public STD clinics are located in every state, every major city, and the majority of smaller cities and counties throughout the United States. Based on published data, the committee's interactions with other health professionals, site visits, results of site assessments conducted by the CDC, and personal experience working with dedicated public STD clinics, the quality of care, scope of services provided, and other characteristics of these clinics are quite variable. Some clinics, commonly those affiliated with academic institutions, seem to offer comprehensive, high-quality STD-related services, whereas other clinics do not provide either comprehensive or high-quality care. In addition, the scope and level of services provided by many clinics are limited by available resources. In some locations, these clinics are high-volume, full-time clinics administered by local health departments or in partnership with medical schools. In contrast, in many rural settings and smaller population centers, dedicated public STD clinics are staffed by individuals who have numerous other responsibilities; these clinics may be open only on a part-time basis, sometimes only a few days a week. Most public clinics charge only a nominal fee or have a sliding fee scale for services.

The services provided in dedicated public STD clinics emphasize diagnosis and treatment, and partner notification for a limited number of STDs (Stein, 1996). Much of this diagnostic effort focuses on gonorrhea, nongonococcal urethritis, clinically defined cervicitis, pelvic inflammatory disease, and genital ulcer disease (i.e., syphilis, chancroid, and genital herpes). These clinics often conduct STD screening for gonorrhea, syphilis, or, more recently, chlamydial infection. Voluntary HIV counseling and testing, which may be offered either in the context of an STD evaluation or as a "stand-alone" service, is offered at most, but not all, clinics.

While there has been increasing interest in, and emphasis on, counseling and health education in dedicated public STD clinics, providers receive little training in techniques and skills for conducting education or counseling (Lewis et al., 1987; Roter et al., 1990). In the fast-paced environment found in most of these clinics, there is little time allocated for, or little emphasis on, counseling (Stein, 1996). "Disease intervention specialists" are often charged with much of the counseling and health education responsibilities in these facilities, as well as with collection of partner information and partner notification. These staff, as discussed later in this chapter, typically emphasize partner notification responsibilities over patient education activities. In dedicated public STD clinics, partner notification activities are primarily focused on patients with syphilis, HIV infection, and, to a highly variable degree, gonorrhea, chlamydial infection, or pelvic inflammatory disease. Ideally, the process of interviewing index patients to obtain both the names and locations of sex partners begins with counseling and education, but it is unclear how consistently this is done. Little or no counseling is provided in dedicated STD clinics for risk reduction or management of chronic or other incurable viral STDs other than HIV infection. One study found that 28 percent of dedicated public STD clinic patients did not receive any information

---

BOX 5-1
STD-Related Services Among Local Health Agencies, 1995

A stratified, random sample of 800 local health departments that were identified as providing STD treatment were sent a questionnaire in September 1995 regarding various characteristics of their programs and policies related to STD-related clinical services. Approximately 77 percent of the eligible agencies responded.

Results indicate that 50 percent of 2,888 local health departments provide treatment for STDs. Of these providers, 74 percent integrate STD-related services with HIV/AIDS-related services; 21 percent offer STD- and HIV-related services in separate programs; and 5 percent provide STD-related services but do not provide HIV screening or testing. Almost half (49 percent) of the local health departments that offer services for STDs offer both dedicated STD sessions and sessions where such services are integrated with other services, such as family planning. An additional 37 percent always integrate STD sessions with other clinic services such as family planning, and 14 percent provide only STD-related services in dedicated sessions. Only 23 percent of agencies offered services after 6 p.m. and only 5 percent had weekend hours.

Regarding testing and treatment services for chlamydial infection, gonorrhea, and syphilis, a greater percentage of agencies reported treating chlamydial infection (97 percent) than testing for it at all or some sites (82 percent). The percentages of agencies testing and treating for gonorrhea and syphilis at all sites were all over 98 percent.

Agencies were also asked to report what type of client history, risk assessment, and educational/counseling services they routinely provide patients making an initial STD visit (Table below). More than 90 percent of agencies reported routinely collecting information on a client's sexual, STD, and contraceptive history. A smaller proportion of agencies routinely query patients regarding any history of substance abuse (78 percent). While approximately 97 percent of STD agencies reported routinely providing educational services regarding risk factors of STDs and HIV, far smaller percentages of agencies reported routinely providing services on how to use contraceptive methods effectively or how to negotiate condom use (66–70 percent). Although more than 70 percent of health departments that provide services for STDs in integrated sessions reported routinely providing education and counseling regarding contraceptive use, less than half (47 percent) of agencies that only provide services in separate sessions provide this service.

---

regarding prevention during their clinic visit (Roter et al., 1990). Several states mandate counseling of patients, using a prescribed content outline, before to HIV testing; however, there is no method for ensuring that these regulations are followed.

Data on the specific types of STD-related services provided by local health departments through public STD clinics are limited. The Alan Guttmacher Institute, with support from the CDC, however, has recently conducted a survey to provide national estimates describing the STD-related activities of local public health agencies in the United States (Box 5-1).

It should be noted that the survey results represent only health departments that offered treatment for STDs and that the quality and consistency of services provided were not evaluated. In addition, most agencies that reported integration of STD-related services with other services were in nonmetropolitan areas with relatively low caseloads.

Distribution of Local Health Agencies Providing STD Risk Assessment and Educational and Counseling Services by Type of Service, 1995

Type of Service	Total No. of Agencies	Routinely Provided (%)	Provided Only on Indication or Request	Not Provided (%) (%)
Client history				
Client sexual history	575	98.9	1.1	0.0
Client contraceptive history	579	93.9	5.9	0.2
Client/partner substance use history	575	77.8	18.6	3.6
Client/partner STD history	578	97.3	2.1	0.6
Education/counseling services				
How to use contraceptive method effectively[a]	577	69.6	26.0	4.4
Risk factors for STDs-HIV	580	97.4	2.6	0.0
Condom negotiation skills	576	66.4	29.6	4.0

[a]This question was generally worded and may have been interpreted by respondents to mean education and counseling regarding contraceptive use generally or to prevent STDs only, or both.

SOURCE: Landry DJ, Forrest JD. Public health departments providing sexually transmitted disease services. Fam Plann Perspect 1996;28:261-6.

Effectiveness

Dedicated public STD clinics provide services to large numbers of patients at little or no cost to the patient. One of the guiding principles of these clinics is that no patient should be turned away because of cost considerations. However, it has been estimated that as many as 25 percent of those presenting for care cannot be accommodated because of inadequate clinic capacity (CDC, DSTD/HIVP, 1992). The performance of these clinics is usually evaluated on the basis of quantitative measures, such as numbers of patients seen and number of cases of specific diseases diagnosed, rather than on quality of care measures. Based on the committee's site visits and personal experience working with dedicated public STD clinics, there is little emphasis on, and almost no reporting of, quality-related indicators such as consistency of risk-reduction counseling or numbers of patients with positive STD screening tests who are successfully treated as opposed to simply having been screened. Systems for evaluation of clinic services tend to be developed in reaction to increasing STD rates or other evidence of perceived failure. This may also be related to the clinics' emphasis on quantitative performance measures. There has been little effort to measure potential positive impact of dedicated STD clinic services on populations using their services. The CDC has not conducted routine on-site quality assessments of public STD clinics and programs since 1993. Federal oversight of quality in such clinics and programs currently consists of a yearly review of written program activities (submitted annually as a requirement for federal funding), periodic telephone and on-site technical assistance consultations, and the work of federal program consultants who are stationed in some project areas.

There are few data regarding the perceptions of care provided to STD clinic patients. In a study by Celum and others (1995), a high proportion of patients attending these clinics stated they would preferentially attend public STD clinics should they need further STD care. The most common reasons cited for preferring to use the public STD clinic were walk-in/same-day appointments, lower costs, privacy or confidentiality concerns, convenient location, and expert care (Figure 5-2). Confidentiality concerns are a primary determinant of whether adolescents seek health care for potential STDs.

Federal Role

As mentioned earlier, nonclinician public health professionals referred to as "disease intervention specialists" (previously known as "contact tracers") have played a special role within state and local STD programs. These personnel include federal employees assigned as field staff in local programs and state and local government employees. The provision of federal field staff is referred to as "direct [federal] assistance" and "in lieu of cash," as opposed to "financial assistance," which is given to the states through the STD prevention cooperative agreements.

Historically, disease intervention specialist positions served as the entry level for all management staff within federal public health programs. Disease intervention specialists initially began at the lowest federal civil service entry levels as personnel in state or local public health field assignments, largely performing provider referral field work. Eventually, many staff were reassigned to new positions and given supervisory responsibilities within other state and local STD programs. Federal public health advisors are typically recruited back to the CDC

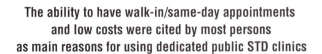

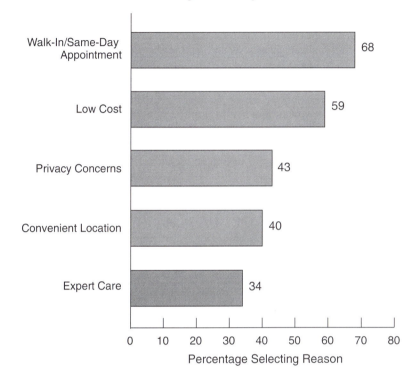

FIGURE 5-2 Reported main reasons for utilizing public STD clinics among clinic users in five U.S. cities, 1995. Categories are not mutually exclusive; respondents were allowed to indicate up to three reasons. SOURCE: Celum CL, Hook EW, Bolan GA, Spauding CD, Leone P, Henry KW, et al. Where would clients seek care for STD services under health care reform? Results of a STD client survey from five clinics. Eleventh Meeting of the International Society for STD Research, August 27-30, 1995; New Orleans, LA [abstract no. 101].

and to other divisions outside of the STD division and seem to have formed a useful managerial infrastructure for the agency.

Many problems existed with the system of management training for federal staff. The mixing of state, local, and federal staff often created conflict in local areas because federal salaries were higher than most local and state salaries, leading to staff resentment. Since management positions were often given to these transient federal assignees, local staff felt that promotional opportunities were hindered by the presence of federal staff, and they questioned the loyalties of the assignees to state or local programs. Because the assignees were part of the federal cooperative agreement, many states and local areas depended, in part or fully on, federal support to maintain core program functions. This federal training program may have inhibited the development of local and state STD program capacity, because states became dependent on federal assignees to fill key service delivery and program management positions, thereby limiting the development and training of local or state staff.

As a result of these problems and the feeling that disease intervention specialist training was too narrow and not flexible enough to adapt to the future role of public health, recruitment and initial training of CDC federal nonphysician field assignees are being restructured in ways currently being defined (CDC, 1995a). CDC is initiating a transitional training program for current disease intervention specialists and has begun to reduce their total number. Thus, the total number of federal field assignees for STD prevention will be reduced by nearly half from 1996 through 2000, but remaining assignees will receive further training and new recruits will have more extensive training. Transition from a direct service delivery role to a technical assistance and local capacity-building role for federal assignees is being planned (CDC, DSTDP, 1996). The CDC is currently developing criteria for evaluating state and local government requests for replacement of federal assignees and conversion of direct assistance funds to financial assistance funds. As a result of federal downsizing, in most cases, direct assistance vacancies will not be filled on a one-to-one basis and requests for converting direct assistance to financial assistance will not result in a dollar-for-dollar conversion.

A major concern of STD program managers is that the former federal disease intervention specialists, whose number is now being reduced, have represented significant support for many STD programs and have served in key STD program management positions. Federal assignees from CDC to state and local governments have decreased in number from 1993 through 1996 as a result of the CDC downsizing program and the freeze on hiring for new positions. This resulted in closing the four training programs for new disease investigation specialists, so that the greatest decrease in federal assignees occurred in Florida, Georgia, the city of Chicago, and California, where these training programs and positions were located. These federal positions have not been replaced by reciprocal federal or state resources to hire or contract for replacement disease intervention specialists or management staff. No state or county resources are currently available to replace these positions, nor could they be used, even if available, where states are currently experiencing a hiring freeze. In essence, a major portion of the federal support that has been provided as direct assignment of disease investigation specialists is being redirected to states for other types of disease control activities (e.g., chlamydia prevention, training, and local recruitment). This may potentially leave state and local STD programs, many in high morbidity areas such as the South, at least temporarily without the resources to conduct adequate STD surveillance and program management activities. To maintain local capacity, it will be essential for state and local governments to use both federal financial assistance and their own resources to develop local capacity as the number of federal assignees is reduced, and not simply withdraw state and local funds as federal financial assistance is received. There is no evidence that initiatives to increase funding from local sources will generate adequate resources to replace federal positions being withdrawn from local agencies.

In an effort to expand prevention efforts beyond those delivered through public STD clinics, the CDC launched the STD Accelerated Prevention Campaigns grant program for selected states and local health departments in 1994 (Noegel et al., 1993). The program seeks to (a) increase links between STD clinic activities and other health programs and community-based programs, (b) promote innovative approaches to STD prevention, (c) encourage commitment of local resources to prevention, and (d) develop cost-effective methods of prevention. Activities funded by the campaign are encouraged to focus on populations that are disproportionately impacted by STDs, including women, infants and adolescents, and certain racial and ethnic groups.

Community-Based Clinics

Many types of community-based clinics, such as family planning clinics, prenatal clinics, youth and teen clinics, homeless programs, community-based health centers, and school-based clinics, also provide STD-related services. Like dedicated public STD clinics, community-based clinics that treat STDs tend to be high-volume clinics that provide services at relatively little or no cost to the patient. STDs are not the primary focus for these clinics, but rather are dealt with in a context of providing general or specific (e.g., family planning) health care services.

Although the populations served by community-based clinics overlap substantially with public STD clinic patients, there is surprisingly little communication between these facilities. Similar to dedicated public STD clinics, community-based clinics generally serve young patients of certain ethnic and racial groups from lower socioeconomic class communities. A major difference between persons attending community-based clinics and those attending dedicated public STD clinics, however, is that some persons attending community-based clinics rely on these clinics for regular health care, that is, they attend on a scheduled basis rather than the episodic, problem-oriented basis that characterizes utilization of dedicated public STD clinics.

Even more so than for dedicated public STD clinics, the scope of STD-related clinical services in these community-based clinics is highly variable. These clinics identify proportionally more STDs through screening activities than by evaluating patients with acute signs or symptoms of STDs. In the past, gonorrhea screening has been funded on the basis of availability of government funds. More recently, publicly funded family planning clinics have become the focus of a national initiative on preventing chlamydial infection coordinated by the CDC. Unlike dedicated public STD clinics that provide services to a disproportionate number of men, most persons who use community-based clinics are women and children. In fact, some family planning clinics will not provide services to men even if they are sex partners of infected women seen in their facility. STD-related clinical services are often provided in the context of other regular health care, and there is often little emphasis on partner notification and treatment as part of care for infected women. These clinics presumably have a strong investment and interest in issues of STD counseling and health education. Federal funds for STD diagnosis and treatment in community-based clinic settings are often restricted to specific uses.

A 1990 survey conducted by the State Family Planning Administrators collected data regarding STD-related services in 410 Title X[2] family planning clinics nationwide (SFPA, 1991). The survey showed that most family planning clinics provided STD-related services to their clients, but the scope of services varied considerably. For example, 82 percent of clinics reported capability for treating gonorrhea, but only 48 percent provided treatment for syphilis. Approximately one-third of clinics reported using staff resources to contact partners for at least one STD, and approximately 60 percent of clinics provided testing for gonorrhea. Virtually all clinics provided some preventive services, and more than 80 percent reported conducting community-based education activities. Half of the clinics surveyed shared family planning and local STD program staff in integrated service settings. Family planning clinics throughout the country have implemented special programs to reach disenfranchised populations, including substance users, inmates, the homeless, disabled persons, and non-English-speaking populations (Armstrong et al., 1992; Donovan, 1996).

Data regarding STD-related services in community-based clinics such as community health centers and clinics for the homeless and migrant workers are more limited than for family planning clinics. This is a result of the failure to collect STD-service-specific data, since such services are often provided as an integral part of primary care. However, in a 1994 survey of Health Care for the Homeless programs (Section 340 of the Public Health Services Act), 68 percent of responding programs offered screening and 67 percent offered STD treatment services directly (UCLA Center for Health Policy Research, unpublished data, 1994). The remainder offered services through parent agencies, under contracts, or did not offer services.

---

[2]Part of the Public Health Service Act that authorizes federal grants to state and local entities to provide for family planning services for low-income women and adolescents.

School- and University-Based Settings

School-based health clinics in elementary and high schools and student health services on university and college campuses often provide STD-related services for their students. The number of school-based health centers has dramatically increased in recent years, from 40 in 1985 to 607 in 1994, in an effort to improve access to primary health services for children (Schlitt et al., 1995). The School Health Services and Policies Study examined school health services and HIV infection policies on a state and school district basis nationwide in 1994 (Leavy Small, et al., 1995). Approximately 60 percent of states fund school-based or -linked clinics, and 12 percent of all school districts have at least one school-based or -linked clinic. Diagnostic and treatment services for STDs were available for 16 percent of all middle and junior high schools and for 20 percent of all senior high schools. School health services are supported in part by state funds and in part by federal funds, primarily through the CDC, the Health Care Financing Administration, and the Health Resources and Services Administration (Leavy Small et al., 1995; Schlitt et al., 1995). Most school-based clinic services are provided by registered school health nurses (Igoe, 1994). For example, in one study, 31 percent of adolescents surveyed cited fear of parental discovery as their reason for not utilizing available health services at family planning clinics (Zabin et al., 1991).

Students at universities and colleges are at high risk for STDs (DeBuono et al., 1990; Reinisch et al., 1995). Recent national data on the scope and quality of STD-related clinical services among university health services are not available. Anecdotal evidence, however, suggests that university student health services at a minimum provide confidential STD diagnosis and treatment services to students (Cindy Launchbaugh, American College Health Association, personal communication, April 1996). Several universities have published descriptions of prevention activities for STDs that generally focus on HIV prevention (McLean, 1994; Turner et al, 1994; Keeling, 1995). Several have shown that specific interventions were successful in improving knowledge and promoting safer sex behavior (McLean, 1994; Turner et al., 1994).

Private Sector Settings

Many private sector health care providers, including private physician offices, health plans, private clinics, and private hospital emergency rooms, provide some STD-related services. Most cases of STDs are diagnosed by private sector health care professionals (Berg, 1990). However, very little is known about the volume, extent, disease prevalence, or spectrum of STDs encountered in private sector settings compared to either dedicated public STD clinics or community-based clinics. Accurate estimates of STD morbidity seen in private sector settings are lacking as a result of underreporting from clinicians in these settings. Nonetheless, available data suggest that the patterns of diseases seen in these settings may be quite different from those seen in public clinics. In 1994, while public STD clinics reported 1.93 times more syphilis than all non-STD reporting sites (including private sector providers and community-based facilities), non-STD clinic sites reported 1.93 times the number of chlamydial infections (CDC, DSTDP, 1995).

In addition to the lack of disease surveillance data from private sector settings, there is limited information regarding the distribution and types of care and the costs and expenditures for STD diagnosis and management in these settings. Undoubtedly, patients with acute STD syndromes may be seen in emergency rooms as well as by private practitioners or other clinics. However, the distribution and allocation of patients among these services are unknown. Similarly, how often and how well patients are screened for STDs is unknown, although the prevailing opinion is that screening for STDs is relatively uncommon in the private sector. For example, a survey of 19 hospital-based emergency centers in Los Angeles County revealed that only 5 implemented a policy for cervical cancer screening (Marcus et al., 1990).

There are few data regarding what proportion of patients seen in private settings are given recommended therapy for STDs or whether partner notification and treatment practices are routinely conducted (Winkenwerder et al., 1993; Celum et al., 1995). One recent study provides some information regarding compliance of primary care physicians in California with the CDC recommendations regarding the management of pelvic inflammatory disease (Hessol et al., 1996). Of 553 physicians responding, 55 percent reported treating at least one case of pelvic inflammatory disease during the previous 12-month period, and of these physicians, 52 percent were either unsure of or did not follow the CDC's treatment guidelines for this STD. Partner notification is not well supported in private sector settings, probably because most private sector clinicians do not accept responsibility for partner notification; there is no reimbursement for care of sex partners; and providers may be reluctant or not trained to interview their patients regarding sexual practices.

Most private practitioners emphasize acute care and provide screening when mandated by standards of practice, but, as discussed previously, most clinicians do not routinely conduct STD risk assessment and many do not provide counseling for behavior change (Lewis and Freeman, 1987; Boekeloo et al., 1991; ARHP and NANPRH, 1995). Complicating private practitioners' management of STDs is that, although there are national treatment guidelines for STDs (CDC, 1993) and practice guidelines for STD clinics (CDC, 1991), there are no generally accepted clinical practice guidelines or standards for STD screening and risk assessment. In addition, private practitioners generally are ill-prepared to assess their patients' risks, educate and counsel them, or notify and treat their sex partners.

Managed Care Organizations and Other Health Plans

Managed care is a method of integrating the organization and financing of health care services.[3] There are various approaches to managed care, including management of care under fee-for-service provider reimbursement (e.g., a preferred provider organization) and primary care case management. Prepayment places the health plan "at risk" financially because it must provide contract services in return for only the monthly premium and any nominal copayments allowed by the contract. This at-risk arrangement imposes financial incentives to control or "manage" the use of health services. Increasingly, managed care organizations are shifting some or all of this financial risk downward through capitation contracts with providers, who receive a fixed monthly sum for each member and earn their retained surplus or income by efficiently managing the clinical care. Most managed care organizations utilize a selected network of providers to help control both cost and utilization of services, thus potentially reducing access for enrolled members to STD-related services. Many plans require all services to be provided or arranged through a primary care clinician, often referred to as a "gatekeeper" or "care manager." The combination of financial incentives to control cost, including capitation, and the reliance on managing access through primary care providers places greater responsibility on managed care organizations than on traditional fee-for-service plans to ensure that beneficiaries receive comprehensive health services.

There are several types of managed care organizations, and more are evolving. Managed care organizations are usually classified by their method of providing services. Staff-model organizations employ providers on salary; group-model organizations contract with a single medical group practice; network-model organizations engage two or more medical groups; and independent practice associations (IPAs) contract with individual physicians or organized associations of independent physicians. Many managed care organizations now offer several of these options and are called mixed, or hybrid, plans. In each case, the contract can provide for payment to the provider in the form of a capitation (fixed monthly fee per member) or a discounted fee-for-service schedule. Point-of-service plans allow services from network providers at the usual copayment, but also permit

---

[3]The committee uses the term "managed care organization" to refer to health plans that are prepaid for the defined benefits of the plan—that is, health plans that provide, or arrange and pay for, all covered health services needed by the enrollee, in return for a specified premium plus any allowed copayments. This definition best describes health maintenance organizations (HMOs). The committee applies the term "managed care organization" only to health plans that use methods similar to those of health maintenance organizations. The committee uses the general term "health plan" to refer to all types of health insurance plans, including managed care organizations and fee-for-service indemnity plans.

members to seek care from any provider, in which case they pay deductibles and copayments similar to traditional indemnity insurance.

The early prepaid group- and staff-model managed care organizations (e.g., Group Health Cooperative of Puget Sound, Harvard Pilgrim Health Care, Kaiser-Permanente Health Plan) are nonprofit. The greatest growth in recent years, however, has been among investor-owned for-profit plans, which are mostly independent practice associations or hybrid plans (e.g., Aetna U.S. Healthcare, United HealthCare). A few managed care organizations, such as the Los Angeles County Department of Health Services' Community Health Plan and the Contra Costa County (California) Health Plan, are publicly owned and operated by local health departments. In 1994, approximately 31 percent of persons enrolled in managed care organizations were in predominantly staff- or group-model organizations, and 69 percent were in network or independent practice association plans (GHAA, 1995).

For-profit managed care organizations are managed somewhat differently from most not-for-profit managed care organizations, and quite differently from publicly operated managed care organizations. Investor-owned managed care organizations are managed to generate profits and increased equity for shareholders. Not-for-profit managed care organizations must reinvest any excess revenue in the organization and provide some type of benefit for plan members. A 1986 IOM report found that not-for-profit health care organizations were more likely than for-profit ones to provide care to uninsured persons and to conduct research and educational activities (IOM, 1986). Publicly operated managed care organizations are usually formed to meet the needs of Medicaid beneficiaries and uninsured residents for whom a local health department has responsibility.

Many managed care organizations have recently formed partnerships or entered into contracts with other community health care providers. For example, several states require or encourage school-based health centers to develop agreements with managed care organizations to improve primary care services for children (Schlitt et al., 1995). Several contractual models for such agreements have been implemented (Zimmerman and Reif, 1995).

Growing Role of Managed Care

Managed care organizations have grown rapidly in the last 10 years; nationwide enrollment in managed care organizations increased from 6 million in 1976 to 51 million in 1994 (GHAA, 1995). These health plans now provide health services to more than 20 percent of all privately insured persons in the United States. In 1994, more than 60 percent of the employed and insured under 65 years of age in 14 major metropolitan areas were enrolled in a managed care organization. As more people become dependent on the services provided only through their health plan, local public health leaders have expressed concerns regarding the effects on the scope, accessibility, and quality of services traditionally provided by, or in conjunction with, public health agencies, such as STD-related services.

One concern voiced by advocates for the poor is the rapid pace at which states are converting their Medicaid programs to prepaid managed care plans, thereby enrolling a population at higher risk for STDs into health plans with little experience managing STDs. For example, as of January 1996, 12 states have statewide managed care programs for Medicaid beneficiaries under 1115 waivers, and 47 states have more limited 1915(b) waivers from the Health Care Financing Agency (National Governors' Association, unpublished data, 1996).[4] In 1994, approximately 7.8 million Medicaid beneficiaries, or 23 percent of all enrollees, were enrolled in managed care plans (The Kaiser Commission on the Future of Medicaid, 1995). The push by states to enroll Medicaid recipients into managed care plans in order to contain costs raises several concerns regarding the design and implementation of these new programs and the accountability of the new managed care plans for quality (Fisher, 1994).

Effect of Managed Care on STD Prevention

There are both opportunities and concerns associated with increased involvement of managed care organizations in the delivery of preventive and public health services (CDC, 1995b). Potential opportunities for managed care organizations to improve prevention of STDs include the following:

• The prepayment arrangement of managed care organizations provides a potential incentive to effectively prevent STDs among enrollees. They are directly responsible for providing their enrollees with comprehensive personal health services, which include care for STDs and their complications.

• The organizational structure of managed care organizations as a system for providing care increases opportunities for effectiveness. For example, group- and staff-model organizations could effectively implement guidelines for STD-related screening and case management across all clinicians in their plan. Less-structured managed care organizations, however, such as independent practice associations, would have more difficulty in consistently implementing guidelines.

• Managed care organizations, because they are responsible for delivering

---

[4] Under section 1115 of the Social Security Act, states can apply to deviate from many federal Medicaid requirements in order to test new Medicaid policy. Section 1115 waivers are also called "research and demonstration" waivers. Under section 1915(b) of the Social Security Act, states can apply to waive certain federal requirements related to "freedom of choice" requirements for beneficiaries in order to enroll them into managed care plans. Section 1915(b) waivers are also called "program" waivers. Section 1115 waivers are typically broader in scope than section 1915(b) waivers.

care to large numbers of plan members, may be more inclined than traditional fee-for-service providers to view their enrollees from a public health perspective, that is, to examine and address their enrollees' health needs as a community or population, rather than as individuals.

• The large size, resources, and complexity of group- and staff-model managed care organizations potentially allow them to support the services of highly trained health professionals, such as physicians trained in infectious diseases, to manage and provide STD-related services.

• The highly developed information systems of many managed care organizations can be used to monitor STD trends among their enrolled population and to assess the quality and adequacy of treatment and case management protocols. These information systems are more common among group- and staff-model organizations than among independent practice associations and network plans.

• Managed care provides opportunities for purchasers, such as employers and government programs, to hold plans accountable for specific performance standards. This is a tremendous potential opportunity to provide and improve STD-related services if purchasers take a strong interest in this issue. Information systems can also help purchasers measure the performance of managed care organizations in STD-related activities through standardized quality assessment tools, such as the Health Plan Employer Data Information Set (HEDIS),[5] if such performance measures include measures of STD-related services.

The potential concerns regarding the increased role of managed care organizations in STD prevention include the following:

• STDs are not a high priority for most managed care organizations or their sponsors. Those that do not serve populations at high risk for STDs, in particular, may not have a strong interest in providing comprehensive STD-related services.

• The mission of the managed care organization is often related to whether the managed care organization is a nonprofit or for-profit organization. The mission of for-profit organizations may be in conflict with providing services that do not provide short-term cost savings to the organization.

• There is a wide spectrum of managed care organizations; consequently, there is a wide range of technical ability among such organizations in delivering services. In general, staff- and group-model managed care organizations are likely to be more effective in STD prevention than health plans that have less infrastructure. Given the limited experience of most managed care organizations in public health activities, however, even some of the best organized managed care organi-

----

[5]This performance measurement tool, developed by the National Committee for Quality Assurance, is utilized primarily by employers and other purchasers of health care to compare and evaluate large managed care organizations.

zations may not have the technical expertise to take on full responsibility for STD prevention. In addition, the types of managed care organizations that currently dominate the market typically do not have highly developed systems for ensuring quality care.

• Many managed care organizations may be reluctant to provide STD-related services that have not been shown to be cost-saving for the organization. For example, the long interval between infection and appearance of consequences of STDs may be years; managed care organizations with high turnover rates may have little incentive to emphasize STD-related services. In addition, capitated payments for services may increase the risk of cost-shifting by managed care organizations. For example, health plans may refer persons in need of STD-related services to public STD clinics to avoid assuming the costs of their care.

• Persons with STDs may prefer to receive care at public STD clinics and may not feel comfortable receiving care through a managed care organization for a variety of reasons. A recent multisite survey of STD clinic patients showed that most persons surveyed chose a public STD clinic over other providers because of the convenience of obtaining care without an appointment and lower costs (Celum et al., 1995). The lack of walk-in services among many managed care organizations may result in delays for evaluation and treatment of STDs.

• Managed care organizations may not provide services to sex partners of plan members if the partner is not a plan member. Many aspects of STD prevention, such as partner notification, screening and case finding, and community education, may involve persons who are not members of the managed care organization.

The billing and claims-processing procedures of some health plans may be a major barrier to confidential STD-related services, particularly for dependent minors. In approximately one-third of managed care organizations surveyed, the employee-beneficiary is likely to be notified of care for their dependents through a copayment bill or other means (Benson Gold and Richards, 1996). Of particular concern are billing procedures among traditional indemnity insurance plans, preferred provider organizations, and point-of-service networks, which often result in lack of confidentiality for dependents because the employee-beneficiary is usually required to be involved in the claims process.

Data regarding the impact of managed care on STD-related services are limited. One study examined the effect of managed care enrollment on the management of three ambulatory conditions (vaginitis, pelvic inflammatory disease, and urinary tract infection) among Medicaid recipients (Carey and Weis, 1990). The authors found that the presence of managed care plans did not reduce diagnostic testing or return visits for the three conditions, compared to fee-for-service providers. Many of the potential concerns mentioned above regarding expanding the role of managed care in STD prevention are similar to those associated with managed care and other controversial health services, such as reproductive health (Delbanco and Smith, 1995) and HIV infection (Aseltyne et al., 1995).

Services and Programs of Managed Care Organizations

Studies show that most managed care organizations provide considerably more comprehensive coverage for reproductive health services than the traditional indemnity insurance plans (Benson Gold and Richards, 1996). Data regarding STD-related services provided or covered by health plans are limited.

Given the lack of published information regarding the potential role of managed care organizations in STD prevention, the committee sponsored a workshop on the role of managed care organizations in the prevention of STDs. A summary of this workshop can be found in Appendix G.

As a follow-up to the workshop, the committee conducted a limited survey of managed care organizations to collect preliminary data regarding STD-related services and programs in these organizations. Results of this survey are presented in Appendix H. Managed care organizations were selected primarily on the basis of their likelihood of serving high-risk populations (i.e., Medicaid, inner city), and therefore their increased likelihood of providing STD-related services. The committee found that 73 percent of responding managed care organizations requested information regarding previous history of STDs or sexual activity, and 65 percent requested information on sexual activity, on patient history forms. More than half (57 percent) of these organizations attempted to define high-risk groups for STDs, and approximately half reported STD prevention or clinical activities that specifically targeted adolescents. Only 26 percent of managed care organizations reported that they provided STD-related services to persons outside their plan, and just 17 percent had a specific individual in charge of STD-related activities.

Examples of programs and activities conducted by survey respondents are provided in Appendix H. Two examples of managed care organizations that have comprehensive prevention and case management programs that extend beyond the boundaries of the plan's enrollees are the Harvard Pilgrim Health Plan and Kaiser-Permanente of Southern California. At the Harvard Pilgrim Health Plan, all levels of services for members with HIV infection and AIDS have been integrated through a central multidisciplinary program. This program is closely linked to local health department services and provides extensive outreach and community services beyond the member population. In Southern California, Kaiser-Permanente has developed an effective system of STD-related services under the direction of an infectious disease specialist; the system includes monitoring of STD trends through reports from its centralized laboratory, implementation of STD treatment and case management protocols among its health professionals, and creation of a prevention and primary care program for STDs that is targeted to adolescents in the plan and in the general community. STD programs such as those mentioned above may have a dramatic impact on reducing STDs and associated costs in managed care organizations. For example, a recent randomized control study conducted at Group Health Cooperative of Puget Sound showed that identifying, testing, and treating women at increased risk for asymptomatic chlamydial infection reduced the rate of pelvic inflammatory disease by more than 50 percent compared to women who received routine care (Scholes et al., 1996).

Government Initiatives Related to Managed Care and STDs

Public health agencies, such as the CDC, have been exploring the impact of managed care on public health services. The CDC recently established a Managed Care Working Group to foster partnerships between public health agencies and managed care organizations to improve public health (CDC, 1995b). The CDC's high-priority areas for collaborative activities with managed care organizations and other health organizations include prevention effectiveness and guidelines, Medicaid and managed care, research, and capacity development in public health agencies. In addition, a CDC epidemiologist is currently assigned on detail to the American Association of Health Plans as a resource on public health issues. As mentioned previously, CDC staff have provided input regarding public health performance indicators, including STD-related indicators, for future versions of HEDIS.

The California Department of Health Services has also recently initiated the California Partnership for Adolescent Chlamydia Prevention. This is a statewide partnership, bringing together government agencies, managed care organizations, academic health centers, and professional associations to address policy issues related to STDs among adolescents. This initiative also seeks to coordinate clinical preventive services for adolescents in managed care settings with community STD prevention activities and to coordinate all categorical state STD-related programs. Other components of this initiative include a media campaign targeted towards teenagers; development of screening, counseling, and education interventions; school-based programs; and training programs for health care providers.

The Los Angeles County Department of Health Services has developed a model contract between the agency and managed care organizations that contract under the Medi-Cal (California's Medicaid program) program (County of Los Angeles, Department of Health Services, 1995). The contract, which covers a wide range of public health services, describes STD clinical services as a "shared responsibility between County and Plan." The contract would require managed care organizations participating in Medi-Cal to "reimburse the County for services provided to Plan beneficiaries at the Medi-Cal [fee-for-service] rate." In turn, the county agrees to "make all reasonable efforts to provide medical records to the Plan relating to STD care billed to the Plan." The county's contract language parallels language required by the California Department of Health Services for all contracts with managed care organizations serving Medi-Cal beneficiaries. Similar provisions in Medicaid contracts have also been adopted by Missouri, Oregon, and Minnesota. Although such an agreement appropriately would provide for plan reimbursement for out-of-plan STD-related services, better methods are needed to document billing of the plan for their enrollees' use of such services. The language included in the Los Angeles County model contract suggests that the health department will divulge confidential patient information to the plan and may inhibit infected persons from seeking care—an outcome that would not be in the best interests of the plan or the larger community.

NATIONAL SURVEILLANCE AND INFORMATION SYSTEMS

Public health surveillance is the process of collecting information regarding the frequency and distribution of disease or other health conditions among specific populations. Data are collected at local, regional, and national levels to (a) monitor trends in diseases and other health conditions, (b) identify problems that need intervention, (c) improve effectiveness of prevention or health care resources, and (d) evaluate the impact of specific interventions. The current national system for STD surveillance is a complex amalgam of different reporting systems from multiple sources.

National Notifiable Disease Reporting

The foundation of STD surveillance is the national public health notifiable disease reporting system, coordinated on a national basis by the CDC. This system is fundamentally a "passive" system, that is, reports are brought to the attention of public health officials when health care providers or laboratories submit a report of a positive laboratory test or clinical diagnosis of a reportable health condition. Active case finding is not routinely conducted. Each of the 50 states has the authority to declare certain diseases or health conditions that are to be reported by clinicians and laboratories. Syphilis and gonorrhea are reportable conditions in all 50 states; and 48 states (New York and Alaska are the exceptions) also require the reporting of chlamydial genital infection (CDC, 1995c). Other bacterial STDs, such as chancroid or lymphogranuloma venereum, are not consistently reported from state to state. Viral STDs, such as herpes simplex virus type 2 infections, are generally not well identified through this system.

In general, initial case reports generated by laboratories or providers are submitted to local public health departments and are, in turn, reported to state public health authorities. All states participate in a voluntary system whereby statewide notifiable disease data are reported to the CDC. National STD data reported by the CDC are compiled from individual reports from states, submitted without name identifiers. Not all states report uniform data to the CDC. For example, California does not report STD morbidity data by race but includes other variables.

Limitations of the Reporting System

The passive reporting system for STDs has several major limitations. Numerous studies have indicated that reporting from public clinics, such as public STD clinics, is more complete than reporting from private providers (Anderson et al., 1994). Reported data actually may underrepresent true STD incidence by 50 percent or more because many cases diagnosed by private providers are not reported. The reporting bias toward public sector providers also skews the demographic characteristics of reported STD rates, since public providers are more likely to see poor or uninsured patients, a greater proportion of whom are from certain racial and ethnic groups (CDC, DSTD/HIVP, 1995). In a comparison of surveillance data collected by the CDC with survey data collected by population-based surveys (i.e., National Survey of Family Growth), one study found that national surveillance data may underrepresent the incidence of STDs among higher socioeconomic groups because they tend to use private sources of health care, whereas survey data may be prone to underreporting of past STDs (Anderson et al., 1994).

Analysis of national data by the CDC requires considerable effort to produce basic reports and often does not systematically assess trends within subpopulations and geographic areas. For example, the increase in heterosexual syphilis that peaked in the late 1980s was not identified in a timely way because national data were aggregated and not systematically analyzed by sex and risk behavior. This was because the decline in syphilis rates among men who have sex with men obscured the increase in syphilis among heterosexual men and women until a year or more into the epidemic.

Since surveillance data are only compiled as diagnosed cases, rather than number of cases per number of persons tested, such estimates are difficult to interpret. This is especially problematic when new diseases are added to the list of notifiable diseases or when new diagnostic technologies become available. This phenomenon occurred most recently with chlamydial genital infection. As more providers became aware of the availability of culture and nonculture diagnostic tests, screening for chlamydial infection among women increased in many health care settings. Reported statistics demonstrated dramatic increases in chlamydial genital infection that reflected increased screening rates rather than true rising disease incidence rates. Similarly, case-definition bias may also confuse interpretation of surveillance statistics. For example, women may be more likely to be tested and identified as laboratory-confirmed cases, whereas men with nongonococcal urethritis will be presumptively treated (treated after a syndromic diagnosis) and never reported as a case, since they were not confirmed by laboratory tests. Furthermore, should nongonococcal urethritis become reportable, this will only partially reflect chlamydial infection among men because, although chlamydia is the most common cause of nongonococcal urethritis, it still accounts for less than half the cases.

Other limitations in these data may not be immediately evident. Reporting to public health agencies is sometimes not carried out in a timely way, so that delays in reporting may result. In addition, surveillance case definitions are often not uniformly followed, leading to misclassification of cases or nonreporting of true cases. This occurred in many areas when the congenital syphilis case definition changed in 1989, but local areas continued to follow the old case definition, thereby severely underestimating the true impact of syphilis on infant health.

Surveillance and Public STD Programs

Publicly funded STD programs, particularly in urban areas, have largely focused on case-finding and partner notification activities rather than development of infrastructure for data management and surveillance data analyses. In areas where syphilis rates remain high (largely in urban areas and in the South), programmatic activity by disease intervention specialists has focused on following up positive laboratory tests for syphilis with tracking and testing of sex partners. In areas of lower syphilis morbidity, this intense outreach program by disease intervention specialists was carried out for other STDs, such as gonorrhea. In all cases, efforts were largely focused on cases identified in public STD clinics, and mechanisms were not developed to uniformly assess the extent of STD diagnosis and treatment in nonpublic STD clinic settings or through private providers. In some STD programs, so little effort is being made to identify gonorrhea or chlamydial infections identified outside publicly funded STD clinics that reports sent to the local health departments from non-STD clinic providers are discarded, and little effort is made to identify broader, community-based morbidity trends. As discussed in Chapter 4, partner notification and follow-up of positive laboratory results for syphilis are labor intensive and result in a heavy emphasis on STD program indicators rather than on true population-based measures of program effectiveness.

Other Surveillance Systems

Other types of data regarding STDs are collected through a multitude of systems, some clinic-based, some local or regional, and others national in scope. Coupled with the national notifiable disease surveillance system, they provide a patchwork of information for inferring the actual scope and impact of STDs nationwide.

Rather than attempting to capture data from all data collection sites, sentinel systems are designed to capture detailed data from a few sites that are considered to be representative of the region or the country. Sentinel surveillance can address the biases from increased screening practices or inconsistent application of case definitions, since the populations under surveillance and participating providers are well defined. Perhaps the best functioning sentinel STD surveillance system is the Gonococcal Isolate Surveillance Project sponsored by the CDC. This project collects data from 21 nationwide sites to assess patterns in gonorrhea isolate antimicrobial resistance.

Coordinated by the National Center for Health Statistics, the National Health and Nutrition Examination Survey (NHANES) collects health-related data from a randomly selected sample of the U.S. population. In addition to data regarding self-reported health behaviors, blood samples collected at the time of interview provide critical information regarding the actual prevalence of diseases through detection of serological markers. This is particularly useful for some viral STDs that are often asymptomatic, including herpes simplex virus infection, hepatitis B virus infection, and HIV infection (McQuillan et al., 1989, 1994; Johnson et al., 1993). For example, using these data, public health officials have estimated that at least one of four European American women and one in five European American men will be infected with genital herpes in their lifetime (Johnson et al., 1993).

Provider-based information systems are used to estimate the scope and frequency of treatment among private sector and other physicians and can provide useful data on STDs to supplement disease surveillance data. The National Disease and Therapeutic Index is a commercially developed provider database that systematically collects patient encounter data from a stratified sample of U.S. private practice physicians. It has been used to follow trends in the diagnosis of some nonreportable STDs, such as genital warts caused by human papillomavirus, genital herpes, vaginal infections, and nongonococcal urethritis. Another potential method for assessing STD trends is by monitoring of the sequelae of STDs. For example, the National Ambulatory Care Survey and the National Hospital Discharge Survey have been used to monitor rates of pelvic inflammatory disease. Physician consultations for infertility and cervical cancer rates within specific populations also may be used as surrogates for underlying STD trends. In addition, disease registries are helpful in documenting the occurrence of STDs in specific communities and in conducting clinical research. For example, a national disease registry collects information regarding infants exposed to herpes simplex at birth and treated with acyclovir. Although limited in scope, these registries provide useful information on treatment of STDs.

Health Behavior Surveys

A crucial but underdeveloped tool for directing and targeting STD prevention programs is the behavioral health survey. Surveys that regularly collect nationally representative information on specific STD-related risk behaviors are important in monitoring national trends and have become more prominent since the advent of the HIV epidemic. The Behavioral Risk Factors Surveillance Survey supported by the CDC was originally developed to ascertain health behaviors related to chronic diseases such as heart disease, but has been modified to include questions regarding HIV/STD-related risk behaviors. A similar survey, the Youth Risk Behavior Surveillance System, designed to determine risk behaviors of teenagers, including sexual activity and alcohol and other drug use, has been developed by the CDC and implemented by schools nationwide. This survey is perhaps the best currently available source of information on the scope and frequency of STD-related behaviors among teenagers and is commonly used to develop effective prevention programs for adolescents (CDC, 1995d).

The National Center for Health Statistics, CDC, also sponsors health interviews with women regarding reproductive health issues. The National Survey of Family Growth provides important information regarding the self-reported prevalence of STDs and STD-related health behaviors among the general U.S. population. The National Survey of Adolescent Males is another federally funded survey that collects data on sexual behavior and contraceptive use from a nationally representative cohort of male adolescents 15–19 years old (Ku et al., 1992). Other health behavior surveys and studies that are not periodically administered have also produced important data regarding sexual behavior. For example, the National Health and Social Life Survey collected information from a probability sample of 3,432 American adults between 18 and 59 years of age in 1992 and produced the most comprehensive nationally representative data on sexual behavior among adults in the United States in many years (Laumann et al., 1994). In addition, a multiyear study, the National Adolescent Health Survey, jointly sponsored by several agencies, recently has completed data collection to examine the influence of family, peers, schools, and the community on adolescent health.

There is no evidence that participating in surveys of sexual behavior has a detrimental effect on sexual behavior. Halpern and others (1994) analyzed multiple study groups from three longitudinal studies of the effect of repeated administration of questionnaires regarding sexual behavior on male adolescents. They found no evidence that such questionnaires had an effect on sexual behavior.

Measuring and Evaluating Program Effectiveness

Data regarding federally supported projects collected by the CDC through state and local health departments consist primarily of output indicators that relate to laboratory reporting, community screening, case investigation, preventive and other clinical services, and gonorrhea, chlamydia, and HIV case detection. Other federal agencies, such as the Health Resources and Services Administration and the Health Care Financing Administration, collect information primarily related to the provision of direct health care services they support.

The committee is not aware of any nongovernmental organizations or associations that routinely collect data regarding STDs. However, the National Com-

---

BOX 5-2
Draft Description of HEDIS Measure for Chlamydia Screening Under Evaluation by the National Committee for Quality Assurance.

Chlamydia Screening

Chlamydia is not widely known, but it is an important health problem. It is the most common sexually transmitted bacterial disease in the United States, with an estimated 2 million new infections in women each year. It is usually a silent illness; about 70 percent of infected women have no symptoms. Left untreated, chlamydia can cause pelvic inflammatory disease, infertility, ectopic pregnancy (where the egg is implanted in the fallopian tube instead of in the womb), and chronic pelvic pain. Regular screening for the infection by testing for it during annual gynecological check-ups is often the only way to detect it so it can be treated before complications arise. Detection and treatment also help keep the person from spreading the disease.

This measure estimates the percentage of women between the ages of 15 and 25 who were screened for chlamydia in the past year. This measure is being evaluated for inclusion in a future reporting set. Since sexually active women are the group of interest for chlamydia screening, a reliable method needs to be developed to distinguish women who are sexually active from those who are not. We also need to assess how reliably chlamydia screening is reported. These issues, among others, will be evaluated during the testing phase.

NOTE: The above text is a direct quote from the primary source. The estimate of 2 million chlamydial infections, presumably for 1996, differs from the estimate of 2.6 million in 1994 cited previously by the committee. These estimates, however, are not necessarily inconsistent.
SOURCE: NCQA, Committee on Performance Measurement. HEDIS 3.0 Draft for public comment. Washington, D.C.: National Committee for Quality Assurance, July 1996.

---

mittee for Quality Assurance, through the Committee on Performance Measurement, is currently evaluating a proposed STD-related performance measure for inclusion in subsequent versions of HEDIS. This performance measure on chlamydia screening, developed and submitted by the CDC, is presented in Box 5-2 and is in the "testing set" of HEDIS 3.0.

Another IOM committee, the Committee on Using Performance Monitoring to Improve Community Health, has evaluated the use of population-based performance monitoring to improve community health (IOM, 1996c). This committee examined capacities and processes for implementing and conducting performance monitoring. The final report, scheduled for release in 1997, will include proposed indicators for a community health profile and prototypical sets of indicators related to specific health issues.

Data Management, Utilization, and Limitations

In addition to uses associated with disease surveillance, data collected regarding STDs are primarily utilized for management of specific publicly sponsored disease control programs and for assessment of clinical performance of federally funded health care providers, such as community health centers. More specifically, with respect to the data collected on a national basis through the Division of STD Prevention at the CDC, existing management information systems are intended to support four primary service objectives in STD prevention: (1) preventing and containing early and congenital syphilis; (2) preventing and containing gonorrhea and pelvic inflammatory disease; (3) preventing and containing chlamydial infection and chlamydia-related sequelae such as pelvic inflammatory disease; and (4) preventing HIV infection through public STD clinics (Alan Friedlob, CDC, Division of STD Prevention, personal communication, February 1996).

To facilitate national data collection, the CDC provides management information software (STD*MIS) to state and local disease control programs to compile morbidity and service delivery output data. These data are intended to help state and local programs (a) track patient disease information and out-of-jurisdiction activity; (b) maintain files related to interview investigations, field investigations, morbidity, and laboratory surveillance; (c) allow electronic submission of data to the federal government; and (d) generate standard and customized reports.

However, while existing data systems may be adequate to support many of the internal management requirements outlined above, it is not clear that these data are adequate for overall program assessment. According to the Division of STD Prevention systems development staff, minimum national standards defining an adequate program for preventing STDs do not exist. STD-related services data and data collection procedures have been characterized as inflexible, relying on historic performance measures and focused on public STD clinics rather than linking data from all sites that provide STD-related services, including family planning agencies, emergency rooms, correctional institutions, substance use treatment programs, and other health care providers (Alan Friedlob, CDC, Division of STD Prevention, personal communication, February 1996). Additional deficiencies in STD-related data include lack of information on population subgroups, transmission-related behavior, services assessment, and outcomes related to specific interventions.

Information Systems Development

STD information systems development is, in concept and in application, inseparable from the larger community health information network development environment. Effective community health information network systems collect both population information and service and encounter data. This allows for (a) integration of data across programs (e.g., tuberculosis, HIV, substance abuse); (b) efficient data-based decision-making; (c) application flexibility and systems compatibility (e.g., software independent of language or platform); (d) confidentiality safeguards; and (e) menus of indicators that are responsive to local needs. It should also be recognized that STD information systems development is occurring within a wider and rapidly changing planning environment, such as the Department of Health and Human Services proposed Performance Partnership Grants, the work of the Public Health Service's Public Health Data Policy Coordinating Committee, and the National Information Infrastructure and High Performance Computing and Communication initiatives (Braithwaite, 1995).

General issues to consider in developing and coordinating community-based information systems initiatives such as those mentioned above include:

1. quality and usefulness of data;
2. coordination with state- and national-level information systems;
3. coordination of data collection processes, including collection of data from public and private sources;
4. capacity to track outcome, process, and capacity measures in a timely manner;
5. assurance of data privacy and security;
6. development of standards for data elements, such as utilization of uniform diagnostic coding;
7. resolution of proprietary concerns or ownership issues related to data;
8. capacity to produce anonymous health data files for public health surveillance and other purposes; and
9. flexibility to utilize grant funds to build and maintain information systems.

Local Data Analysis Capacity

The Division of STD Prevention at the CDC currently provides technical assistance to state and local programs implementing the division's management information software, "STD*MIS." Rather than technical assistance related to initiating or implementing information systems, it has been suggested that technical assistance is needed to develop local data analysis capacity so that data can be used to improve the effectiveness and efficiency of local STD programs (Alan Friedlob, CDC, Division of STD Prevention, personal communication, February 1996). With respect to analytic capacity, a survey of 65 STD project areas in December 1994 found that half had one half-time or less position dedicated to data analysis activities (CDC, Division of STD Prevention, unpublished data, 1995). Only 20 percent of projects surveyed had one or more full-time staff with master's or doctoral level training in epidemiology. The survey also found that 48 percent of STD programs derived epidemiological support exclusively from HIV/

AIDS programs. Finally, 44 percent of STD program managers stated that epidemiological support for their activities was inadequate.

Local capacity in data management and analysis is required if surveillance data are to be used as a program management tool. For example, the decline in rectal gonorrhea rates in many areas of the United States could be interpreted to be a result of the efficacy of HIV prevention activities among gay men. In order to make this assessment, however, local health districts need to have sufficient data management capacity both to collect data on gonorrhea incidence and STD-related behaviors, and to analyze data systematically.

A possible explanation for the lack of data analysis capacity is the dependency of information systems, such as STD*MIS, on state and local resources for maintenance and enhancement. The Council of State and Territorial Epidemiologists has reported that less than half of data resources at state and local levels is provided through federal resources (CSTE, 1995). The council further observed that almost one-half (46.4 percent) of all federal funding for state and local activities related to communicable disease data management was directed towards HIV/AIDS and that one-third of all federal funding was designated for HIV/AIDS. In addition, the council found that, with respect to data management, state and local governments were supporting 59 percent of funding for tuberculosis, 40.8 percent of funding for STDs, 44.2 percent of funding for vaccine-preventable diseases, and 86.7 percent of funding for all other communicable diseases.

TRAINING AND EDUCATION OF HEALTH PROFESSIONALS

The spectrum of health care providers who are responsible for providing STD-related services includes physicians, nurse practitioners, nurses, physician assistants, and other professionals. The intensity and content of training and educational activities for health professionals vary considerably. Training may occur as part of the formal professional curricula or as part of continuing education activities.

Medical School and Medical Graduate Education

Two national committees in the United States have previously expressed concern regarding the adequacy of education in the area of STDs (Kampmeier, 1975; Work Group on Sexually Transmitted Disease, 1979). In addition, a 1980–1981 study indicated that medical school instruction regarding STDs was generally inadequate (Stamm et al., 1982). This survey of the infectious disease divisions of 122 U.S. medical schools and 15 Canadian medical schools collected information on preclinical and clinical training of medical students and clinical training of medical residents and other resident groups. Of the 127 infectious disease divisions responding to the survey, almost all offered preclinical training consisting mostly of lectures on STD pathogens. Only 30 percent of U.S. medical schools had access to hospital-based or dedicated public STD clinics for teaching purposes. At these schools, only 30 percent of medical students received clinic-based training and the clinical experience offered to these students averaged only six hours. Thus, approximately 1 in 10 students received clinic-based STD training, and even this training was brief. Similarly, only 23 percent of internal medicine residencies in the United States offered specific clinical training in STD management and, even where available, this training only averaged 12 hours. Residents in other programs (dermatology, family practice, obstetrics and gynecology, pediatrics, and urology) were even less likely to be offered STD clinical training.

In 1991, 126 U.S. medical schools were again surveyed concerning clinical training offered medical students in the areas of STDs, including HIV infection (MacKay, 1995). The responses from 102 schools indicated that over the previous 10 years, the amount of clinical training of medical students in STDs had decreased at 6 percent of schools, remained the same at 17 percent, and increased at 77 percent of schools. Despite the increase in the number of schools that provided additional clinical training in STDs, several areas of STD-related education require improvement. For example, links to a clinic devoted specifically to STDs existed in only 42 percent of schools, and only 37 percent of schools offered students a clinical elective in STDs or HIV/AIDS. Programs for improving medical school and medical graduate training that focus on communication skills and involve a series of lectures, workshops, and role-playing have been developed (Steinberg et al., 1991; Ross and Landis, 1994).

Clinical training in dedicated public STD clinics, therefore, remains the exception rather than the rule for medical students in the United States. While infrequent encounters with patients with STDs in other ambulatory settings such as primary care, general medicine, or family medicine clinics (Berg et al., 1984) have been cited as reasons for difficulty in ensuring comprehensive training in STD management and prevention in these environments, there remains relatively little training in other aspects of STD prevention such as risk assessment or screening practices.

Primary Care Health Professional Training

Programs to train medical students, physicians, physicians assistants, nurse practitioners, nurses, and other primary care professionals in STD prevention are critical in increasing the capacity of the primary care system to address public health problems. The current system of clinical training for health care professionals is inadequate to produce effective primary care providers. For example, an IOM committee, charged to provide direction on improving primary care, came to the following conclusion regarding graduate medical education in the United States (IOM, 1996a:186-7):

Based on its public hearing and site visits, the committee shares with many medical educators and medical directors of integrated health care delivery systems concerns about traditional GME [graduate medical education], especially about the extent to which such training is preparing tomorrow's doctors for the new ways and settings in which they will be expected to function. Graduates of residency programs often lack knowledge of population-based health promotion and disease prevention, evidence-based clinical decisionmaking, and patient interviewing skills (particularly communication and consultation skills).

The IOM committee on primary care recommended that primary care provider training be based on a common core set of clinical competencies, regardless of their disciplinary background, to be defined by a coalition of educational and professional organizations and accrediting bodies. Two specific areas of suggested emphasis were communication skills and cultural sensitivity (IOM, 1996a).

Primary care professionals (including family practitioners, internists, obstetrician/gynecologists, and pediatricians) see the majority of STDs in the United States (Berg, 1990), yet little research has been performed about STD management in primary care settings. It is likely that primary care clinicians in the private sector will be called upon to assume a greater role in STD prevention, including case management. However, because of the limited data regarding the knowledge, skills, and training needs of primary care professionals in these settings, an assessment of these issues is critical.

Primary care professionals often do not receive special training in STD risk assessment, diagnosis, and treatment. Such training, when it does exist, is often based within dedicated public STD clinics, and is not accessible to primary care professionals. Some of the federally funded STD training centers require a lengthy time commitment that limits participation by primary care providers. Further, diagnostic and management strategies and physician responsibilities appropriate for dedicated STD clinics often require modification for primary care practice (Berg, 1990).

Some primary care practices, such as community health centers in inner-city urban areas or programs for high-risk migrant populations, are the primary source of STD-related care in communities with high rates of STDs. Based on a chart review of all patient encounters in an inner-city Atlanta community health center during a four-week period in 1994, 10 percent of all patient encounters, and nearly all encounters among young men, were related to STD diagnosis and treatment (Kathleen Toomey, Georgia Department of Human Resources, Division of Public Health, unpublished data, 1996). However, patients frequently received inappropriate or inadequate treatment not consistent with published STD treatment guidelines. For example, half of all women with clinical diagnosis of pelvic inflammatory disease were treated inadequately for simple cervical infection. Clinicians in this clinic included nurse practitioners, internists, pediatricians, and family practitioners without specific training in STD clinical management. However, all staff expressed willingness to participate in training in STD diagnosis and treatment and adopted STD treatment guidelines when they were made available. As previously mentioned, lack of physician compliance with standard practice for prevention and management of STDs has been documented (Gemson et al., 1991; Hessol et al., 1996) and additional training of clinicians in STD-related skills has been recommended (Boekeloo et al., 1991; Gemson et al., 1991; Steinberg et al., 1991; Hessol et al., 1996).

Federal Efforts in STD Training

Federal efforts to provide STD training have focused almost exclusively on training health professionals who provide services in the public sector. Since 1979, the CDC has funded 10 to 12 regional STD Prevention Training Centers. These centers have provided instruction composed of didactic lectures and clinic-based experiences to nearly 100,000 nurse practitioners, physician assistants, and physicians working in public health or family planning clinics throughout the United States. These centers are comanaged by medical schools and local or state health departments, but have not, until recently, specifically provided training to medical students or residents in training. In contrast, the AIDS Education and Training Centers funded by the Health Resources and Services Administration have focused on training primary care providers, but have not generally offered STD-related training. The Health Resources and Services Administration puts most of its sexuality-related training funds into programs related to family planning and HIV infection to the exclusion of other STDs. Generally, the National Institutes of Health's funding for STD-related training is primarily directed at training researchers, not clinicians.

To strengthen training of health professional students and trainees, the CDC plans a new initiative to support faculty positions in a limited number of medical centers to initiate clinical training of students and residents. However, the existing Regional STD Prevention Training Centers have not been adequately utilized to provide clinical training to health professional students and residents, who are often strongly motivated to obtain elective training in STDs. For example, the Seattle STD Prevention Training Centers cannot accommodate most of the medical and physician assistants and residents who seek training and have actually reduced training for these groups during the past year (King Holmes, University of Washington, personal communication, August 1996). To the committee's knowledge, no specific agency is responsible for training medical or other health professional students. Medical school curricula, which address human sexuality, do so from a perspective of sexual dysfunction and sexual "deviance" rather than from a perspective of healthy sexuality. The CDC also supports training of disease intervention specialists, who generally coordinate HIV testing, provide patient education, and conduct partner notification for STDs, including HIV infection. This type of training support, however, is changing as described previously.

Advances in Information Technology

Advances in information technology are having a dramatic impact on how health-related information is disseminated among health professionals and have increased opportunities for their education. Telemedicine is rapidly being employed, especially in rural areas, to increase access of primary care providers to the expertise of specialists in medical centers (IOM, 1996b; Crump and Pfeil, 1995). The proliferation of the Internet has dramatically increased access to information that was previously only accessible at libraries and information reference centers. In addition, information technology has enabled many primary care professionals to learn new skills or improve current practice through distance learning activities such as televised courses. The CDC has recently initiated distance learning activities employing teleconferencing, use of the Internet, CD-ROM, and other information technologies to improve STD education.

FUNDING OF SERVICES

Federal, State, and Local Government Funding

Publicly funded STD programs have had several notable successes (CDC, DSTDP, 1995). Beginning in the late 1940s, and continuing through the early 1950s, aggressive national programs against syphilis succeeded in nearly eliminating early syphilis in the United States. Only 10 years after the number of cases of primary and secondary syphilis peaked at 94,957 cases in 1946, cases were reduced to 6,392 in 1956 (CDC, DSTDP, 1995). At that time, the apparent success of the program may have led to an assumption that syphilis was no longer a problem, with the result that funding was sharply reduced (CDC, DSTD/HIVP, 1995). Four years later, the number of cases of primary and secondary syphilis in the United States nearly tripled (CDC, DSTDP, 1995). In the early 1970s, and continuing through the early 1980s, national programs against gonorrhea were also initiated. Along with a number of other factors such as the decreasing proportion of the population in the age groups at greatest risk, safer sexual practices related to HIV concerns, and changes in contraceptive methods, this national program contributed to a substantial decline in gonorrhea cases. The number of reported cases dropped 59 percent from 1,013,436 cases in 1978 to 418,068 in 1994 (CDC, DSTDP, 1995).

In fiscal year 1995, the federal budget for the CDC's Division of STD Prevention, the lead federal agency for STD prevention, was $105.2 million. Of that amount, approximately $91.8 million (87 percent) was awarded in grants by the CDC to states and cities for STD prevention activities.[6] The National Institute of

---

[6] The remaining amount of the appropriated funds ($13.4 million) supports CDC overhead costs and Division of STD Prevention staff salaries and activities, such as technical assistance and intramural research.

Allergy and Infectious Diseases and other divisions at the National Institutes of Health, which are responsible for supporting most STD-related biomedical and clinical research activities in the federal government, invested approximately $105.4 million in the same year for biomedical and clinical research in STDs. In addition, other federal agencies, such as the Health Resources and Services Administration, Office of Population Affairs, the Health Care Financing Administration (primarily through its Medicaid program), and the Indian Health Service, all directly support or provide STD-related clinical services. The amount of funds that support STD-related services in these agencies, however, is unclear because such services are provided in the context of primary care or other programs and are not allocated or accounted for separately. The proportion of federal funds that is used to support prevention activities versus other services is likewise unclear, but it is reasonable to broadly categorize funds allocated for the Division of STD Prevention at the CDC and National Institutes of Health STD-related grants as related to noncurative prevention services and to research, respectively, and funds originating from the other federal agencies as primarily used to support clinical services for STDs.

The precise amount of financial support for STD-related programs, including both curative and noncurative services at the state and local levels, is unknown because there is no matching requirement for most federal funding. State and local governments vary widely in their financial support for STD-related programs. Some jurisdictions spend several times more than they receive from the CDC, while others only provide a small proportion of the total funding for such programs in their area. Based on an informal CDC survey of state and local health departments regarding their contributions to STD program funding in 1994, the total state and local contribution to STD-related programs was approximately $125.6 million or approximately 58 percent of combined state, local, and federal funding (CDC, Division of STD Prevention, unpublished data, April 1994). State and local contributions, as a percentage of combined state, local, and federal funding in the respective area, ranged from 0 percent ($0) to 90 percent ($22.7 million). These estimates are sensitive to variability in how STD program funding is categorized in state and local government budgets. However, in order to provide a rough estimate of public investment in STD prevention (including STD treatment),[7] it is reasonable to use the estimated state and local contribution in 1994 ($125.6 million) and the actual CDC contribution to state and local STD programs in federal fiscal year 1995 ($91.8 million).

---

[7] The term "STD prevention," as used in this report, refers to all interventions, behavioral, curative, or otherwise, that are needed to reduce the spread of infection in a population. Therefore, the estimate provided here represents public funding for all these types of interventions. The formula used for estimating public investment in STD prevention is as follows: Public investment = the CDC contribution to states/local governments plus the CDC staff support funds plus the estimated state/local contribution. Therefore, total public investment in 1994 = $91.8 + $13.4 + $125.6 = $230.8 million.

Given the assumptions mentioned above, the total national public investment in STD prevention in fiscal year 1995 was approximately $230.8 million, and approximately $105.4 million was invested in biomedical and clinical research in STDs. Comparing these estimates to the estimated total costs of selected STDs, excluding AIDS ($9.954 billion), the total cost associated with STDs in the United States in 1994 was approximately 43 times the total national public investment in STD prevention and 94 times the total national investment in STD-related research (Figure 5-3). Again, it should be noted that the estimate of public investment in STD prevention and research does not include all publicly funded prevention or research programs that are related to STDs or STD-related programs funded by the private sector.[8] Similarly, the estimate of total costs for STDs does not include costs for all STDs. Even if the true public investment in STD prevention and research is several times higher than that estimated by the committee, the public investment would still be extremely low compared to the total costs of STDs in the United States.

Categorical Funding

Funding for state and local health departments comes from the CDC cooperative agreements and state and local governments. The legislative authority for the prevention of STDs in the United States stems from Section 318 of the Public Health Service Act, which authorizes the Department of Health and Human Services to make grants to and assist states, their political subdivisions, and public and nonprofit private entities for STD prevention research, demonstrations, public information and education programs, and training, education, and clinical skill improvement of health care providers. The Department of Health and Human Services is also authorized to make grants to states and their political subdivisions to carry out prevention programs. A list of prevention programs funded by the CDC's Division of STD Prevention in fiscal year 1996 is presented in Table 5-1.

The Preventive Health Amendments of 1992 modified Section 318 and authorized the CDC to make grants and provide assistance for activities to reduce STDs that can cause infertility in women. These amendments also authorized grants for the purpose of conducting research to improve the delivery of STD-related infertility prevention services.

Reimbursement for STD-related services in the private sector comes from

---

[8]For example, public investment in cervical cancer or hepatitis B prevention programs was not included because, as for many STDs that can be also transmitted by other means, it is not possible to determine the proportion of the program that is focused on prevention of sexually transmitted infections versus infections acquired by other means. In the case of hepatitis B, for example, vaccination programs are intended to prevent both sexually transmitted infections and nonsexually transmitted cases.

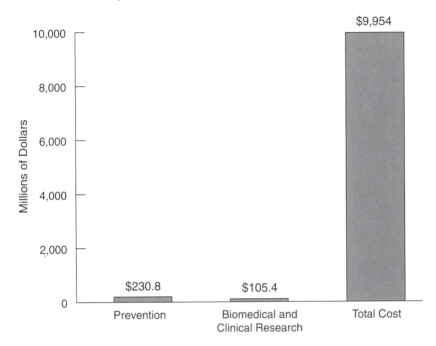

The estimated total costs associated with STDs were more than 43 and 94 times greater than the national public investment in STD prevention and research, respectively, in 1994

FIGURE 5-3 Comparison of estimated annual direct and indirect costs for selected STDs and their complications in 1994 versus national public investment in STD prevention and research in federal fiscal year 1995. NOTE: The estimate for investment in STD prevention provided here represents public funding for all interventions, behavioral, curative, or otherwise, that are needed to reduce the spread of infection in a population. SOURCES: Total cost of illness estimate was calculated by the IOM Committee on Prevention and Control of STDs; estimate of federal, state, and local investment in STD prevention was based on unpublished data from the CDC, Division of STD Prevention, 1996; and estimate of national investment in research was based on unpublished data from the National Institutes of Health, 1996.

third party reimbursement, such as private health insurance and Medicaid. STD-related care provided in community-based health facilities, such as family planning clinics and community health centers, receive federal and other support. Local health departments receive reimbursement for services provided by public STD clinics to persons with private insurance only to the extent allowed by law or under written contract.

TABLE 5-1 STD Prevention Programs Funded by the Division of STD Prevention, Centers for Disease Control and Prevention (CDC), Fiscal Year 1996

Program	Funding Level ($)
Preventive Health Services	
STD Accelerated Prevention Campaign	69,954,310
Prevention of Infertility Caused by STDs	9,798,309
Intra-agency Agreement: Office of Population Affairs and the CDC	1,700,000
The National AIDS, STD, and National Immunization Program Hotline	715,390
Intra-agency Agreement: Indian Health Service (IHS) and the CDC	325,000
Human Resources Development	
STD/HIV Prevention Training Centers	4,008,547
Public Health Graduate Training Certification Program	2,965,623
Sexually Transmitted Diseases Faculty Expansion Program	648,070
Association of Schools of Public Health (ASPH)	400,000
Association of Teachers of Preventive Medicine (ATPM)	22,500
Extramural Research and Demonstrations	
STD Accelerated Prevention Campaign Enhanced Projects	1,463,510
Research and Evaluation Issues in Prevention of Infertility Due to STDs	1,275,000
STD Accelerated Prevention Campaign: Enhanced Projects for STD Prevention in High-Risk Youth	1,025,188
Innovations in Syphilis Prevention in the United States: Reconsidering the Epidemiology and Involving Communities	1,000,000
Development and Feasibility Testing of Interventions to Increase Health-Seeking Behaviors in, and Health Care for, Populations at High Risk for Gonorrhea	750,000
STD APC Enhanced Projects: Jail STD Prevalence Monitoring	125,000
Total Program Funding	96,176,447

SOURCE: CDC, Division of STD Prevention. Unpublished data, October 1996.

Block Grant Proposals

Current proposals from the Department of Health and Human Services would consolidate many federal categorical programs into block grants that each state would allocate among competing health needs and among local public and private sector agencies. A Senate legislative proposal would consolidate and replace 12 CDC categorical programs with 1 or 2 block grants. The Department of Health and Human Services advocates consolidating these CDC programs into three new public health "Performance Partnership Grants," including one for HIV/AIDS, STD, and TB. Performance Partnership Grants are essentially block grants that require states to set health objectives in an interactive process with the Department of Health and Human Services, providing some federal oversight but few constraints on state policies, programs, or funding.

Arguments for Block Grants

Proponents of block grants argue that categorical funding has forced programmatic rigidity and excess administrative costs on local programs. Categorical funding, proponents of block grants argue, imposes a bureaucratic straitjacket on public health and safety-net programs, forcing local programs and services into one-size-fits-all national models, ignoring local conditions and slowing innovation. In addition to restraining innovation and modifications to meet local needs, grant applications for federal funding are time-consuming, imposing substantial administrative costs on local agencies. State allocation of block grant funds may simplify the application process.

Categorical funding also encourages narrowly defined programs even when it is logical to merge staff and services. For example, many states have kept HIV and STD prevention programs completely separate, although most observers acknowledge that it is logical to coordinate programs to prevent HIV infection and other STDs because they share common modes of transmission and risk groups and many common interventions. By measuring accountability in terms of the number of persons who receive a service or educational program, federal categorical funding encourages state and local agencies to keep programs separate.

Some observers believe that block grants will free local communities from the rigidity and administrative burdens of categorical funding. States, they argue, will allocate funds based on locally and professionally determined health and social needs and will be responsive to state and local conditions. Whereas categorical programs subordinate local needs to uniform federal requirements imposed by distant bureaucrats, block grant supporters believe state officials will allocate federal and state moneys guided by the technical assessments of state health agencies, the judgments of the public health professionals, and the views of local communities.

Arguments Against Block Grants

Opponents of consolidating STD funding into a block grant along with other public health programs believe that STDs will suffer in competition with less controversial public health problems or other state priorities. In the real world of allocating budgets and setting priorities, they are concerned that elected state officials will make funding decisions based more on political considerations than on assessments by public health professionals and agencies. STD programs traditionally have weak political constituencies and will suffer in competition with programs that have powerful constituencies. As discussed in Chapter 3, advocacy for STD funding has been traditionally weak because many patients infected with STDs are unaware of the infection, and those who are rarely want to disclose their infection in public, let alone organize public support for STD funding.

Opponents of block grants are particularly concerned that socially conservative interest groups will prevail in lobbying against STD programs at the state level. Allowing states to set funding allocations would also increase the already wide variability in STD programs among the states, because some states may seriously neglect STD programs. In addition, consolidating STD funding into a block grant may also result in the dissolution of the relatively weak constituency groups fighting for STD funding. The Coalition to Fight STDs, an alliance of more than 40 groups organized by the American Social Health Association, monitors public sector efforts against STDs and advocates at the national level for funding for STD prevention, treatment, and research. STD coalitions at the state or local level are rare, although they are emerging in some states, such as North Carolina, to improve STD funding.

Lastly, opponents suggest that past experience with other block grants may portend the fate of STD programs in a consolidated state grants program. For example, in 1981, the categorical Lead-Based Paint Poisoning prevention program was folded into the newly created Preventive Health and Health Services block grant, and the Urban Rodent Control program was folded into the new Maternal and Child Health block grant. These efforts lost funds in virtually all states after the federal categorical programs that funded these services were folded into the block grants. Both of these programs were widely viewed as federal "big-city" programs that found little support in state legislatures dominated by rural representation. Programs that had state support before the advent of federal categorical programs fared better than those that previously had little or no state funding (U.S. General Accounting Office, 1984; Peterson et al., 1986; Elling and Robins, 1991).

CONCLUSIONS

Current STD prevention services comprise several disjointed components, including provision of clinical services, disease surveillance and information collection activities, training and education of health care professionals, and funding of activities and programs. Although these components are largely publicly sponsored programs, they involve all levels of government and the private sector.

Dedicated public STD clinics have been instrumental in public efforts against STDs since they were established several decades ago. The quality and effectiveness of services delivered in these settings, however, are extremely variable and clearly need significant improvement. Until universal health care coverage is implemented in the United States, the function of public clinics as providers of care to the uninsured will need to be preserved. Unlike dedicated public STD clinics, community-based clinics and private health plans provide STD-related services in the context of primary care. However, the scope and quality of services provided in these environments are unknown. It is evident that clinical preventive services in both public and private health care settings need to be expanded and improved. Risk assessment and counseling to effect behavior change remain underutilized by primary care professionals, in part because the providers are poorly trained in their use.

Data regarding the scope and quality of STD-related services among managed care organizations and other health plans are limited, but data collected by the committee and other information suggest that, with several notable exceptions, even managed care organizations that serve high-risk populations are not providing comprehensive services to infected persons and their partners in a consistent manner. Most managed care organizations and other health plans do not currently give STDs sufficiently high priority. One of the more notable potential advantages of increasing the role of managed care organizations in providing STD-related services is the opportunity to increase accountability, particularly with the support of employers and other purchasers of health care. The traditional role of dedicated public STD clinics and some of the functions of public health agencies will likely change given the national trend towards managed care, especially the increasing enrollment of Medicaid beneficiaries into managed care plans. This change in the health care delivery environment is both an opportunity to improve services and a cause for concern that the "safety net" for essential public health services will be eroded.

Surveillance and information systems provide the basis for public health decision-making and function as the backbone for an effective system of STD prevention. An extensive system of data collection has been developed based on passive surveillance (with biases and incomplete data), sentinel surveys, and population-based surveys. However, specific improvements in these components are needed. Improvements are also needed in the current system for training and educating health professionals to deliver high-quality STD-related clinical services.

Even in an era of shrinking federal and state budgets, the current investment in STD prevention is extremely low when compared to the enormous economic consequences of these diseases. Proposals to consolidate federal funding for STD programs to the states in the form of block grants have serious flaws, given the lack of adequate accountability. The current system of categorical funding, however, needs to be substantially improved.

REFERENCES

Anderson JE, McCormick L, Fichtner R. Factors associated with self-reported STDs: data from a national survey. Sex Transm Dis 1994;21:303-8.

Armstrong K, Samost L, Bencivengo M. Integrating family planning services into drug treatment programs. In: Epidemiologic trends in drug abuse. Proceedings Community Epidemiology Work Group. Rockville, MD: National Institute on Drug Abuse, June 1992:548-59.

Aseltyne WJ, Cloutier M, Smith MD. HIV disease and managed care: an overview. J Acquir Immune Defic Syndr Hum Retrovirol 1995;8[Suppl 1]:S11-22.

ARHP, NANPRH (Association of Reproductive Health Professionals and National Association of Nurse Practitioners in Reproductive Health). STD counseling practices and needs survey: a national survey of primary care physicians and other health care providers. Conducted by Schulman, Ronca, and Bucuvalas, Inc., Silver Spring, MD. June 28, 1995.

Benson Gold R, Richards CL. Improving the fit. Reproductive health services in managed care settings. New York: Alan Guttmacher Institute, 1996.

Berg AO. The primary care physician and sexually transmitted diseases control. In: Holmes KK, Mårdh PA, Sparling PF, Wiesner PJ, Cates W Jr, Lemon SM, et al., eds. Sexually transmitted diseases. 2nd ed. New York: McGraw-Hill, Inc., 1990:1095-8.

Berg AO, Heidrich FE, Fihn SD, Bergman JJ, Wood RW, Stamm WE, et al. Establishing the cause of genitourinary symptoms in women in a family practice. Comparison of clinical examination and comprehensive microbiology. JAMA 1984;251:620-5.

Boekeloo BO, Marx ES, Kral AH, Coughlin SC, Bowman M, Rabin DL. Frequency and thoroughness of STD/HIV risk assessment by physicians in a high-risk metropolitan area. Am J Public Health 1991;81:1645-8.

Bowman MA, Russell NK, Boekeloo BO, Rafi IZ, Rabin DL. The effect of educational preparation on physician performance with a sexually transmitted disease-simulated patient. Arch Intern Med 1992;152:1823-8.

Braithwaite WR. Health information systems. Presentation delivered at the Conference on Strengthening Public Health Infrastructure, July 28, 1995, Chicago.

Brandt AM. No magic bullet: a social history of venereal disease in the United States since 1980. New York: Oxford University Press, Inc., 1985.

Carey TS, Weis K. Diagnostic testing and return visits for acute problems in prepaid, case-managed Medicaid plans compared to fee-for-service. Arch Intern Med 1990;150:2369-72.

CDC (Centers for Disease Control and Prevention). Sexually transmitted diseases. Clinical practice guidelines. Department of Health and Human Services, Public Health Service. Atlanta: Centers for Disease Control, May 1991.

CDC. 1993 Sexually transmitted diseases treatment guidelines. MMWR 1993;42(No. RR-14):56-66.

CDC. The future role of CDC field assignees. Internal memo from Dr. David Satcher, Director of CDC, May 25, 1995a.

CDC. Prevention and managed care: opportunities for managed care organizations, purchasers of health care, and public health agencies. MMWR 1995b;44:(No. RR-14):1-12.

CDC. Summary of notifiable diseases reporting, United States, 1994. MMWR 1995c;43:1-80.

CDC. Youth risk behavior surveillance—United States, 1993. MMWR 1995d;44:(No. SS-1).

CDC, DSTD/HIVP (Division of STD/HIV Prevention). Annual report 1991. U.S. Department of Health and Human Services, Public Health Service. Atlanta: Centers for Disease Control, 1992.

CDC, DSTD/HIVP. Annual report 1994. U.S. Department of Health and Human Services, Public Health Service. Atlanta: Centers for Disease Control and Prevention, 1995.

CDC, DSTDP (Division of STD Prevention). Sexually transmitted disease surveillance 1994. U.S. Department of Health and Human Services, Public Health Service. Atlanta: Centers for Disease Control and Prevention, 1995.

CDC, DSTDP. Guidance for requesting direct and financial assistance personnel. Draft document, October 1996.

Celum CL, Hook EW, Bolan GA, Spauding CD, Leone P, Henry KW, et al. Where would clients seek care for STD services under health care reform? Results of a STD client survey from five clinics. Eleventh Meeting of the International Society for STD Research, August 27-30, 1995; New Orleans, LA [abstract no. 101].

CSTE (Council of State and Territorial Epidemiologists). Blueprint for a national health surveillance system for the 21st century. Washington, D.C.: CSTE, May 1995.

County of Los Angeles Department of Health Services. Draft proposal of the agreement between the County of Los Angeles and plan. March 29, 1995.

Crump WJ, Pfeil T. A telemedicine primer. An introduction to the technology and an overview of the literature. Arch Fam Med 1995;4:796-803; discussion 804.

DeBuono BA, Zinner SH, Daamen M, McCormack WM. Sexual behavior of college women in 1975, 1986, and 1989. N Engl J Med 1990;322:821-5.

Delbanco S, Smith MD. Reproductive health and managed care—an overview. West J Med 1995;163[3 Suppl]:1-6.

Donovan P. Taking family planning services to hard-to-reach populations. Fam Plann Perspect 1996;28:120-6.

Elling RS, Robins LS. The politics of federalism and intergovernmental relations in health. In: Litman TJ, Robins LS, eds. Health politics and policy. Albany, NY: Delmar Publishers, 1991:200-5.

Fisher RS. Medicaid managed care: the next generation? Acad Med 1994;69:317-22.

Gemson DH, Colombotos J, Elinson J, Fordyce EJ, Hynes M, Stoneburner R. Acquired immunodeficiency syndrome prevention. Knowledge, attitudes, and practices of primary care physicians. Arch Intern Med 1991;151:1102-8.

GHAA (Group Health Association of America [currently American Association of Health Plans]). 1995 National directory of HMOs. Washington, D.C.: Group Health Association of America, 1995.

Halpern CT, Udry JR, Suchindran C. Effects of repeated questionnaire administration in longitudinal studies of adolescent males' sexual behavior. Arch Sex Behav 1994;23:41-57.

Hessol NA, Priddy FH, Bolan G, Baumrind N, Vittinghoff E, Reingold AL, et al. Management of pelvic inflammatory disease by primary care physicians: a comparison with Centers for Disease Control and Prevention Guidelines. Sex Transm Dis 1996;23;157-63.

Igoe, JB. A closer look: a preliminary report of some of the findings from the national survey of school nurses and school nurse supervisors. Denver: University of Colorado Health Sciences Center, Office of School Health, 1994.

IOM (Institute of Medicine). For-profit enterprise in health care. Gray BH, ed. Washington, D.C.: National Academy Press, 1986.

IOM. Primary care: America's health in a new era. Donaldson MS, Yordy KD, Lohr KN, Vanselow NA, eds. Washington, DC: National Academy Press, 1996a.

IOM. Telemedicine. A guide to assessing telecommunications in health care. Field MJ, ed. Washington, DC: National Academy Press, 1996b.

IOM. Using performance monitoring to improve community health: exploring the issues. Workshop summary. Durch JS, ed. Washington, D.C.: National Academy Press, 1996c.

Johnson R, Lee F, Hadgu A, McQuillan G, Aral S, Keesling S, et al. U.S. genital herpes trends during the first decade of AIDS—prevalences increased in young whites and elevated in blacks. Proceedings of the Tenth Meeting of the International Society for STD Research, August 29-September 1, 1993, Helsinki [abstract no. 22].

The Kaiser Commission on the Future of Medicaid. Medicaid and managed care: lessons from the literature. Menlo Park, CA: The Henry J. Kaiser Family Foundation, 1995.

Kampmeier RH. The national commission on venereal disease. J Am Vener Dis Assoc 1975;1:99-104.

Kassler WJ, Zenilman JM, Erickson B, Fox R, Peterman TA, Hook EW 3rd. Seroconversion in patients attending sexually transmitted disease clinics. AIDS 1994;8:351-5.

Keeling RP. College health responds to HIV; hard lessons and a rich heritage. J Am Coll Health 1995;43:271-2.

Ku L, Sonenstein FL, Pleck JH. Patterns of HIV risk and preventive behaviors among teenage men. Public Health Rep 1992;107:131-8.

Laumann EO, Gagnon JH, Michael RT, Michaels S. The social organization of sexuality: sexual practices in the United States. Chicago, IL: University of Chicago Press, 1994.

Leavy Small M, Smith Majer L, Allensworth DD, Farquhar BD, Kann L, Pateman BC. School health services. J Sch Health 1995;65:319-26.

Lewis CE, Freeman HE. The sexual history-taking and counseling practices of primary care physicians. West J Med 1987;147:165-7.

Lewis CE, Freeman HE, Corey CR. AIDS-related competence of California's primary care physicians. Am J Public Health 1987;77:795-9.

MacKay HT, Toomey KE, Schmid GP. Survey of clinical training in STD and HIV/AIDS in the United States. Proceedings of the IDSA Annual Meeting; September 16-18, 1995, San Francisco [abstract no. 281].

Marcus AC, Crane LA, Kaplan CP, Goodman KJ, Savage E, Gunning J. Screening for cervical cancer in emergency centers and sexually transmitted disease clinics. Obstet Gynecol 1990;75:453-5.

McLean DA. A model for HIV risk reduction and prevention among African American college students. J Am Coll Health 1994;42:220-3.

McQuillan GM, Khare M, Ezzati Rice TM, Karon JM, Schable CA, Murphy RS. The seroepidemiology of human immunodeficiency virus in the United States household population: NHANES III, 1988-1991. J Acquir Immune Defic Syndr 1994;7:1195-201.

McQuillan GM, Townsend TR, Fields HA, Carroll M, Leahy M, Polk BF. Seroepidemiology of hepatitis B virus infection in the United States. 1976 to 1980. Am J Med 1989;87:5S-10S.

NCQA (National Committee for Quality Assurance), Committee on Performance Measurement. HEDIS 3.0 Draft for Public Comment, Washington, D.C.: National Committee for Quality Assurance, July 1996.

Noegel R, Kirby J, Schrader M, Wasserheit J. Sexually transmitted disease accelerated prevention campaigns. Opportunities to expand prevention efforts in the United States. Sex Transm Dis 1993;20:118-9.

Peterson GE, Bovbjerg RR, Davis BA, Davis WG, Durman EC, Gullo TA. The Reagan block grants: what have we learned? Washington, D.C.: The Urban Institute, 1986.

Rabin DL, Boekeloo BO, Marx ES, Bowman MA, Russell NK, Gonzalez Willis A. Improving office-based physicians' prevention practices for sexually transmitted diseases. Ann Intern Med 1994;121:513-9.

Reinisch JM, Hill CA, Sanders S, Ziemba-Davis M. High-risk sexual behavior at a Midwestern university: A confirmatory study. Fam Plann Perspect 1995;27:79-82.

Ross PE, Landis SE. Development and evaluation of a sexual history-taking curriculum for first- and second-year family practice residents. Fam Med 1994;26:293-8.

Roter DL, Knowles N, Somerfield M, Baldwin J. Routine communication in sexually transmitted disease clinics: an observational study. Am J Public Health 1990;80:605-6.

Russell NK, Boekeloo BO, Rafi IZ, Rabin DL. Unannounced simulated patients' observations of physician STD/HIV prevention practices. Am J Prev Med 1992;8:235-40.

Schlitt JJ, Rickett KD, Montgomery LL, Lear JG. State initiatives to support school-based health centers: a national survey. J Adolesc Health 1995;17:68-76.

Scholes D, Stergachis A, Heidrich FE, Andrilla H, Holmes KK, Stamm WE. Prevention of pelvic inflammatory disease by screening for cervical chlamydial infection. New Engl J Med 1996;334:1362-6.

SFPA (State Family Planning Administrators). Family planning clinic provision of STD and HIV services: national questionnaire findings. Seattle, WA, February 1991.

Stamm WE, Kaetz SK, Holmes KK. Clinical training in venereology in the United States and Canada. JAMA 1982;248:2020-4.

Stein ZA. Editorial: family planning, sexually transmitted diseases, and prevention of AIDS—divided we fail? Am J Public Health 1996;86:783-4.

Steinberg JK, Wellman J, Melrod J. A proposal for strengthening medical school training in STD prevention techniques. Public Health Rep 1991;106:196-202.

Turner JC, Garrison CZ, Korpita E, Waller J, Addy C, Hill WR, et al. Promoting responsible sexual behavior through a college freshman seminar. AIDS Educ Prev 1994;6:266-77.

Upchurch DM, Farmer MY, Glasser D, Hook EW. Contraceptive needs and practices among women attending an inner-city STD clinic. Am J Public Health 1987;77:1427-30.

U.S. General Accounting Office. Maternal and child health block grant: program changes emerging under state administration. Washington, D.C.: General Accounting Office, 1984.

Weinstock HS, Sidhu J, Gwinn M, Karon J, Petersen LR. Trends in HIV seroprevalence among persons attending sexually transmitted disease clinics in the United States, 1988-1992. J Acquir Immune Defic Syndr Hum Retrovirol 1995;9:514-22.

Winkenwerder W, Levy B, Eisenberg JM, Williams SV, Young MJ, Hershey JC. Variation in physicians' decision-making thresholds in management of a sexually transmitted disease. J Gen Intern Med 1993;8:369-73.

Work Group on Sexually Transmitted Disease. Conference on preventing disease/promoting health—objectives for the nation: sexually transmissible diseases. Sex Transm Dis 1979;6:273-7.

Zabin LS, Stark HA, Emerson MR. Reasons for delay in contraceptive clinic utilization. Adolescent clinic and nonclinic populations compared. J Adolesc Health 1991;12:225-32.

Zenilman JM, Hook EW 3rd, Shepherd M, Smith P, Rompalo AM, Celentano DD. Alcohol and other substance use in STD clinic patients: relationships with STDs and prevalent HIV infection. Sex Transm Dis 1994;21:220-5.

Zimmerman DJ, Reif CJ. School-based health centers and managed care health plans: partners in primary care. J Public Health Manage Pract 1995;1:33-9.

6

Establishing an Effective National System to Prevent Stds

The committee concludes that prevention of Stds is technically feasible today in the United States, but an effective national system for STD prevention currently does not exist, and, as a result, Stds are a severe health burden in the United States. Many components of an effective system for STD prevention (described in Chapters 4 and 5), such as a surveillance system to measure STD incidence, public and private sector clinical services, and public education programs, exist in many areas in various stages of development, but these and other components are neither adequate nor coordinated locally, statewide, or nationally.

As outlined in the previous chapters, the current strategy for preventing Stds is based primarily on categorical STD programs run by state and local health departments with guidance and funding from the CDC. Other federal agencies, including the U.S. Department of Justice (Bureau of Prisons), the Agency for Health Care Policy and Research, the Food and Drug Administration, the Health Care Financing Administration, the Health Services and Resources Administration, the Indian Health Service, the National Institutes of Health, the Office of Population Affairs (Department of Health and Human Services), and the Substance Abuse and Mental Health Services Administration, also provide or support STD-related services or research, as do their state and local counterparts.

Public health agencies, private practitioners and medical groups, and community-based clinics all provide STD-related services, but many providers work in relative isolation. Dedicated public STD clinics, family planning clinics, and other community-based clinics serve the uninsured and other populations at high risk for Stds, but often do not coordinate their services. Publicly sponsored STD programs consider containment of STDs to be their primary mission, but collaborate with other public sector health programs infrequently and even less often with private sector health programs. Federal demonstration projects to prevent infertility associated with chlamydial and gonococcal infections, however, are beginning to improve service coordination among family planning clinics, dedicated public STD clinics, and public sector laboratories. In addition, private sector health care professionals often do not recognize the importance of their role in preventing STDs.

The lack of an effective system is particularly acute for noncurative prevention programs for STDs, which are far less developed than programs for curative services. In addition, despite the interrelationship between STDs, HIV infection, unintended pregnancy, and cancer, prevention programs for these health conditions are typically neither integrated nor coordinated.

The fragmented system of STD-related services directly hinders effective prevention of STDs in many ways. For example, as described in Chapter 5, the national surveillance system collects information regarding reportable STDs among persons who use public STD clinics and community-based services. However, information about the privately insured population is incomplete because many private clinicians do not report STD cases and some cases are presumptively treated. Without a comprehensive system for surveillance that involves all potential caregivers for STDs, it is difficult to accurately monitor disease trends or effectiveness of interventions.

A fragmented system of clinical services can result in lapses in coverage and ineffective treatment. As documented in Chapter 5, STD-related clinical care is provided by a variety of clinicians in many settings, and the training of these clinicians, including physicians, in diagnosis, treatment, and prevention of STDs is inadequate. Despite the growing role of private sector primary health care professionals in delivering services, there are large gaps in health professional school training and continuing education regarding STD-related skills. Inadequate training and poor awareness of STDs perpetuates the lack of involvement in prevention activities, such as evaluation and treatment of sex partners, by health plans and private practice clinicians. Inadequate training and poor awareness of STDs among health care professionals also result in clinicians who may fail to diagnose and treat STDs or do not have the skills or confidence to promote behavior change in their patients. The failure to adequately diagnose and treat STDs or become involved in certain prevention activities, therefore, leads to lost clinical opportunities to prevent STDs, and thus, to incomplete or fragmented clinical services.

As discussed in Chapter 5, because health plans do not assume responsibility for those who are not plan members, there is no assurance that sex partners of infected plan members will receive appropriate evaluation and treatment. In prisons and jails, prisoners may be screened and found to be positive for an STD, but may be released before treatment is given. Without linkages to community providers, their infections will likely go untreated and spread to others in the community at large. As a final example, a fragmented system of information and educational services for STDs can result in inadequate awareness and misperceptions of risk. Data presented in Chapters 3 and 4 show that awareness of STDs in the United States is low and misperceptions of risk are common, even among those at highest risk for STDs. This is likely a result of the lack of open public education about STDs and the failure of the mass media to provide accurate information regarding the consequences of high-risk sexual behavior.

To develop an effective system for STD prevention, many existing programs need to be redesigned and improved through innovative approaches and closer collaboration. In addition, new programs and initiatives that address important gaps in the current fragmented system of prevention services need to be designed and implemented. In this chapter, the committee proposes an effective national system of STD prevention that can be developed from the currently fragmented set of services and funding streams for STDs. Unless otherwise indicated, the background and support for the committee's strategic plan for reducing the adverse health and economic impact of STDs in the United States are found in Chapters 2 through 5.

LAYING THE FOUNDATION FOR A NATIONAL SYSTEM

In formulating a national strategy to prevent STDs, the committee developed the following vision statement and principles to guide its deliberations (Box 6-1). To realize this vision, the committee recommends that:

• **An effective national system for STD prevention be established in the United States.**

The committee uses the word "system" to describe an interacting or independent group of services and organizations that function as a whole. By an "effective" system, the committee means a system that is coherent, comprehensive, and coordinated. A coherent system is founded on a clear strategy for prevention that ensures that the components of the system are logically consistent and synergistic. A comprehensive system fully utilizes all types of relevant approaches and effective interventions. A coordinated system ensures that the components of the system relate to each other in order to maximize efficiency and effectiveness. By a "national" system, the committee means a system that is based on a national policy coordinated at all levels and composed of local, state, and national (including federal) programs. A nationally coordinated system is necessary because STDs are a threat to the nation's health and do not recognize geographic borders. In addition, many interventions are most effectively or efficiently developed and implemented at the national level. It is expected that state and local systems will be developed and implemented concurrently and coordinated at all levels. Coordination of interventions for HIV infection and other STDs, in particular, is an important aspect of an effective national system.

An effective national system for STD prevention should: (a) provide comprehensive curative and noncurative preventive services; (b) provide STD-related services in the context of primary care; (c) coordinate public and private sector services; (d) coordinate local, state, and federal programs; and (e) ensure universal access to STD-related services for all persons in the United States. The committee proposes a model for carrying out the functions of a national system for prevention in the context of community and individual roles and responsibilities in Figure 6-1.

In the context of the model, the term "community" refers to all persons and entities that have a potential role in STD prevention besides the individual. The committee's model is based on the recognition that both individuals and the community have a role and responsibilities in preventing STDs. In some cases, such as reducing high-risk behaviors, the degree of individual responsibility may exceed that of the community. Even then, however, the community plays a role in setting social norms and providing the knowledge and resources needed for behavior change to occur. In other cases, such as ensuring access to health care, the community's responsibility is clearly greater. Many responsibilities and functions are best shared; many overlap and are related; and some will likely change as the system evolves or as conditions warrant. In addition, responsibilities for specific functions need to be tailored to the local community environment. In the case of STDs, the committee believes that communities have a special responsibility to become involved because STDs and other communicable diseases threaten the health of the community at large, not just the infected individual. In addition, many of the underlying factors that contribute to the STD epidemic, such as lack of awareness, lack of access to health care, and unbalanced messages regarding sexual behavior, are most effectively addressed through community-based interventions.

The committee believes that it is inappropriate to advocate that the STD epidemic be solved by individuals without the support of community interventions. It is the community's responsibility to provide individuals with the support, information, and tools that are needed to prevent STDs. Many factors that are often beyond the control of the individual, especially sociocultural factors, directly influence individual behavior and risk of STDs (Wasserheit, 1994).

It has been proposed that the various biomedical and behavioral health professionals currently involved in STD prevention, including clinicians, epidemiologists, public health workers, microbiologists, psychologists, and social scientists, develop and participate in interdisciplinary approaches to prevention (Sparling and Aral, 1991). The committee proposes that an even wider range of individuals and institutions is needed. In addition to the professionals mentioned above, health plans, pharmaceutical and medical device companies, educators, and other individuals and entities that have not traditionally been involved in

---

BOX 6-1
Vision and Guiding Principles for a National System for STD Prevention

Vision
An effective system of services and information that supports individuals, families, and communities in preventing STDs including HIV infection, and ensures comprehensive, high-quality STD-related health services for all persons

Guiding Principles

Prevention
STDs can be prevented by implementing individual- and population-based interventions that:
• decrease exposure to infected persons by delaying sexual intercourse among adolescents and by reducing the prevalence of high-risk sexual behaviors;
• decrease the probability of STD transmission during sexual intercourse by promoting the use of barrier methods, especially condoms; and
• decrease the duration of infection by improving knowledge and promoting awareness of STDs and their consequences; promoting utilization of health care services for symptoms of STDs; encouraging early detection and effective treatment; and ensuring access to essential clinical services.

Responsibility
In an effective system for STD prevention:
• individuals and the community share responsibility for prevention;
• the community has a responsibility to promote social norms that encourage

---

STD prevention should also become involved. These include mass media companies, social service agencies, employers and businesses, labor unions, religious organizations, and other community-based organizations. A list of potential stakeholders in the community envisioned in the model system is presented in Table 6-1. Given the wide spectrum of stakeholders in STD prevention, the committee advocates a substantial emphasis on coordination and collaboration (IOM, 1996a).

The committee's proposed system is founded on the simple infectious disease prevention model of (a) preventing exposure to infection, (b) preventing acquisition of infection when exposed, and (c) preventing transmission to others once infected. In this system, there are multiple points at which to intervene and multiple approaches or interventions at both the individual and the community levels. Programs that focus only on preventing exposure, acquisition, or transmission are unlikely to succeed because no single intervention is totally effective in isolation. Although existing interventions are not perfect, they can have an additive impact in reducing the risk of STDs in the population (Cates, 1996). There-

healthy sexual behaviors and to provide access to education, services, and resources that enable individuals to adopt these behaviors;
- individuals must have the necessary knowledge, skills, and resources to practice healthy behaviors in order to assume full responsibility for their health; and
- the public sector is ultimately responsible for preventing transmission of communicable diseases in the population.

Implementation/Operational Issues
An effective system for STD prevention should have:
- strong leadership;
- integrated and coordinated components;
- programs for monitoring access and performance and for ensuring quality of services;
- comprehensive educational programs for all persons;
- interventions that are multisectoral (e.g., involve both private and public sectors in health, education, and other sectors), multidisciplinary (e.g., involve health professionals from various disciplines as well as nonhealth professionals), and multifaceted (e.g., involve coordinated behavioral and biomedical approaches); and
- partnerships among the various stakeholders in the community.

Access and Financing
An effective system for STD prevention should have:
- curative and other preventive services that are confidential, comprehensive, of high quality, and accessible to all, particularly the uninsured, adolescents, and disenfranchised groups;
- no financial disincentives for accessing essential services, especially those that have a potential impact on the spread of disease; and
- adequate and reliable funding.

fore, resources committed to multiple intervention points are necessary. An effective system must have both behavioral and biomedical approaches that are complementary and intertwined. Biomedical interventions may be ineffective without behavioral components to support them, and behavioral approaches must incorporate biomedical tools for prevention.

The committee's model is consistent with the multifaceted, holistic approaches for STD and HIV prevention previously advocated by several experts in STDs (Sparling and Aral, 1991; Wasserheit, 1994; Stryker et al., 1995; Cates, 1996). Similar approaches cited in Chapter 4, such as Wisconsin's comprehensive chlamydia prevention program, have been successful. While primarily a screening program, this initiative included public-private partnerships, leadership from legislators, expanded laboratory services, expanded screening in family planning and STD clinics, education of health care professionals, and integrated information systems. Another example of a successful multifaceted program implemented on a national level is the Thai "100% Condom Program" as de-

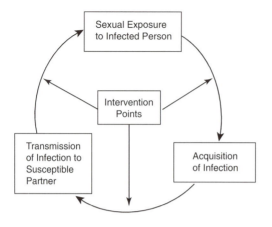

FIGURE 6-1 A model for community and individual roles and responsibilities in STD prevention.

Roles and Responsibilities of:	
Community	**Individuals**
Promote healthy behaviors • promote delay in onset of sexual intercourse for adolescents • promote safer sex behaviors • promote use of and increase access to barrier methods (e.g., condoms) **Increase public awareness and knowledge of STDs and their symptoms and consequences** • reduce unbalanced mass media messages • provide health information and access to resources • promote health-care-seeking behavior for symptoms of STDs **Reduce prevalence of contributing social factors and other barriers to STD prevention** • reduce substance use, sexual abuse, and other contributing factors • address fundamental social problems **Reduce prevalence of sexually transmitted infections in population** • reduce prevalence in "core" transmission groups • screen and treat high-risk groups • conduct partner notification and follow-up treatment • improve vaccination coverage for STDs (i.e., hepatitis B vaccine) **Improve access to health care** • provide universal access • develop capacity to deliver care • minimize barriers to care • promote early health-seeking behavior **Improve diagnosis and treatment of STDs** • improve diagnostic test characteristics • provide laboratory services • develop new treatments and improve existing treatments • improve training of health professionals **Improve effectiveness and access to essential biomedical interventions for STDs** • improve effectiveness of barrier methods • develop and implement vaccines and other biomedical interventions **Improve the knowledge base** • improve surveillance and information systems • improve behavioral and biomedical research	**Avoid high-risk behavior** • seek health information • delay onset of sexual intercourse • reduce number of partners • avoid high-risk sexual practices • avoid high-risk partners • avoid drug and other substance use • use condoms consistently and other barrier methods and microbicides as appropriate **Seek medical care promptly for symptoms of STDs** **Reduce likelihood of infecting partners** • assist in partner notification and follow-up • avoid sexual intercourse until cured

TABLE 6-1   Potential Community Stakeholders in STD Prevention

Academic Health Centers
Schools of medicine, dentistry, nursing, pharmacy, public health, allied health, and related other health-disciplines

Biomedical and Social Science Researchers
Universities; private industry; government agencies

Biomedical Industry
Pharmaceutical, biotechnology, and medical device companies

Businesses and Organized Labor
Small businesses; corporations; labor unions

Clinical Laboratories
Public sector laboratories; hospital and private laboratories

Community-Based Organizations
Voluntary organizations; churches, synagogues, and other religious organizations; private social service agencies and programs for women, children, runaways, homeless, migrants

Government Agencies and Programs
Federal agencies (e.g., AHCPR, CDC, FDA, HCFA, HRSA, IHS, NIH, SAMSHA, Department of Justice); state and local health departments; government social service agencies and programs for special populations (e.g., women, children, runaways, homeless, migrants)

Health Care Professionals and Organizations
Physicians, nurses, pharmacists and other health care professionals; managed care organizations and other health plans; hospitals (emergency rooms); community health centers; health professional

organizations, including medical societies and member organizations

Health Programs for High-Risk Populations
Juvenile detention health services; jail and prison health services; drug and alcohol treatment programs; migrant health programs; health programs for the homeless

Individuals and Families

Mass Media
Television; radio; print and electronic media; commercial sponsors and advertisers

Policymakers
Federal, state, and local legislators; government health agency leaders; private health care sector leaders

Private Foundations

Purchasers of Health Services
Private employers; government employee benefits groups; purchasing coalitions; Medicaid and other publicly sponsored programs

School-Based Programs
K–12 school-based programs; educators; school administrators; school boards; college and university health services

STD-Related Programs and Clinics
Dedicated public STD clinics; family planning clinics, prenatal clinics, HIV clinics

scribed in Chapter 4. With a mass media advertising campaign to change risky sexual behaviors, increased access to condoms, and environmental interventions, this initiative seemed to be highly successful because it involved high-level government and community leaders, different sectors of government (e.g., health, education, and law enforcement agencies), and businesses (owners of commercial sex establishments). Coupled with programs to provide STD-related services, this initiative led to substantial positive behavior change among young men, and the incidence of HIV infections declined.

Formulating a National Policy and Strategy

A national system for STD prevention must be based on sound national policy and a coherent strategy. Currently, a comprehensive national policy regarding STD prevention does not exist. The elements of a national strategy to prevent bacterial STDs are more fully developed than those needed to prevent viral STDs, for which a national strategy for prevention is not well articulated. Furthermore, a national strategy to prevent STD risk behaviors has not been developed. Since almost all sexually transmitted pathogens that infect people do not have animal reservoirs, many STDs can theoretically be eradicated. Although this goal is probably not attainable in the near future for many STDs, it may be an appropriate intermediate-term goal for some STDs. For example, Sweden has virtually eliminated transmission of three major STDs (syphilis, gonorrhea, and chancroid) among the native population, and several U.S. states have reduced transmission of syphilis and chancroid to very low levels. The committee believes that elimination of ongoing transmission of syphilis within the United States is an attainable goal that should now be attempted.

To establish a national system for STD prevention, the committee recommends four major strategies for public and private sector policymakers at the local, state, and national levels:

1. Overcome barriers to adoption of healthy sexual behaviors.
2. Develop strong leadership, strengthen investment, and improve information systems for STD prevention.
3. Design and implement essential STD-related services in innovative ways for adolescents and underserved populations.
4. Ensure access to and quality of essential clinical services for STDs.

The establishment of an effective national system for STD prevention and implementation of these strategies is a difficult, long-term process that involves intermediary steps. Efforts consistent with these strategies should be initiated immediately and concurrently. The committee suggests that the Department of Health and Human Services consider the goals and strategies outlined in this report in developing and updating its national health objectives (e.g., Healthy People 2000) related to STDs.

In the committee's strategic plan for an effective national system for STD prevention, four strategies and a number of tactics are presented. Because of the comprehensive nature of the committee's approach, implementation of all the recommended tactics may seem daunting to some communities. While the committee believes that each component of the national system identified in its deliberations is essential to preventing STDs, it recognizes that not all communities will be able to, or need to, implement every tactic described in this chapter. In addition, it is likely that many communities will need to adapt some of the committee's recommendations to maximize their effectiveness under local conditions. The committee purposely has not prioritized the recommendations in this report because it believes that this process should be locally driven. Which interventions are most effective for a particular community will vary depending on the local epidemiology of STDs, the status of STD-related services, and the prevalence of STD risk behaviors. For example, in areas where rates of STDs and risky behaviors are low and access to clinical services for STDs is problematic, improving training of and access to primary care providers and interventions to maintain low rates of risky behaviors may be emphasized. In contrast, in communities where rates of STDs and risky behaviors are high, outreach to health plans, improving public STD clinics, and community-based behavioral interventions may be priorities. The committee proposes that the local health department and community representatives collaboratively prioritize the recommended tactics in this chapter.

The committee's recommendations for accomplishing its vision for STD prevention are presented in the remainder of this chapter. Before turning to these recommendations, however, the committee first discusses and makes recommendations about two important concepts that need to be considered in formulating a national strategy for STD prevention: the impact of STDs on HIV transmission and the impact of STDs on cancer.

Recognizing the Impact of STDs on HIV Transmission

Studies cited in Chapter 2 show that STDs increase the risk of HIV acquisition and transmission. Individuals infected with an STD are more likely to acquire HIV infection when exposed, and individuals coinfected with HIV and another STD are more likely to transmit HIV to their sex partners. Mathematical models and epidemiologic and biologic data collectively provide strong evidence that improved prevention of STDs would reduce sexual transmission of HIV in this country. A major study has shown that improved management of STDs through extensive training of primary health workers, ensuring treatment for STDs, and promoting health-seeking behavior for STDs can significantly reduce the incidence of HIV infection in communities (Grosskurth et al., 1995). Although initial studies documenting the impact of STD prevention on HIV transmission have been conducted in other countries, current estimates suggest that a large proportion of heterosexually transmitted HIV infections could be prevented by reducing the prevalence of STDs in the United States.

The interrelationship between HIV infection and other STDs is clearly documented and supports the concept that prevention of other STDs should be an essential component of HIV prevention programs. As discussed in Chapters 2 and 3, many of the populations at high risk for STDs are also at high risk for HIV infection. Interventions designed to increase awareness of HIV infection or other STDs and to reduce high-risk sexual behavior (such as condom promotion) are likely to have a positive impact on prevention of both HIV infection and other STDs. Therefore, programs for HIV and STD prevention, especially those focused on similar populations, need to be coordinated to maximize the effectiveness and efficiency of both intervention efforts. Educational programs for HIV prevention should disseminate information related to other STDs without making the message too diffuse. Examples of public messages that may not be widely known include: (a) HIV infection is not the only STD with serious health consequences, (b) other STDs increase the risk for HIV infection, (c) condoms and safer sex behaviors prevent both HIV infection and other STDs, (d) the cardinal signs of STDs (e.g., genital sores or discharge or pelvic pain in women), and (e) prompt treatment for STDs prevents complications. Similarly, STD and HIV surveillance systems and research studies need to improve monitoring and assessment of the impact of interventions on both HIV infection and other STDs. For example, population-based serosurveys for HIV infection should also include testing for other STDs, and both HIV and other STD infection rates should be used as outcome measures when evaluating effectiveness of interventions as appropriate. The committee also believes that greater access to STD-related services in clinical HIV programs could reduce sexual transmission of HIV.

During the past several years, far more attention has been given to developing HIV prevention than to other STD prevention programs. The strong interest in HIV prevention is justified, but inadequately addresses the prevention of other STDs. HIV prevention programs should support the incorporation of STD prevention activities into HIV prevention efforts. It is important to integrate and coordinate STD and HIV prevention activities without weakening either effort. The intent of the committee is not to divert resources away from HIV prevention efforts to prevention of other STDs, but rather to increase investment in prevention of all STDs.

Therefore, the committee makes the following recommendation:

• **Improved prevention of STDs should be an essential component of a national strategy for preventing sexually transmitted HIV infection.** As part of this effort, federal, state, and local health agencies should review current HIV and STD programs and should coordinate STD and HIV activities related to health education and prevention, clinical services, surveillance, and research and evaluation that focus on similar populations. The Health Resources and Services Administration and the CDC should develop financial incentives for communities to demonstrate coordination of STD- and HIV-related services. At a minimum, health agencies should ensure that:

1. educational activities for STD and HIV prevention focused on similar populations include information on both HIV infection and other STDs;
2. HIV prevention programs incorporate STD prevention activities and commit necessary resources to improve these activities;
3. program managers of STD- and HIV-related programs develop a formal mechanism for regular communication and for coordinating program planning, implementation, and evaluation;
4. STD and HIV program staff are educated regarding the relationship between STDs and HIV transmission;
5. clinicians are educated about the importance of early diagnosis and treatment of STDs to reduce the risk of sexually transmitted HIV infection;
6. public STD and HIV clinics, including HIV testing and counseling sites, provide both STD- and HIV-related clinical services to the extent appropriate for the clinical setting;
7. HIV and STD surveillance and data collection activities gather information on both HIV and other STDs when appropriate;
8. epidemiological, behavioral, and biomedical studies examine the relationship between HIV infection and other STDs;
9. evaluations of STD and HIV interventions examine the impact of the interventions on both HIV infection and other STDs; and
10. HIV/AIDS clinical programs in health plans are encouraged to provide clinical services for other STDs, and HIV prevention programs in health plans also provide interventions for other STDs.

Recognizing the Impact of STDs on Cancer

Several cancers, including cervical, liver, and other cancers, are associated with sexually transmitted infections that are typically acquired during adolescence or early adulthood. The association between STDs and cancer supports the incorporation of STD prevention information, especially information regarding human papillomavirus and hepatitis B virus infection, into appropriate cancer prevention programs. Specific strategies now available for preventing STD-associated cancers that should be expanded include behavioral interventions to prevent risky sexual behaviors, Pap smears for early detection of cervical cancer in women not currently reached by existing programs, and hepatitis B vaccination. Supporting STD prevention as a strategy for preventing cancer is indicated because many STD-related cancers are not curable and are potentially fatal. In addition, preventing and treating STDs is less costly than treatment for cancer.

The role of STDs in cervical, liver, and other cancers is not well recognized by health professionals and the public, and information regarding this link needs to be disseminated widely.

Therefore, the committee makes the following recommendation:

• **Government agencies and private organizations concerned with cancer prevention should support STD prevention activities as an important strategy for prevention of STD-related cancers.** Agencies and organizations that fund research and other activities in cancer prevention (e.g., the National Cancer Institute at the National Institutes of Health, the American Cancer Society) should support biomedical and prevention-oriented research and programs related to STDs, and they should expand their public education efforts to include prevention of STDs as a means of preventing cervical, liver, and other STD-related cancers. As with the prevention of many cancers, prevention efforts for STD-related cancers should focus on the challenge of linking behaviors initiated during adolescence and young adulthood with health consequences that manifest much later in life.

The committee's discussion of, and recommended tactics for implementing, its four strategies for establishing a national system for STD prevention are now presented.

STRATEGY 1: PROMOTE HEALTHY SEXUAL BEHAVIORS

Strategy 1 is to overcome barriers to adoption of healthy sexual behaviors. Barriers to effective STD prevention efforts include biological, social, and structural factors. Biological factors reviewed in Chapters 2 and 3 include preexisting or concurrent STDs, the impact of asymptomatic infections, the long lag time to clinical complications, increased susceptibility of women and female adolescents to sexually transmitted pathogens, lack of curative treatment for viral STDs, lack of vaccines against most STDs, and immunological factors. Many of these factors are difficult to alter. In addition, some social factors, such as poverty, inadequate access to health care, substance use, sexual abuse, and violence, are enormously complex issues, with solutions beyond the scope of this committee. However, the committee believes that the major social factor that contributes to the STD epidemic—the reluctance of American society to openly confront issues regarding sexuality and STDs—can eventually be overcome by a concerted long-term national effort. This issue is a major focus of Strategy 1. Tactics for addressing structural factors, such as the organization of clinical services, are described under Strategy 4.

Under Strategy 1, the committee recommends that (a) a new social norm of healthy sexual behavior be established, (b) knowledge and awareness of STDs be increased; (c) the mass media assist in efforts to reduce risky sexual behaviors;

(d) clinicians and others be trained to address sexual health issues; and (e) research regarding sexual health behaviors be supported.

Catalyzing Change Through Open Discussion

A new social norm of healthy sexual behavior should be the basis for long-term prevention of STDs. This is because, as discussed in Chapter 4, in one way or another, all interventions to prevent STDs are partly dependent on, and must be integrated with, healthy behaviors. Despite the progress made in improving awareness of protective behaviors as a result of HIV prevention efforts in recent years, there is still a substantial gap between current practices and the desired social norm of healthy sexual behavior.

The committee expects that the definition of "healthy sexual behavior" and its interpretation will vary substantially among individuals and communities. The National Commission on Adolescent Sexual Health has identified the characteristics and behaviors of a "sexually healthy adolescent" in the context of the adolescent's relationship to self, parents and other family members, peers, and romantic partners (NCASH, 1995). The committee believes that many of the attributes and characteristics of a "sexually healthy adolescent" that are described in this consensus statement, which has been endorsed by 48 national organizations, also are relevant in considering the parameters and components of a social norm of healthy sexual behavior for adults.

It is clear that a new social norm regarding healthy sexual behavior is a long-term goal, and cannot occur without intermediate steps and bold initiatives. In order for societal norms regarding sexual behavior to change, open discussion of and access to information regarding sexual behaviors, their health consequences, and methods for protecting against STDs must occur. These issues need to be openly discussed in both private (between partners and among families) and in public arenas. Open discussion is important because history has shown that moralistic approaches against STDs, including censorship, have hindered the ability of public health officials and programs to successfully prevent these diseases. The means to achieve a new norm of healthy sexual behavior include mass media interventions, school-based programs, and population- and individual-based interventions. The committee makes specific recommendations regarding these efforts later in this chapter. In Chapter 3, the committee showed how constraints on acknowledging and discussing issues related to sexuality impede sexuality education programs for adolescents, hinder communication regarding protective behaviors between sex partners, promote misleading messages from mass media, and hamper education and counseling activities of health care professionals. Little is known about the basis for the reluctance of many in American society to acknowledge and openly discuss sexuality and its health consequences. In addition, lack of open communication and information regarding sexuality fosters misperceptions and may actually encourage high-risk sexual behaviors.

The committee believes that a significant national Campaign to catalyze social change toward a new norm of healthy sexual behavior in the United States is necessary. Highly visible leadership and active participation of nationally recognized opinion leaders are particularly important in promoting open public discussions regarding healthy sexual behaviors and STDs. These opinion leaders are also essential as role models for social change. Leadership at the highest levels, especially from elected officials, is also needed to ensure that a national Campaign to change social norms of sexual behavior is sufficiently visible.

The committee recognizes that the CDC is the primary federal agency with responsibility for STD prevention on a national level, and believes that the CDC should continue to be a leader in federal agency efforts in this area. However, the committee is concerned that the CDC or any other government agency would be unable to fully promote public awareness of healthy sexual behaviors and establish a comprehensive national system of prevention services. Political constraints too often prevent government agencies from adequately addressing controversial issues associated with STD-related programs. Based on experience with past initiatives, limitations on government agencies regarding public education programs related to sexuality are particularly problematic. Therefore, an independent entity is needed to promote a social norm of healthy sexual behavior. Because of their independence, nonpartisanship, and resources, private foundations are particularly well suited to provide leadership and support for a bold national campaign in this area.

There are several examples of independent, nonpartisan organizations that have been established around other controversial health issues and appear to be successful in developing wide support for their missions. Two major recently established initiatives include the National Campaign to Prevent Teenage Pregnancy and the National Center for Tobacco-Free Kids. The campaign was formed "to prevent teen pregnancy by supporting values and stimulating actions that are consistent with a pregnancy-free adolescence." The center was founded to prevent tobacco use among children and has a mandate "to change the social environment and public policies to reduce tobacco use by children." These organizations were established in 1996 with initial funding primarily from private foundations and other organizations. Both the National Campaign to Prevent Teenage Pregnancy and the National Center for Tobacco-Free Kids have attracted a broad range of participants, including representatives from a wide array of health, religious, business, and community organizations, as well as political leaders. An example of an independent, nonpartisan organization that was effective in changing social norms around a major social health problem is MADD (Mothers Against Drunk Driving). Since 1980, this organization has successfully promoted both social (e.g., improving public knowledge, awareness, and practices) and structural changes (i.e., legislation) to reduce the practice of driving under the influence of alcohol. It seems that this behavior recently has become socially unacceptable.

The spectrum of agencies and organizations involved in STD prevention and the controversial nature of STD-related programs require that the proposed Campaign be nonpartisan and independent, especially from special interests and political constraints. The Campaign's work would be developed by its participants, and it is the committee's hope that the Campaign will use this report as a blueprint for its initial efforts.

Therefore, the committee makes the following recommendation:

• **An independent, long-term, national Campaign should be established to serve as a catalyst for social change toward a new norm of healthy sexual behavior in the United States.** This Campaign should:

1. provide new, highly visible leadership to promote healthy sexual behaviors and the implementation of a national system for STD prevention;

2. promote public discussion and awareness of healthy sexual behaviors and STDs among all population groups;

3. provide assistance to local community efforts to promote a new norm of healthy sexual behavior;

4. advocate for additional public and private investment in STD prevention;

5. work collaboratively with existing campaigns and other activities to prevent HIV infection, unintended pregnancy, and STD-associated cancers;

6. include nationally recognized public opinion leaders such as entertainment industry representatives, sports figures, business and labor leaders, elected officials and other policymakers, and mass media executives as members;

7. represent the spectrum of perspectives on STDs and sexual health issues; and

8. be funded by a broad range of sponsors, including private foundations, private sector health plans, the biomedical industry, employers, and the Department of Health and Human Services. The Campaign should be funded primarily by a coalition of private foundations with an interest in STDs; these foundations should provide leadership for initiating and maintaining the Campaign and provide "seed" money to establish it.

Promoting Knowledge and Awareness

As shown in Chapter 2, the scope of STDs and their consequences is broad. STDs infect all population groups in the United States. They can cause health problems for all infected persons, but the complications are most severe for women and their infants. Surveys cited in Chapter 3 show that there is little recognition of the spectrum of health consequences of STDs. In particular, the contribution of STDs to severe health complications, such as genital and liver cancer, pelvic inflammatory disease, ectopic pregnancy, infertility, chronic liver disease, neurological disorders, and perinatal illness, is not well known or understood by policymakers, many health professionals, or the general public.

In Chapter 3, the committee found that a major barrier to healthy sexual behavior is the lack of awareness regarding STDs and misperception of individual risk, especially among adolescents and young adults. The committee also found that accurate information is important in preventing misperceptions of risk. Programs to promote STD awareness and education, therefore, should result in increased motivation to prevent STDs. Increasing awareness of STDs among health professionals is important because it encourages clinicians to evaluate their patients for STDs when appropriate, thus improving the likelihood of early detection and treatment.

A national initiative to increase public awareness of STDs requires active participation of, and support from, various agencies and organizations from both the private and public sectors. Because of the sensitive nature of effective STD education programs, and the potential constraints upon government-run educational campaigns, an independent organization should develop and implement an appropriate STD education initiative. Along with a national educational initiative, however, it should be recognized that barriers to implementing healthy behaviors also must be reduced. Public health agencies and private health care professionals have a responsibility both to educate and to provide accurate public health information to the community, because providing disease prevention information is an essential component of clinical practice.

Innovative methods for increasing awareness and reaching the public need to be developed. Recent advances in information technology will have a great impact on access to health information among both health professionals and segments of the public. These new technologies should be harnessed to improve awareness and knowledge of STDs and ways to avoid them. Appropriate methods of disseminating information on STDs and local health services include the use of hotlines and evolving information technology, such as the Internet and other electronic methods of disseminating information. The Internet may be an especially effective method for disseminating information to adolescents and young adults because many users of such technology are young.

Therefore, the committee makes the following recommendation:

• **The independent Campaign to establish a new norm of healthy sexual behavior should support and implement a long-term national initiative to increase knowledge and awareness of STDs and to promote ways to prevent them.** The initiative should:

1. be coordinated with HIV- and pregnancy-prevention campaigns;
2. include a substantial mass media component;
3. provide information both on how to implement health-protective behaviors and on STDs;

4. provide information regarding the association of STDs and specific cancers and incorporate STD information into current cancer awareness and education activities;

5. focus on specific groups and audiences, including public and private sector policymakers, health care and public health professionals, employers and other purchasers of health care, health plans, and the public, particularly women and adolescents;

6. include an evaluation component; and

7. use new information technology to disseminate information. As part of this initiative, the CDC, the Health Resources and Services Administration, and the National Institutes of Health should increase support for innovative ways to educate and train health care professionals through the use of new information technology.

Promoting Balanced Mass Media Messages

The mass media do not portray sexuality in a healthy way, and mass media messages supporting healthy sexual behavior are rare. Changes in social norms regarding healthy sexual behaviors will be difficult to achieve unless the content of programming in mass media supports these behaviors. As discussed in Chapter 3, children and adolescents are most influenced by mass media messages. Adolescents spend a large amount of time watching television and participating in other forms of mass media, and they undoubtedly are influenced by the explicit and implicit messages in such media. Many adolescents are not receiving appropriate information regarding STDs and healthy sexual behavior from their parents, peers, public health officials, or family doctors to counter misleading mass media messages. Therefore, the committee believes that mass media companies should incorporate messages regarding STDs and healthy sexual behaviors, including delaying sexual intercourse and using condoms, in television and radio programming and the print media, with a special focus on reaching adolescents and young adults.

In spite of advertisers' use of sexually suggestive advertisements to promote their products, and in spite of polls showing that most Americans support promoting condoms on television, most mass media companies still refuse to allow STD-related public service announcements and condom advertisements on prime-time television or in widely read publications. The committee calls on mass media and advertising executives to recognize the hypocrisy of this practice and to help promote healthy sexual behaviors.

It is important that mass media and other public health messages regarding STDs be clear. The public should be informed that the only sure way to prevent STDs is either not to have sexual intercourse or to have intercourse only with an uninfected partner who is also monogamous. Adolescents should be encouraged to delay sexual intercourse. Despite these messages, however, many individuals will engage in unprotected sex. Therefore, media messages also must provide information regarding the methods for safer sex, including the correct and consistent use of condoms. Such messages should be comprehensive and incorporate public health messages regarding HIV and other STDs, sexual abuse, and unintended pregnancy.

As reviewed in Chapter 4, mass media methods of educating and increasing the awareness of the general public have been shown to be effective. Innovative media programs that use popular media, such as those developed by the Harvard School of Public Health related to drinking and driving, can complement public service announcements or more targeted public health campaigns. Although there have been few evaluations of such programs, they can reach audiences not touched by traditional approaches and should be evaluated further. The Media Project, described in Chapter 3, is a potential model for developing material regarding STDs. In addition, initiatives such as the STD Communications Roundtable, which functions as an expert resource on STDs for mass media companies, are important to ensure that mass media messages regarding STDs and safer sex behaviors are accurate. The STD Communications Roundtable could be used as a model for a standing committee of experts to facilitate the development of sexual health messages in mass media.

Therefore, the committee makes the following recommendations:

• **The independent Campaign to establish a new norm of healthy sexual behavior should develop a standing committee comprised of public health experts, mass media and advertising executives, public communications experts, and consumer representatives to function as an expert resource and to develop guidelines and resources for incorporating messages regarding STDs and healthy sexual behaviors into all forms of mass media.** Public health officials, including the CDC and state and local health departments, should also function as expert resources for mass media companies in developing and incorporating such messages.

• **Television, radio, print, music, and other mass media companies should accept advertisements and sponsor public service messages that promote condom use and other means of protecting against STDs and unintended pregnancy, including delaying sexual intercourse.** Adolescents are at high risk for STDs and are susceptible to mass media messages; therefore, such advertising and public service messages should be permitted to air during times when adolescents are likely to be watching or listening or should appear in print media that adolescents commonly read. Commercial advertisers and sponsors should support mass media companies in such efforts.

Improving Professional Skills in Sexual Health Issues

The committee believes that many individuals in the community should become more involved in educating others regarding STDs. These key individuals include parents, educators, health professionals, persons in the mass media, and religious leaders. It is important that clinicians, educators, and researchers become more skilled at discussing sexuality and learn more about sexuality. Improved skills in these areas will not only improve the effectiveness of behavioral interventions for STDs, but also for reproductive health problems in general. Clinicians, in particular, need to understand the context in which high-risk sexual behaviors occur, as well as the social and cultural factors that reinforce these behaviors. It is often difficult for professionals to remain objective during clinical interactions because sexuality is an emotionally charged issue, especially when the professional's own beliefs and behaviors differ from those of the patient.

Research on sexuality provides the basis for understanding the determinants of risky sexual behaviors. Two formidable barriers to strengthening and developing social and behavioral research in sexuality and STD-related risk behaviors are the lack of comprehensive research training in sexuality and inadequate funding of both basic (e.g., research on determinants of behavior change) and applied (e.g., behavior change interventions) research. The continuing fragmentation of the social science fields in sexuality research, the low status given to sexuality research, and lack of sufficient research funding all hinder training in this area. Inadequate dissemination of existing data has also hampered development of interventions and policy initiatives.

All appropriate clinical opportunities to counsel patients regarding healthy sexual behaviors should be utilized. To improve effectiveness of behavioral interventions, clinicians, educators, and researchers need training and skills to deal with issues related to human sexuality and STDs among their patients and students. Providing new, and enhancing existing, continuing education courses for clinicians, educators, and researchers will help these professionals become more comfortable working with sexual health issues. Courses designed to educate all these professionals about sexuality, attitudes, alternative lifestyles, and cultural factors will provide a fuller understanding of sexual behavior.

Therefore, the committee makes the following recommendation:

• **The Health Resources and Services Administration, health professional schools and associations, and schools and associations for training educators should support comprehensive sexuality training for health care professionals, educators, and researchers in order to increase their comfort in working with sexual health issues and to increase their effectiveness in sexual behavior counseling.** Health professional schools and associations should sponsor continuing education courses in sexuality for clinicians and incorporate appropriate instruction in undergraduate and graduate education programs. The focus of these programs should be to provide instruction in basic, effective intervention counseling and clinical skills that are appropriate for any setting or population.

Supporting Sexual Health Behavior Research

Health behavior research provides the basis for developing interventions to prevent high-risk sexual behaviors. Population-based surveys mentioned in Chapter 5 that collect information on STD-related health behaviors are critical for monitoring trends in health behaviors among the general population and in developing effective interventions. In addition to improving STD prevention efforts, research on sexual behavior has direct benefits in improving prevention programs for HIV and unintended pregnancy. To address the barriers to adoption of healthy sexual behaviors, there needs to be considerably more research regarding the psychological and sociocultural, including religious, factors responsible for the secrecy surrounding sexuality and additional evaluation of approaches (that are respectful of individual beliefs) to successfully overcome these barriers. There is limited information available regarding the origins of sociocultural strictures on open discussion of sexuality and STDs. Understanding this factor should be useful in developing strategies to overcome societal constraints on preventing STDs.

Population-based surveys and studies to assess STD-related health behaviors are not only justified but are necessary for the development of effective interventions to prevent high-risk behaviors. Such surveys, particularly those for adolescents, have been severely criticized by some policymakers and interest groups. This committee, while recognizing the sincere concerns expressed by some of these groups, strongly believes that collecting information on STD-related health behaviors, especially among adolescents, is critical to STD prevention, because sexual behaviors are usually initiated during adolescence. The committee found no evidence to support the belief that asking questions about sexual activity in any way promotes or increases sexual activity among survey respondents or changes attitudes of respondents regarding these activities (Halpern et al., 1994). Without data on sexual behaviors, it is more difficult to prevent the very behaviors that concern the critics of such surveys.

Federal legislation has been introduced that would require prior written parental consent for minors to participate in federally funded survey research if the survey or questionnaire contains questions in several specific areas, including sexual behavior.[1] The committee strongly believes that such restrictions would seriously jeopardize both behavioral research and the ability to prevent high-risk behaviors among adolescents. Requiring parental consent or prior written consent for a minor's participation in survey research would make it practically impossible to conduct research in settings where minors obtain confidential health services, such as STD and family planning clinics, because parents could not be notified. Yet it is precisely in these types of settings that it is particularly impor-

---

[1]H.R. 1271, The Family Privacy Protection Act of 1995, 104th Congress, 1st session.

tant to collect information regarding sexual behavior. The committee believes that current federal and state regulations are adequate to protect the interests of minors in survey research. Current federal regulations allow for waivers of parental permission in cases where acquiring such permission would be considered unreasonable. Consensus guidelines for adolescent health research have been developed to clarify these regulations and to ensure that research involving adolescents has adequate mechanisms to protect minors (SAM, 1995). The committee believes that these guidelines appropriately balance the potential risks and benefits of health research that involve adolescents. In addition, the committee believes that it is critical to preserve the peer-review process for scientific research. It is potentially very damaging to the objectivity and integrity of this process specifically, and to scientific research in general, if external forces are allowed to influence the outcome of peer review.

Therefore, the committee makes the following recommendation:

• **The National Institutes of Health and other federal agencies should continue to support research on health behaviors, including sexual behaviors, and their relationship to STDs.** Both basic and applied research on sexual behavior and determinants of behavior change should be supported. Research should include study of the origins and maintenance of current societal strictures against open discussion of sexuality and STDs. Such research initiatives should be coordinated among federal agencies by the National Institutes of Health. Findings of these studies and surveys should be widely disseminated to policymakers, health care professionals, educators, community leaders, and the general public. In addition, these data should be used to promote appropriate behavior change and prevention. Under the conditions specified in the consensus guidelines for adolescent health research, the committee strongly believes that waivers of parental consent for a minor's participation in research that poses minimal risk to the participant should be preserved.

STRATEGY 2: DEVELOP LEADERSHIP

Strategy 2 is to develop strong leadership, strengthen investment, and improve information systems for STD prevention. Building a national system for STD prevention requires active participation from both the public and private sectors, and requires strong leadership at the national, state, and local levels. Public and private health agencies, especially those concerned with adolescent, women's, and reproductive health; communicable diseases; cancer prevention; delivery and financing of health services; community health; and public health in general, should strongly advocate for an effective system for STD prevention. National and state health professional societies and organizations and organizations with a special interest in STDs and adolescent, women's, and reproductive health also should work together to ensure that STDs are a priority in both the private and public sectors. Advocacy by the above public and private organizations is important because, unlike many other health problems, there are virtually no patient-based constituent groups for STDs other than HIV infection. As discussed in Chapter 3, this is because having an STD is still perceived as socially unacceptable.

Developing Leadership in the Private Sector

Traditionally, public health agencies have led the efforts to improve STD-related services and have assumed most of the responsibility for STD prevention because private sector clinicians refused or were reluctant to provide STD-related services. The committee believes that the private sector needs to assume more responsibility and leadership (Showstack et al., 1996), and that the organizational norms of some private sector organizations regarding responsibility for STD prevention need to change. This is because, although the public sector must continue to play a major role in preventing STDs, the public sector does not have the resources or the organizational reach to fully implement a national system of STD-related services. Developing leadership in the private sector may be a challenge, given the heterogeneity of the organizations potentially involved in STD prevention. As mentioned previously, independent private nonprofit organizations, such as foundations, may be key in bringing these disparate organizations together.

Therefore, the committee makes the following recommendation:

• **Private sector organizations and clinicians should assume more leadership and responsibility for STD prevention.** The committee proposes the following major responsibilities in STD prevention for private sector organizations and clinicians:

1. *Health Plans and Clinicians.* Provide confidential, comprehensive, high-quality STD-related clinical services to enrollees/patients and their sex partners; implement clinical practice guidelines for management of STDs; and ensure complete and accurate reporting of surveillance information.

2. *Employers and Purchasers of Health Services.* Ensure that comprehensive STD-related services are available to employees/beneficiaries and their sex partners.

3. *Health Plan Accrediting Organizations.* Develop and promote health plan performance measures for STD-related services.

4. *Mass Media Companies, Commercial Sponsors, and Advertisers.* Improve public awareness and knowledge of STDs and promote healthy sexual behaviors.

5. *Health Professional Membership Organizations.* Improve awareness and

knowledge of STDs among the membership and support and sponsor training of health care professionals in STD-related clinical management.

6. *Private Foundations.* Sponsor initiatives and provide independent, nonpartisan leadership for activities that improve collaboration among various organizations and encourage universal participation in STD prevention efforts.

7. *Health-Related Nonprofit Organizations.* Improve public awareness and knowledge and integrate STD prevention efforts into other relevant disease prevention strategies.

8. *Academic Health-Related Institutions.* Sponsor continuing education activities for clinicians and provide adequate STD-related training to health professional and other students; collaborate with health agencies to improve STD-related services; and conduct STD-related research.

9. *Biomedical Industry.* Develop and improve biomedical interventions for diagnosis, treatment, and prevention (e.g., vaccines, microbicides) of STDs; ensure that new and existing interventions are affordable for publicly sponsored STD programs; and assist in efforts to educate health care professionals.

10. *School-Based Programs (including public sector programs).* Provide confidential, comprehensive, high-quality STD-related clinical services for students and provide instruction regarding STDs and healthy sexual behaviors.

11. *Community-Based Social Service Organizations.* Improve public awareness and knowledge of STDs and promote healthy sexual behaviors.

12. *Laboratories.* Ensure high-quality diagnostic services for STDs.

Discussion of the rationale for the above recommendations and more specific recommendations for private sector organizations are presented later in this chapter.

Developing Leadership in the Public Sector

In this section, the committee proposes a set of responsibilities and functions for which federal, state, and local public health agencies should assume leadership. The committee believes that the proposed functions are most effectively and efficiently performed by government agencies in collaboration with private sector organizations.

Promoting Federal Leadership

Government agencies have the ultimate responsibility for ensuring the public health. At the national level, the Public Health Service Act gives the Secretary of Health and Human Services legislative authority to assist states in preventing communicable diseases. Ultimate responsibility for coordinating government efforts to establish a national system for STD prevention most logically rests in the office of the Secretary because the Secretary has authority over most of the federal health agencies with activities in this area. The Secretary needs to charge these agencies to develop and implement the public sector components of the proposed national system and to provide these agencies with sufficient resources to do so. From a technical expertise and program implementation perspective, the CDC is the appropriate agency to provide national leadership in many aspects of STD prevention. The leadership of the Department of Health and Human Services, especially the CDC, must give higher priority to STD prevention programs. For example, in its fiscal year 1997 budget proposal to Congress,[2] the administration requested reduced funding for STD prevention at a time when the CDC lacks the capacity to adequately provide technical assistance to states. Other health agencies, such as the National Institutes of Health, the Health Resources and Services Administration, the Health Care Financing Administration, the Substance Abuse and Mental Health Services Administration, the Agency for Health Care Policy and Research, the Food and Drug Administration, and the Indian Health Service, also need to assume leadership roles in their areas of responsibility. The Department of Health and Human Services needs to ensure that the agencies within its purview collaboratively provide bold innovative standards, guidance, technical assistance, and resources to state and local health departments and appropriate community-based organizations.

Therefore, the committee makes the following recommendation:

• **Federal government efforts in STD prevention, under the leadership of the Secretary of Health and Human Services, should:**

1. provide guidance for STD-related clinical services and provide guidance and financial and technical assistance to states and local communities for STD prevention programs;

2. develop scientifically based standards for STD-related services, including clinical services, such as screening and counseling, diagnosis and treatment, laboratory services, and prevention programs; such standards should be sufficiently flexible and applicable to all states and communities and to all types of practitioners and programs that provide STD-related care;

3. develop and coordinate a comprehensive national surveillance system that collects STD-related data from public, private, and community-based providers and programs;

4. ensure that high-quality STD-related services, including all supporting disease prevention activities, and effective community-based prevention programs are coordinated and integrated as appropriate and are available and accessible to every person, regardless of insurance status, income, state of residence, or urban or rural location;

---

[2]The Budget of the United States Government Fiscal Year 1997.

5. improve public and health professional awareness and knowledge of STDs and promote healthy behaviors on a national basis;

6. ensure that health professionals are appropriately and adequately trained to provide STD-related services, including clinical services, disease prevention activities, and community-based prevention programs;

7. ensure that STD prevention activities are an integral part of national HIV and cancer prevention programs;

8. support and conduct research to improve strategies for STD prevention;

9. coordinate STD prevention programs, including research activities, among states and relevant federal agencies, including the CDC, the National Institutes of Health, the Health Resources and Services Administration, the Health Care Financing Administration, the Substance Abuse and Mental Health Services Administration, the Agency for Health Care Policy and Research, the Food and Drug Administration, and the Indian Health Service; and

10. expand and maximize existing funding streams and develop new and increased resources from both public and private sources to support this system at all levels.

Promoting State Leadership

Within state and local governments, the health department is responsible for implementing STD-related programs and is the logical agency to lead STD prevention efforts. Other agencies and state and local elected officials, however, need to support the efforts of these health departments, because the health department may not have sufficient authority or resources to implement interventions. In cases where direct responsibility for some aspects of STD-related clinical care is under the purview of another agency, the health department needs to assume a coordinating role.

State and local health departments vary considerably in their capacity and technical ability to provide clinical and outreach services and to conduct disease surveillance, quality assurance, and training activities. Most state and local health agencies, however, will require substantial additional funding and technical assistance to fully establish an effective system of STD prevention in their jurisdiction.

Therefore, the committee makes the following recommendation:

• **State government efforts in STD prevention, through the leadership of the state health department and with support and technical assistance from the CDC, should:**

1. develop, implement, and support a comprehensive STD prevention system throughout the state;

2. provide guidance and financial and technical assistance to local health

departments to ensure that STD-related services are appropriately provided and coordinated among the various private and public community-based providers;

3. collect information on reportable STDs from local health departments and private sector health care providers, analyze the information to monitor statewide trends in STDs, and report these data to the CDC;

4. assess the need for STD-related services in the state;

5. ensure that STD-related services are of high quality and are accessible to all state residents;

6. improve public and health professional awareness and knowledge of STDs and promote healthy behaviors statewide;

7. ensure that adequate funds are available to support provision of STD-related services to the uninsured; and

8. provide training and technical assistance to all local jurisdictions to improve the quality and effectiveness of clinical services and prevention programs.

Promoting Local Leadership

Regarding local government leadership, the committee makes the following recommendation:

• **Local government efforts in STD prevention, through the leadership of the local health department, with support and technical assistance from the state health department and the CDC, and in collaboration with community representatives, should:**

1. coordinate all providers of STD-related clinical services and prevention programs, including private providers, schools, and other community-based programs, to develop a comprehensive prevention system in the community;

2. collect information on reportable STDs from all public and private providers, analyze the data to monitor trends in STD incidence and prevalence, and identify high-risk groups and areas for special interventions;

3. assess the need for STD-related services in the community;

4. ensure that STD-related services are appropriate and are accessible to every member of the community;

5. improve public and health professional awareness and knowledge of STDs, and promote healthy behaviors in the community;

6. ensure that adequate funds are available to provide STD-related clinical services to the uninsured; and

7. provide training and technical assistance to providers of STD-related clinical services and prevention programs.

The proposed responsibilities and functions of federal, state, and local governments and health departments are similar to those proposed by special committees of the Association of State and Territorial Health Officials (ASTHO, 1995a, b, c) and the National Association of County and City Health Officials (NACCHO, 1994), and a previous IOM committee (IOM, 1988). Many state and local governments have already addressed some or many of the responsibilities outlined above; the committee, however, believes that state and local government efforts generally need to be more consistent, more innovative, and better supported.

The monitoring and assessment role of government agencies requires them to monitor the prevalence of STDs in the community, identify high-risk populations or communities, and assess the adequacy of treatment and prevention efforts. This role also requires these agencies to monitor and ensure compliance with minimum standards of quality and accessibility of services. Effective performance of these roles requires collaborative relationships among local health departments and community-based health services, private sector health care professionals, health plans, laboratories, and others in the community. STD services and programs in most local health departments currently are relatively isolated from other providers in the community. Such isolation reduces opportunities for collaborative efforts, such as sharing of disease surveillance data, to improve STD prevention. The performance of local and state government agencies in ensuring and improving STD-related services should be monitored by consumer groups, elected officials, health professional organizations, and the federal government as appropriate (IOM, 1997).

Catalyzing Change Through Partnerships

The barriers to an effective national system for STD prevention are found in government, private sector organizations, and political factors and social norms. Overcoming these barriers is a challenge that requires the active participation of all levels of government, the private health care sector, businesses, labor leaders, the mass media, schools, and many community-based organizations. Many of the committee's recommendations regarding health agencies and private sector organizations involve sharing of responsibility and technical expertise and information; coordination of programs; and forming partnerships both within agencies and organizations and between the public and private sectors. In developing and implementing a national system for STD prevention, it is important that stakeholders be involved in all steps of the process; however, a formal mechanism for collaboration among agencies and organizations does not exist. Therefore, a neutral forum is needed to maximize the range of participants and to catalyze the collaborative process.

To establish an effective national system for STD prevention, the committee believes that a long-term national Roundtable for public agencies and private sector organizations is needed to catalyze the development and implementation of a comprehensive system of STD prevention in the United States. Independence of the Roundtable from special interests and political constraints is especially critical. As with the Campaign to catalyze social change toward a new norm of healthy sexual behavior, while the committee recognizes the important role of government agencies in establishing a comprehensive system of STD prevention, it believes that political constraints on such agencies may sometimes impede the development of collaborations between the public and private sectors. In addition, some potential Roundtable participants may be reluctant to join in a government-agency-led activity. To maximize the range of Roundtable private sector participants, the committee believes that ensuring that all potential Roundtable members have an opportunity to participate on an equal basis is important. The Roundtable would not have bureaucratic functions or be an administrative hurdle for agencies or the private sector, because it would not have administrative authority over government agencies or private organizations. The Roundtable's work would be determined by its participating agencies and organizations. Although the Roundtable's activities should be coordinated with the activities of the previously proposed national Campaign (e.g., through regular joint meetings and appointed liaisons), the two entities would be independent. Independence of the two entities is necessary because, in the case of the Campaign, government agency participation is likely to constrain the effectiveness of its work; in the case of the Roundtable, the participation of government agencies is critical.[3] The activities of the two entities, however, must be coordinated to ensure that they are not only complementary, but synergistic.

An example of a roundtable that brought disparate agencies and organizations together toward a common, although more limited, goal was the IOM Roundtable for the Development of Drugs and Vaccines Against AIDS that operated from 1988 through 1994. The purpose of this roundtable was to identify and help resolve the impediments to the rapid availability of effective drugs and vaccines for HIV infection and AIDS. Roundtable participants included leaders from government, the pharmaceutical industry, academia, and affected communities.

Leadership is needed to establish and maintain a Roundtable on STD prevention. At the current time, there is a lack of leadership among private health care sector organizations in this area. The Department of Health and Human Services, therefore, is the logical agency for ensuring the establishment of the Roundtable because of its mission and its oversight of the major government activities and agencies involved in STD prevention. These include: the CDC (prevention services, technical assistance, and surveillance); the National Institutes of Health (biomedical and behavioral research); the Agency for Health Care Policy and

---

[3]In developing this recommendation, the committee considered the advantages and disadvantages of many types of potential structures for the Campaign and the Roundtable. The committee believes that, of the options considered, the proposed structures are most likely to succeed and are practical based on the experiences of other campaigns and the roundtable cited.

Research (health services research); the Health Resources and Services Administration, the Indian Health Service, and the Substance Abuse and Mental Health Services Administration (primary care and other health services); the Health Care Financing Administration (financing mechanisms for some STD treatment), and the Food and Drug Administration (drug, biologic, and medical device evaluation and approval).

Therefore, the committee makes the following recommendation:

• **An independent, long-term national Roundtable should be established as a neutral forum for public and private sector agencies and organizations to collaboratively develop and implement a comprehensive system of STD-related services in the United States.** The Roundtable should:

1. coordinate public and private sector STD-related services;

2. disseminate information on, and promote implementation of, "best practices" and quality standards in STD prevention;

3. develop consensus regarding the appropriate roles and responsibilities of the various providers of STD-related services;

4. promote partnerships and dialogue among public and private sector agencies and organizations on the state and community level;

5. recruit and involve public agencies and private organizations, including health plans, employers and other purchasers of health services, health professional organizations, pharmaceutical and medical device companies, and other providers of STD-related services;

6. seek input from, provide guidance to, actively involve, and communicate with providers of STD-related services on local and state levels; and

7. be funded by a broad range of sponsors, including private foundations, private sector health plans, the biomedical industry, employers, and the Department of Health and Human Services, but primary funding should come from the Department of Health and Human Services. The Secretary of Health and Human Services should take responsibility for initiating and provide ongoing support for the Roundtable, but it should be housed at a private, nonprofit institution that can ensure a neutral environment for Roundtable participants.

Strengthening Investment in STD Prevention

STDs are a tremendous economic burden on the people of the United States, but the costs of STDs are largely unrecognized. As discussed in Chapter 2, the committee estimates that approximately $10 billion is spent on costs associated with major STDs in the United States annually. The committee's cost estimate is not precise because it is based on incomplete data regarding the incidence and costs of STDs. Not all STD-related costs are accounted for; thus, the true cost of STDs is likely to be much higher than the committee's estimate. For example, this estimate does not include costs associated with newly described STD-related syndromes such as premature delivery in pregnant women and low birth weight associated with bacterial vaginosis. Comprehensive and accurate data regarding the economic costs of STDs are essential for cost-effectiveness analyses of prevention programs, but cost and morbidity data are not currently available for many STDs and related syndromes. Therefore, the CDC or other appropriate federal agency should conduct or support a comprehensive analysis of the economic consequences of STDs and associated sequelae. This analysis should include estimates of direct and indirect costs and appropriate cost-benefit and cost-effectiveness analyses of interventions.

The current national response to STDs is not commensurate with their health and economic costs. STDs are a formidable health problem and should be a national public health priority. An effective national system requires additional investment to avert the much higher long-term costs of STDs. Current public resources allocated for STD prevention are extremely low. As discussed in Chapter 5, the committee estimates that only $1 is invested in STD prevention for every $43 spent on the costs of STDs and their complications every year. Similarly, only $1 is invested in biomedical and clinical research for every $94 spent on the costs of STDs. Studies cited in Chapter 4 show that STD prevention efforts are cost-effective and sometimes cost-saving. Investing in preventive services will avert substantial human suffering and save billions of dollars in treatment costs that result from the costly complications of STDs and lost productivity. The CDC estimates that for every $1 spent on early detection and treatment of chlamydial and gonococcal infection, approximately $12 in associated costs could be saved (CDC, DSTD/HIVP, 1995).

There is a widespread belief among clinicians and researchers who work in STDs that the social and economic costs of STDs in the United States justify expenditures of much more money and effort than currently are devoted to this area. This type of statement often is made for many types of prevention, but the committee is of the opinion that the situation is worse in STDs than in many other areas. The committee also recognizes, however, that devoting resources to prevention programs is not always cost-effective (Russell, 1994). Unfortunately, there is surprisingly little data either on absolute expenditures for STD prevention or the cost-effectiveness of different types of expenditures. Thus, the committee recommends that rigorous analyses of the cost-effectiveness of different types of prevention programs be conducted. This kind of research should be supported by the National Institutes of Health, the Agency for Health Care Policy and Research, and other agencies.

The committee recognizes that establishing a national system for STD prevention requires additional funding and that this may be very difficult in an era of shrinking federal and state budgets. The committee proposes that additional funding to establish a national system for STD prevention come from all levels of government and the private sector. Regardless of whether additional funds can be found for STD programs, it is clear that more efficient and effective use of existing resources is also needed. By providing STD-related services in primary care settings and coordinating public and private sector programs, a more effective and efficient system for prevention can be achieved.

Who Is Currently Paying and Who Should Pay?

Who is currently paying for the substantial economic costs of STDs? The answer is all Americans. Local, state, and the federal governments pay STD-related costs by funding services through the Medicaid and Medicare programs (for STD-related complications that manifest among older persons, such as cancer), public STD clinics, family planning clinics, community health centers, and other publicly sponsored health care programs. Businesses pay for STD-related costs through higher health insurance premiums for their workers and lost productivity of employees with STDs. Hospitals pay for uncompensated STD-related care. Managed care organizations pay STD-related costs by providing expensive treatment for the complications of STDs that can be averted. In short, all Americans eventually pay for the costs of STDs through their tax dollars and through increased health insurance premiums. Therefore, all public and private health-related agencies and organizations, including federal, state, and local governments, employers and other purchasers of health care, businesses, and health plans should invest in and support STD prevention efforts. It is in both the national and local community interest to invest in STD prevention.

Public funding for STD prevention is justified because STDs are communicable diseases that, when left unchecked, potentially endanger the health of the community. Public investment in STD prevention is especially important because the stigma associated with these diseases may hinder availability of clinical services in the private sector, especially for disenfranchised groups who represent a reservoir of infection for other members of the community, as described in Chapter 3.

The committee believes that the financial responsibility for supporting STD prevention is currently not equitable since both the private and public health care sectors benefit from lower STD rates. The private sector, including health plans, employers and other purchasers, and health care providers, needs to assume more responsibility for supporting public health services, including STD-related services, that benefit "the insured" population and ultimately benefit their financial results. Health plans, therefore, should provide their enrollees with access to STD-related services in the public sector through equitable reimbursement agreements. Reasons why the private sector should become more involved in preventive services and provide STD-related services to sex partners of infected persons and prevent STDs in the general community are presented in later discussions.

Aral and colleagues (1996) have proposed a way of thinking about the issue of who should pay for STD prevention according to the emphasis placed on prevention efforts. If preventing acquisition of STDs by susceptible individuals in a community is emphasized, then the entire community assumes the financial costs of the interventions and the intangible costs associated with appropriate behavior change. In this situation, the community also receives the benefits of avoiding STDs. In the case where preventing transmission of STDs from infected individuals to the community is emphasized, members of the highest-risk groups primarily incur the costs associated with behavior change, and the community benefits from avoiding acquisition of STDs and averting future STD-associated public health costs. Therefore, in both cases, the entire community directly benefits from preventing STDs and should assume financial responsibility for STD prevention. Specific potential mechanisms for ensuring funding for STD-related services may include allowing public STD clinics to be contract providers for health plans, requiring health plans to reimburse STD and other public health clinics for out-of-plan use of services, and imposing an assessment on health plans for services and programs that benefit the broad community. Economists recognize the need for public support when "externalities" (e.g., the potential for widespread transmission of disease from an infected individual) transcend the market system for allocating services based on supply and demand. It is important to recognize the fundamental public responsibility for preventing communicable diseases such as STDs.

Increased support should be given to effective prevention programs, including the programs to change STD-related risk behaviors that are described in Chapter 4. Support for education and counseling in publicly sponsored programs is needed. Education and counseling in private health care settings may be covered or reimbursed through either capitation or fee-for-service payments. In addition, community- and school-based interventions that target high-risk groups require a broad funding base that reflects the benefits they generate for the entire community. Finally, a secure source of funding for STD-related services for uninsured persons is essential. Cutbacks in state and local funding for indigent health care have dramatically reduced the availability and accessibility of public health services for the uninsured. Federal funding is essential to enable state and local governments to maintain and improve their STD prevention programs. The fragile successes in containing bacterial STDs in much of the country are endangered by reductions in access to services and underscore the importance of retaining categorical federal funding for STDs.

State and local governments traditionally have had full responsibility for supporting STD-related clinical services and also share responsibility with the federal government for supporting STD prevention efforts. However, state and local governments vary significantly in their investment in STD-related programs and generally need to increase their support of such programs. The CDC's STD Accelerated Prevention Campaigns program, which seeks to encourage collaboration between dedicated public STD clinics and community-based health care professionals, has an enhanced component that requires the grantee to partially

match federal funds. Such matching requirements should be encouraged to expand local commitment of resources to STD prevention.

A common question relates to the appropriate criteria for reducing funding
for public health programs. In the case of STD-related programs, while it is
possible that funding could be reduced without harmful consequences as STDs
are reduced in the distant future, the committee believes that the United States is
far from reaching this stage. In addition, sustained funding for programs are
necessary because STDs operate under a dynamic equilibrium—the nature of the
most effective interventions and the focus on different population groups will
change with time and the phase of the epidemic (Wasserheit and Aral, 1996). For
example, as the prevalence of STDs decreases in a population, there would be
less emphasis on screening programs, but increased emphasis on population-
based interventions to maintain healthy sexual behaviors in the community. In all
cases, surveillance of STDs and assessment of health behaviors are important in
providing feedback to the program planning and implementation process.

Therefore, the committee makes the following recommendation:

- **Federal, state, and local elected officials should provide additional
funding for STD prevention.** Local health departments, in particular, will require additional funding and technical assistance from the CDC and the state
health department to fully assume the responsibilities of ensuring access to STD-
related services. If federal staff assistance to states and localities is reduced,
resources should be redirected back into state and local STD programs to ensure
that the state and local infrastructure can be incrementally shifted from reliance
on federal direct assistance to a state and locally directed program.

Evaluating and Improving Categorical Funding

The advantages and disadvantages of categorical funding and block grants
are summarized in Chapter 5. Categorical funding for STDs has encouraged
programmatic rigidity and excess administrative costs for local agencies, fostered
services that often ignore local conditions and other health problems, and discouraged innovation. Federal funding rules have resulted in local programs adapting to federal requirements rather than local programs adapting to community
needs. This is an unintended effect of a policy intended to maintain high national
standards for services. In addition, categorical funding has encouraged narrowly
defined programs because of the traditional methods used to measure program
effectiveness.

Despite the problems in the current system of categorical funding, the committee strongly believes that moving to a system of block grants for STDs would
have a devastating impact on STD prevention and that categorical funding for
STDs should be preserved. In an ideal world, funding decisions would be based
on assessments of public health need, but past experience suggests that state

politics, rather than objective consideration of public health or social needs, may determine funding for public health programs, especially those with a limited political constituency such as STDs. Because STDs are often perceived to be a problem of marginalized groups, they will fare poorly in competing with other more visible and "acceptable" health conditions for their share of decreasing state health budgets. In many states, STD prevention programs may end up as political orphans because STDs are problems that public officials are reluctant to acknowledge. Funding for these programs is likely to be challenged by well-organized, powerful interest groups that are opposed to open discussion and public education regarding STDs. Many states have weak public health and health policy infrastructures and limited economic resources. Therefore, the likelihood that they will successfully evade pressures to limit or eliminate funding for STD prevention is reduced. With no enforceable national standards and substantial variability in the use of public-health-based decision-making in state legislatures, some states are likely to reduce or eliminate funding for STD programs. In the absence of national standards and mandates, block grants would create wide variability and unevenness in program quality and effectiveness among the states that could undermine a cohesive national system for prevention. Block grant funding is also more vulnerable to budget reductions at the national level. The diffuse purposes of block grants make them more vulnerable to reductions in congressional funding than most categorical programs.

Moving from categorical programs to block grants or Performance Partnership Grants (which the committee considers to be a form of a block grant, as described in Chapter 5) would also dramatically change both funding and accountability relationships among federal, state, and local governments. States would have more flexibility regarding resource allocation for public health. They also would be less accountable to federal agencies and would receive less guidance and support from the federal government. In addition, state and local health agencies may end up with less money than they currently have for STDs, unless state and local governments increase funding. Many elected state officials favor block grants because it gives them more discretion over resource allocation. However, state and local public health officials and STD program managers throughout the nation—the very people whose programs are supposed to benefit from block grants—warned the committee that block grants are likely to weaken and undermine STD prevention efforts.

Federal categorical funding programs can be improved by redesigning, rather than abandoning, current categorical programs. Performance standards that focus on health outcomes and process, rather than on program inputs, can help communities and states set priorities and objectives and measure their progress in achieving specific goals (IOM, 1997; NRC, in press). Process measures that are known to be characteristic of high-quality programs can help communities and states evaluate the quality of their programs. Process measures should focus on cardinal characteristics of prevention systems, such as awareness of and access to programs, consistency of follow-up, quality of prevention advice and treatment services, and continuity of care. Currently, there are no validated measures of these characteristics for prevention systems, but the development and implementation of such measures would greatly increase the capacity to monitor and improve the efficiency and quality of public health programs for STD prevention. It would be most logical for state and local governments to conduct performance monitoring under federal guidelines.

Performance standards would also give the federal government a more meaningful method of holding states accountable for federal funds. Accountability should focus on reducing STDs, including HIV infection, among high-risk populations and the community at large. The Department of Health and Human Services should develop and provide incentives for states and local governments to make substantial financial contributions to STD prevention and to make progress in containing STDs in their jurisdictions. Funding of programs can also be made responsive to local needs by providing more options for local modifications and flexibility. In addition, waivers should be granted for promising innovative programs that may not comply with all federal requirements. With current HIV and STD categorical programs, however, states should be encouraged to coordinate, integrate, and consolidate services and education programs.

Therefore, the committee makes the following recommendation:

• **The CDC should retain and immediately redesign categorical funding for STD programs.** New accountability measures that monitor performance toward achieving community health objectives and outcomes and new process measures should be developed and implemented. In addition, mechanisms should be established to increase local flexibility and program innovation and to encourage integration and coordination of local programs. Regardless of the type of funding mechanism, the CDC should ensure that all state and local governments, as a condition of receiving federal funds:

1. maintain current funding levels for STDs or provide matching funds, whichever amount is greater, and set aside a specified minimum proportion of funding for essential programs and services, and for high-risk populations;

2. develop performance objectives in collaboration with local communities and health departments;

3. meet minimum national quality standards for STD-related services (see recommendations for improving the quality of dedicated public STD clinics for more details); and

4. report federally recommended morbidity data as part of a national surveillance system.

In addition, as an incentive for state and local governments to expand their efforts in STD prevention, the CDC should provide whatever technical assistance is required and match new state and local funds allocated toward these efforts. Because the CDC currently does not have sufficient resources to provide comprehensive technical assistance to state and local health departments, the agency will require additional funding for STD prevention.

Strengthening Global STD Prevention Efforts

STDs are emerging infections and a global public health problem. As discussed in Chapter 2, new STDs with a potentially devastating impact are likely to emerge and become established in the United States. This is a consequence of increasing global travel, inadequate international public health safeguards, and continuing high-risk sexual practices. In addition, inappropriate treatment practices may be leading to the rise of antibiotic resistance among certain sexually transmitted pathogens. Current STD surveillance systems are not adequate to monitor the emergence of new infections or the resurgence of recognized STDs. International travel has enabled persons with infectious diseases to expose persons on different continents within hours or days. Strategies to prevent STDs in the United States should consider the potential impact of global STD rates. The reason for emphasizing the emerging nature of STDs is to strengthen global surveillance, improve international efforts against STDs, and promote behavioral and ecological changes to decrease pressures for the emergence of new infections. Many STDs, such as syphilis and gonorrhea, can survive only in the human host, and theoretically can be eradicated. Eradication or elimination of any STD will require substantial international investment and collaboration. The United States, therefore, has a national interest in preventing STDs worldwide in order to minimize the likelihood of emerging STDs in this country.

Therefore, the committee makes the following recommendation:

• **The federal government, through the Department of Health and Human Services and the U.S. Agency for International Development, and international organizations, such as the World Health Organization and the World Bank, should provide resources and technical assistance to global efforts to prevent STDs.** The CDC should provide more technical assistance in these international efforts.

Improving Surveillance and Other Information Systems

Surveillance and other information systems are necessary to monitor and evaluate the components of a national system for prevention. Data from these information sources are critical to long-term program planning as well as to day-to-day management of programs.

Surveillance and population-based survey data are important in monitoring the status of STDs and STD-related behaviors. These data are the basis for developing and targeting interventions, prioritizing resources, detecting epidemics, and evaluating program effectiveness. As discussed in Chapter 5, current surveillance systems do not give accurate estimates of disease incidence because not all persons with STDs seek medical care and because surveillance data do not reflect all clinical encounters with community health care professionals, especially those in private sector health care settings. The limitations of the current surveillance system are summarized in Chapter 5.

Enhancing the Current System

Certain limitations and weaknesses of the current passive notifiable diseases surveillance system are inherent in passive disease reporting systems, but several enhancements to the current system are indicated. It is critical that a systematic, comprehensive evaluation of the national surveillance system be conducted to describe the attributes of the system and to provide guidance for future improvements. STD surveillance systems need to include and link information from public sector, community-based, and private health care professionals. In particular, public health agencies need to work with the private health care professionals to improve compliance with disease reporting. Private practice clinicians and laboratories should understand that disease reporting and feedback of local epidemiological surveillance information concerning STDs and other emerging infections will greatly assist them in their clinical practice. By minimizing the time delay in reporting of cases from clinicians and laboratories to the local health department, and then to the state health department and the CDC, local and multistate outbreaks can be detected promptly.

Local health departments, with both the skills and the responsibility for collecting health data from a wide array of sources, will continue to be the pivotal agency in monitoring the health of communities. With technical assistance from the CDC and state health departments, they will need to develop effective reporting systems and actively work with community-based and private health care professionals to ensure accurate and complete reporting. Their responsibilities should include feedback regarding local STD trends to health care professionals to inform and engage them in STD prevention efforts. Although not widespread, some local health departments have already taken a collaborative approach to surveillance by developing relationships with private clinicians. One specific disease reporting issue that needs to be resolved at the national level is the lack of reporting guidelines for laboratories that confirm STD diagnoses among out-of-state persons.

The ideal surveillance system for STDs should be robust enough to accurately and promptly identify national and local trends in STD incidence, and flexible enough to provide state and local health officials with necessary data to direct local activities and evaluate interventions. In the future, as resources permit, STD information systems should identify and incorporate data elements that permit surveillance of infection rates within communities and allow assessment of the effectiveness of STD-related services. This information, which requires reliable population-based data as well as data from STD-related clinical services, is necessary to identify and focus on high-risk groups and areas and to evaluate broader public policies.

As mentioned in Chapter 5, sentinel surveillance projects are valuable tools for supplementing and validating information from the national notifiable disease reporting system. For example, the CDC-sponsored Gonococcal Isolate Surveillance Project is a model for how other sentinel systems might operate with close collaboration and communication among local and state STD programs, state laboratories, and the CDC. Another sentinel surveillance system of potential benefit could be developed by collecting and analyzing the results of prenatal testing for gonorrhea, syphilis, and chlamydial infection. Testing of pregnant women for such infections is already being performed in most states, but the resulting data are not systematically captured or analyzed by STD surveillance systems. Such data could provide age-specific rates of STDs (number found infected per number tested) in women. Infection rates among young pregnant women may be good, although not perfect, surrogates for STD rates among the general population of women who do not use contraception. Trends in STD prevalence among young pregnant women also may be particularly sensitive to STD interventions. This sentinel surveillance system would have increasing coverage of the U.S. population over time and could be coordinated with prenatal HIV surveillance systems. In addition, surveillance of STDs within correctional systems and drug treatment facilities could help motivate and evaluate interventions to prevent STDs in these settings.

Therefore, the committee makes the following recommendation:

• **The CDC should lead a coordinated national effort to improve the surveillance of STDs and their associated complications and improve the monitoring of STD prevention program effectiveness.** Specific areas for improvement include the following:

1. The CDC and the states should improve reporting from private sector health care professionals and laboratories and collect data on the number of persons tested for STDs through the national surveillance system. In addition, the CDC should systematically assess the attributes of the current surveillance system, including validity, sensitivity, representativeness, acceptability, and timeliness, in relation to alternative approaches to active or sentinel surveillance. This effort should take into account the potential impact of changes in clinical practice patterns, such as changes in utilization of diagnostic tests or types of tests used, and changes in reimbursement for clinical services on reported STD rates and surveillance for emerging antimicrobial resistance.

2. Disease surveillance systems should be better coordinated with the information systems of community-based clinics, private sector providers and laboratories, and public STD clinics. Special emphasis should be placed on educating clinicians about reporting and collaborating with, and collecting data from, private sector providers, including managed care organizations and other health plans. Training is also needed at all levels of the surveillance system to improve data collection, management, analysis, and dissemination. The use of new information technology to improve surveillance by minimizing reporting delays should be supported.

3. The current passive surveillance system should be supplemented with active surveillance components as appropriate. These activities should include serosurveys or testing of urine and saliva using nationally representative health surveys, including the National Health and Nutrition Examination Survey (NHANES) and the National Survey of Adolescent Males, to estimate rates of STDs and to assess the attributes of passive surveillance systems.

Utilizing Health Services Performance Measures

Surveillance data can be used to evaluate program effectiveness, but current systems to monitor effectiveness, as described in Chapter 5, are inadequate. If surveillance data are to be used as a program management tool, state and local health departments need to develop greater capacity in data management and analysis. The current capacity is inconsistent among local health departments, and is often limited even at the state health department level. Therefore, federal technical assistance to improve data management and analysis capacity at the local and state level is needed.

In addition to disease surveillance, health indicators that measure program effectiveness and support program evaluation are important components of a comprehensive information system for STDs. Disease prevention programs will continue to require timely data to support decision-making in programmatic areas (e.g., prevention and education, partner notification and follow-up, clinic services) and outcome measures to assess the effectiveness of interventions on both individual and community levels. Performance measures and information systems need to be designed to collect data from a variety of health care settings in addition to public STD clinics. These settings include family planning clinics, community health centers, hospital emergency rooms, correctional institutions, substance abuse programs, health plans, and other private sector health care providers. Performance monitoring should not be used exclusively to allocate funding, but also as a tool for program management (IOM, 1997). The ability of public STD clinics and health departments to effectively monitor arrangements or contracts with private health plans will be contingent upon the capacity of STD-related information systems to generate relevant and timely information on program performance measures. Existing data systems of STD programs are not adequate for overall program assessment. In addition, it is important that performance measures be valid and reflect the quality and health impact of services. For example, it can be expected that reported STD rates will rise with expansion of screening efforts. Potential areas for which STD clinical practice performance measures should be developed include:

1. patient reports regarding care;
2. access, availability, and utilization of services;
3. cost and affordability of services;
4. time interval between seeking of care and examination, time interval between initial examination and treatment, and percentage of diagnosed persons treated;
5. incidence of reinfections or persistent infections; and
6. appropriateness of clinician diagnosis, treatment, and counseling; knowledge and compliance with treatment protocols; compliance with precautions and management of adverse reactions; and disease reporting.

The automated information systems of many managed care organizations and other health plans are a valuable source of data on patient encounters, disease diagnoses, and clinical outcomes. The Health Plan Employer Data Information Set (HEDIS), in particular, and other health services performance measures will be particularly valuable as new indicators related to preventive and public health services are developed and implemented. These data represent an excellent opportunity to conduct outcomes research and evaluate the effectiveness of interventions. Not all managed care organizations, however, are currently using such performance monitoring tools; STD-related data from other health plans will also need to be captured.

STD-related information systems should be developed and planned in the context of, and be consistent with, broader information system development initiatives to monitor a range of community health issues (IOM, 1997). Information systems should take into account evolving disease prevention management requirements and opportunities; promote and support cost containment and efficient resource allocation; optimally utilize current and evolving technology; and consider the analytic capacity necessary to maximize available information.

Therefore, the committee makes the following recommendations:

• Federal, state, and local STD programs should encourage and provide technical assistance to employers and other purchasers of health care (including Medicaid programs), managed care organizations and other health plans, and other health care professionals to develop and utilize information systems that effectively integrate preventive services performance data with community health status indicators and STD program data. STD-related information systems should support assessment and evaluation of anticipated system impacts from changes in health program structure and funding such as managed care, Medicaid changes, and block grants. The information system should also monitor the capacity of state and local health departments to execute essential public health functions and services. The CDC should provide adequate technical assistance to state and local health agencies to support the development of STD-related surveillance and other information systems and data analysis capacity at the local level.

• **STD-related performance measures should be included in the Health Plan Employer Data Information Set (HEDIS) and other health services performance measures to improve quality-assurance monitoring of STDs.** The National Committee for Quality Assurance and other relevant organizations, in conjunction with public health agencies and health plans, should continue to develop and promote performance measures related to STD prevention.

STRATEGY 3: FOCUS ON ADOLESCENTS AND UNDERSERVED POPULATIONS

Strategy 3 is to design and implement essential STD-related services in innovative ways for adolescents and underserved populations. Specific populations requiring special emphasis in an effective national system for STD prevention include adolescents and disenfranchised populations. Reasons for the greater risk of STDs among these groups and their importance in prevention strategies are documented in Chapters 2 and 3. Many members of these groups lack access to STD-related services and are difficult to reach through traditional clinical settings and approaches. Under Strategy 3, the committee recommends that prevention of STDs be a central focus in designing interventions for these populations and that innovative methods for delivering STD-related services to such populations be immediately implemented.

Focusing on Prevention

Ultimately, social norms regarding sexual behavior need to change before a sustained reduction in STDs can be realized. Population-based preventive services are the primary means for changing social norms and attitudes by creating an environment that supports such changes. A national strategy for STDs needs to emphasize prevention because averting illness is desirable, many STDs are incurable, and STD-related complications may be irreversible. As summarized in Chapter 4, there are many existing prevention-oriented approaches that are effective in averting long-term health problems and costs. The committee believes that an approach to STD prevention involving multiple interventions at the individual and the community levels is critical. This is because many interventions are highly effective, but no single intervention is sufficient on its own. Complementary behavioral and biomedical approaches to STD prevention are essential. Interventions to promote healthy sexual behavior need to be complemented by access to clinical services, training and education of health professionals, surveillance and research, and community-based programs. Many prevention efforts, such as community- and school-based programs, remain underfunded and weak because of social and political constraints. The committee believes that population-based interventions should be objectively evaluated for funding and implementation based on their scientific merit and potential public health impact.

Prevention programs must address the roles of both men and women in transmitting infection. Many screening programs are appropriately targeted toward women and conducted in facilities exclusively providing services to women. In order to interrupt the transmission cycle of STDs, however, infections among men also need to be addressed. STD prevention efforts should include both screening programs for asymptomatic men and male-specific behavioral interventions, such as promotion of responsibility for condom use. In addition, programs providing health services to women should ensure that sex partners are appropriately evaluated and treated.

Expanding Prevention-Related Research

New research may be used to develop effective prevention programs, but such programs need to be modified regularly based on continuous evaluation of existing programs and changes in the epidemiology of STDs and the health care environment. Prevention-related research allows program managers to maximize the effectiveness of interventions and policymakers to maximize available resources. Professionals responsible for STD prevention efforts should ensure that regular program evaluation and quality improvement activities are integral parts of their programs.

There are many available interventions for STD prevention, but some have not been fully evaluated, and new interventions need to be developed. Wasserheit and Hitchcock (1992), in their assessment of future directions in STD prevention research, concluded that a multidisciplinary approach to research is necessary; prevention research should be given top priority; the long-term sequelae of STDs should be given greater emphasis; and communication and coordination within the research infrastructure should be improved. A recent panel charged to evaluate the social, behavioral, and prevention research areas for the National Institutes of Health found that only 3.4 percent of the total National Institutes of Health budget for research on AIDS was devoted to prevention and intervention research in the behavioral and social sciences (NIH, 1996). The panel recommended the following: intervention and behavioral research be given the highest priority and coordinated with biomedical research; a paradigm shift to develop models that are domain-specific with regard to sexuality (and drug use) and recognition that risk behavior is embedded within personal, interpersonal, and situational contexts; research on individual differences in human sexuality (and drug use) that takes into account cognitive, affective, cultural, and neurophysi-ological variables; studies on direct effects of intoxicants on self-regulatory mechanisms; and studies regarding maintenance of behavior change.

The committee agrees with the above assessments and recommends that general areas of additional research in STD prevention include behavioral, bio-medical, and operational research. In addition, the committee recommends that the following specific topics be studied: determinants of sexual behavior and sustained behavior change on an individual and community level; determinants of initiation of sexual intercourse among adolescents; influence of social and other community-related factors on risk of STDs; interventions to improve con-dom use and reduce high-risk behaviors; effectiveness of sexual risk behavior assessment and counseling; biomedical interventions that do not rely primarily on individual behavior, such as vaccines; female-controlled prevention methods; cost-effectiveness of preventive interventions, including partner notification and treatment techniques; methods for preventing STDs among disenfranchised popu-lations; interventions for preventing STDs among persons of all sexual orienta-tions; and methods to measure prevention program effectiveness.

Therefore, the committee makes the following recommendation:

• **The National Institutes of Health and the CDC should continue to support and expand both basic and applied research in STD prevention.** Research results should be made widely available and should be used by govern-ment agencies, public and private health programs, and health professional orga-nizations to improve STD prevention services.

Developing Female-Controlled Methods for Protecting Against STDs

Although women bear the larger burden of disease associated with STDs, the most effective means for preventing transmission of STDs during intercourse (i.e., the male condom) is largely dependent on the behavior of men. Except for the female condom, there are no female-controlled methods that are sufficiently protective against STDs. Additional methods of protection over which women have greater control need to be made available, and additional effective mechani-cal and chemical methods for protection against STDs need to be developed. Dual protection (i.e., use of one method to protect against pregnancy and one method to protect against STDs) is important because, as discussed in Chapter 4, no single method of preventing STDs or pregnancy confers the maximum level of protection for both conditions.

Therefore, the committee makes the following recommendation:

• **The National Institutes of Health, the Food and Drug Administra-tion, and pharmaceutical, biotechnology, and medical device companies should collaboratively develop effective female-controlled methods for pre-**

venting STDs. Clinicians and STD (including HIV) prevention programs, like family planning programs, should teach that use of a condom (male or female) along with an effective contraceptive for pregnancy is necessary to obtain maximum protection against both STDs and unintended pregnancy. This should be the standard approach for both men and women who are not in a mutually monogamous relationship with an uninfected partner.

Focusing on Adolescents

Many of the severe health consequences of STDs, such as cervical, liver, and other cancers, manifest themselves among older adults because they may not appear until decades after infection. This phenomenon contributes to the under-recognition of the impact of STDs among older adults. These complications, however, usually result from infections acquired or health behaviors initiated during adolescence or early adulthood. Therefore, STD prevention programs need to focus on adolescents. The committee's proposed focus and recommendations regarding appropriate policies to prevent STDs among adolescents are similar to those of numerous health professional and other organizations (AMA, 1996).

Ensuring Effective, Early Interventions and Confidentiality

As outlined in Chapters 2 and 3, three million teenagers acquire an STD each year and high-risk sexual activity among adolescents has become more common during the past two decades, increasing the number of adolescents and young adults at risk for STDs. Current data indicate that almost 40 percent of adolescents in the ninth grade have already had sexual intercourse (CDC, 1995). Adolescents are at greater risk of exposure to and infection with STDs than are adults. This is due to high-risk sexual behavior, increased biological susceptibility of the adolescent cervix to infectious diseases, and the greater likelihood of exposure to the social factors contributing to STD risk.

Many opponents of education for adolescents about sexuality and STDs believe that adolescents should only be told not to have sexual intercourse and that other forms of education are not appropriate. At the other end of the spectrum, some advocate that adolescents should be assumed to be sexually active and given appropriate education regarding STDs, without any messages regarding the appropriateness of sexual intercourse among adolescents. The committee believes that some aspects of both perspectives are valid and should be part of a national initiative to prevent the initiation of high-risk sexual activity among adolescents. Adolescents should be strongly encouraged to delay sexual intercourse until they are emotionally mature enough to take responsibility for this activity. In spite of messages to delay intercourse, most individuals will initiate sexual intercourse during adolescence. They should have access to information and instruction regarding STDs, unintended pregnancy, and methods for preventing both. As reviewed in Chapter 4, such instruction does not increase sexual activity among adolescents. Because information is a necessary but not always sufficient condition for behavior change, interventions and policies to facilitate development of behavioral skills are also necessary.

To prevent STDs among adolescents, it is necessary to provide them with accurate, comprehensive information and give them instruction in ways to implement healthy sexual behaviors. As discussed in Chapter 3, adolescents experience a large information gap regarding STDs. Surveys show that they receive much of their information regarding sexuality and STDs from their peers, the mass media, or other unreliable sources of information rather from their parents or health care professionals. Studies cited in Chapter 4 show that many school-based programs and mass media education campaigns are effective in improving knowledge about STDs and in promoting healthy sexual behaviors. Therefore, the committee believes that school-related programs (including school-based and school-linked programs) and mass media campaigns should comprise two major components of an effective prevention strategy for adolescents.

Although school-based prevention programs should be a major means for preventing risky sexual behaviors among adolescents, it is not realistic to expect that such programs will be successful in all situations or that they will be effective in isolation. This is because such programs cannot control other influences on adolescent health behaviors, such as the mass media and peer and community norms regarding sexual behavior. In addition, the wide variability in the quality of and support for school-based programs in communities is a barrier to effectiveness of programs. Therefore, as with other interventions proposed by the committee, school-based programs must be implemented along with individual- and community-based interventions to promote healthy sexual behaviors. In evaluating school-based programs and other behavioral interventions to prevent STDs, it should be recognized that the outcomes of interest (e.g., reduction in STDs, reduction in risky sexual behaviors) are influenced by factors other than the intervention being studied. Therefore, evaluations of program effectiveness should account for other influences that exist under real world conditions.

Clinical services for adolescents need to be more accessible for reasons outlined in Chapter 3. Adolescents are one of the age groups least likely to have health insurance coverage: they infrequently present to regular health care facilities, and confidentiality is a major concern for them. In addition, the cost of health services may be a significant barrier. Many adolescents are seen at routine exams, including physical examinations for participation in sports, in school-related and family planning clinics, and by primary care professionals. Clinicians should utilize these and other appropriate clinical encounters to educate all and screen sexually active adolescents for STDs. For example, all adolescents should be counseled regarding methods to protect against STDs when prescriptions for nonbarrier contraceptives are given and when they are evaluated for an unintended pregnancy.

As discussed in Chapters 4 and 5, ensuring confidentiality of services is extremely important, especially for adolescents. Given that most adolescents are unwilling to seek medical attention for an STD unless confidentiality is ensured, adolescents should be able to consent to STD-related services without parental knowledge. Forty-nine states and the District of Columbia currently have laws that give a minor explicit authority to consent to diagnostic and treatment services for STDs (AGI, 1995). Of these states, 16 allow physicians to notify parents of treatment provided. Pending federal legislation may interfere with a minor's ability to consent to STD-related services and could have a harmful impact on efforts to prevent STDs among adolescents.[4] As discussed in Chapter 5, billing and claims-processing procedures of some health plans may be a major barrier to confidential STD-related services. The committee believes that parental notification of treatment for an STD, either by providers or indirectly through billing or claim-processing procedures, is likely to discourage adolescents from seeking health care for potential STDs, and thereby increase the potential for STD-related complications and transmission to others.

There are significant numbers of adolescents who are disenfranchised. As documented in Chapter 3, a substantial number of adolescents live in detention facilities and group homes, or are sex workers or runaways or otherwise homeless persons. In addition, a substantial number of these adolescents were sexually abused as children. As a result, these youth often behave in a high-risk manner that puts them at increased risk for STDs and other health problems. All of these young people have significant problems obtaining health care and need access to comprehensive, high-quality health services in general and STD-related services in particular. Although school-based programs will reach the overwhelming number of adolescents, interventions for those who do not attend school should also be developed and implemented.

Therefore, the committee makes the following recommendations:

• **A major part of a national strategy to prevent STDs should focus on adolescents, and interventions should begin** *before* **sexual activity is initiated, which may be before adolescence is reached. Interventions should focus on preventing the establishment of high-risk sexual behaviors.**

• **All health plans and health care providers should implement policies in compliance with state laws to ensure confidentiality of STD- and family-planning-related services provided to adolescents and other individuals.** The following actions should be taken to ensure confidentiality of services:

---

[4]S. 984, H.R. 1946, Parental Rights and Responsibilities Act of 1995, 104th Congress, 1st session.

1. health plans should review billing or claims-processing procedures to ensure that they preserve confidentiality of services;

2. the National Committee for Quality Assurance and other organizations that accredit health plans should ensure that a health plan's ability to ensure confidential access to STD-related services is appropriately assessed;

3. state and local health professional organizations should disseminate information regarding the importance of maintaining patient confidentiality to their members; and

4. the Academy of Pediatrics and other health professional organizations should educate pediatricians and other clinicians who provide health services to adolescents regarding the negative impact of parental notification for STD-related services.

Expanding School-Based Programs

Schools are critical venues for STD prevention activities. Survey data show overwhelming public support for school-based HIV/STD education programs. Studies cited in Chapter 4 show that school-based education programs are effective in improving knowledge regarding STDs, delaying adolescent initiation of sexual intercourse, and increasing use of condoms. Most teenagers indicate that the school is their primary source of information regarding STDs; this indicates that other sources of information are lacking.

Scientific studies and evaluations of school-based programs for STD prevention do not support the contention that such programs encourage students to have sex. Unfortunately, these programs have become highly controversial and efforts to provide STD-related education outside the home have been consistently resisted by certain groups. The committee recognizes that some parents and interested groups have sincere, deeply held personal beliefs regarding sex and STD education in schools that prevent them from supporting such programs. However, the committee believes that the scientific evidence presented in Chapter 4 in support of school-based educational programs for STD prevention is strong; that adolescence is the critical period for adopting healthy behaviors; and that school is one of the few available venues for reaching adolescents.

The committee believes that it is important to distinguish opposition to school-based programs and other STD prevention efforts that are primarily based on religious and personal beliefs from that based on systematic evaluations of program effectiveness or scientific research. Understanding the underlying reasons for such opposition can help communities resolve differences. Because of the controversial nature of the issue, health departments and other agencies and organizations desiring to implement a school-based STD prevention program should work closely with school administrators, health educators, teachers, parents, and students throughout the planning and implementation process.

Surveys cited in Chapter 4 show that many states specifically require schools to offer instruction on HIV and/or STD prevention, and most health education teachers reported teaching STD prevention. However, studies indicate that instruction, when it exists, is not consistently implemented at an early enough age. In addition, teaching materials for STDs need to be developed. Current instruction is of inconsistent quality and effectiveness, and variable content and time is devoted to it. Besides providing information, school-based education programs need to provide students with the skills to implement healthy sexual behaviors. The committee believes that it is possible to increase knowledge, change attitudes, and influence behavior of adolescents by expanding the use of school-based health education curricula and by providing the training and support necessary to improve existing programs.

Given the high rates of sexual intercourse among adolescents and the significant barriers that hinder the ability of adolescents to purchase and use condoms (as cited in Chapter 4), the committee believes that the current evidence is sufficiently strong to recommend expansion of condom availability in schools. Definitive data regarding the effectiveness of condom availability programs in schools are limited, because such programs are relatively new and few have been designed for measurements of effectiveness. However, available data regarding school- and community-based condom availability programs cited in Chapter 4 suggest that such programs are effective. Data also show that both parents and students are highly supportive of such programs and believe that they have a positive effect on prevention of HIV infection and other STDs among adolescents. None of the studies reviewed by the committee suggests that access to condoms in schools results in increased sexual activity among students. Legal challenges to these programs based on constitutionality arguments have been found to be largely without merit. Because of the sensitive nature of this issue, it is clear that schools, school boards, public health officials, health plans, parents, and students will have to work closely together in establishing condom availability programs.

As discussed in Chapters 3 and 5, students in universities and colleges also are at high risk for STDs. The scope and quality of STD-related services in these institutions, however, are unclear. Because many adolescents and young adults do not have private health insurance, school and student health clinics should ensure that confidential and comprehensive STD-related services are available.

Hepatitis B vaccine is highly effective and recently has been recommended for all infants and adolescents (11- and 12-year-olds), as well as for other adolescents and adults at high risk for hepatitis B virus infection. Many adolescents and adults at high risk for this infection, however, have not been vaccinated. Immunizing adolescents is difficult because of their relatively infrequent encounters with health care professionals and inadequate access to health care. Until childhood hepatitis B immunization ensures that all adolescents are protected, all clinical opportunities to immunize adolescents against hepatitis B virus infection need to be utilized. This includes school-based and school-linked clinics and dedicated public STD clinics. Ideally, all adolescents should be immunized before they become sexually active.

Therefore, the committee makes the following recommendations:

• **All school districts in the United States should ensure that schools provide essential, age-appropriate STD-related services, including health education, access to condoms, and readily accessible and available clinical services, such as school-based clinical services, to prevent STDs.** Ultimately, parents, teachers, health professionals, and others in the community should decide what kinds of instruction and services are most appropriate for specific grade levels. Specifically, school districts should:

1. require that information regarding the prevention of STDs, including HIV infection, and unintended pregnancy be part of required health education instruction for all students. Such instruction should be part of a comprehensive health education curriculum that is sequential, age appropriate, and given every year. Instruction regarding STDs, including HIV infection, and unintended pregnancy should start *before* adolescents in the school become sexually active. Because the quality of health education in schools is currently variable, schools should modify and implement model programs, such as those identified and evaluated by the CDC or other organizations. Public health departments and nongovernmental, voluntary organizations should assist departments of education in developing or modifying health education curricula for local needs and in evaluating and disseminating effective school-based curricula and other interventions to reduce high-risk sexual behaviors. In addition, state and local departments of education should support or provide training for teachers and school administrators involved in instructing or advising students regarding STDs;

2. ensure that condoms are available to students as part of a comprehensive STD prevention program. Condoms should be made available along with information regarding sexual decision-making, including delaying of sexual intercourse. Condom availability programs should also include instruction on proper use of the condom and should have an evaluation component to assess effectiveness. Local health departments, health plans, and other private sector organizations should form partnerships with schools to establish and maintain these and other STD prevention programs; and

3. ensure that school-based and school-linked health clinics provide STD-related clinical services, such as counseling for high-risk sexual behaviors; screening, diagnosis, and treatment of STDs; and hepatitis B immunization for all students. Health plans should develop collaborative agreements with school-based and school-linked clinics, including payment for confidential STD-related services for plan enrollees that are provided by such clinics. Schools should work with local health plans to ensure fair reimbursement rates and confidentiality of

services. In addition, universities and colleges should ensure that their student health services provide the above services.

• **All health plans, clinicians, and publicly sponsored health clinics should provide or arrange for hepatitis B immunizations for their infant, adolescent, and adult patients according to the Advisory Committee on Immunization Practices (ACIP) guidelines. Given the difficulty in reaching adolescents in health care settings, public health officials should ensure that adolescents who are not immunized in health care settings are immunized through school-based or other community programs.** Additional infrastructure and programs for vaccinating adolescents and adults at risk for hepatitis B virus infection, through settings such as public STD clinics, should be developed and implemented. This infrastructure may also be used when vaccines against other STDs become available. In addition, communities should consider including hepatitis B immunization for adolescents and children in the local immunization campaigns that have traditionally focused only on vaccines for young children.

Establishing New Venues for Interventions

The risk of STDs among disenfranchised groups can be significantly reduced through appropriate innovative interventions. Venues for intervention need to be expanded because these groups are difficult to reach through traditional health care settings. Health services for disenfranchised persons do not have popular support; as a result, such services have been marginalized and underfunded. However, because these groups represent reservoirs of infection for the community, and for other reasons, it is important that they receive appropriate STD-related services.

Currently, knowledge of sociocultural factors related to transmission of STDs is not sufficient to fully explain why some ethnic and racial groups in the United States have higher STD rates than the general population. As discussed in Chapter 2, poverty and sexual behavior do not entirely explain the higher rates of STDs in some groups. Other potential explanations, discussed in Chapter 3, that are associated with increased risk of STDs and their associated complications are known to vary across racial or ethnic groups. These explanations include inadequate access to health care, lack of awareness and knowledge of STDs, and substance use behaviors. Further research is needed to evaluate the role of sociocultural and other factors in STD transmission among different ethnic and racial groups.

It is important to recognize that the underlying cause of STDs is high-risk sexual behavior that is common among all racial and ethnic groups in the United States. Therefore, in this report, the committee proposes an approach to STD prevention that is focused on the specific behaviors and ecological factors that put all individuals at risk. Race- and ethnic-specific rates of STD should not be used to stigmatize specific groups as high-risk populations, but rather they should be used to justify adequate attention and allocation of resources to reduce STD rates among these population groups. The committee recognizes that by its emphasis on behaviors common among all groups, it is possible that funds may be diluted and redirected away from certain high-risk communities to more general, lower-risk populations. The committee, however, does advocate focusing interventions on certain high-risk groups as discussed later in this section. The notion of focusing on behaviors that put all persons at risk rather than certain high-risk groups is reflected in current health policies. For example, the recommendation to screen all pregnant women for HIV, rather than screen only certain groups of pregnant women, reflects the notion that all pregnant women have had unprotected sexual intercourse. In order to appropriately address target behavioral risk factors, however, surveillance of sexual behaviors and STDs is essential.

Most of the research regarding drugs, alcohol, and STD transmission cited in Chapter 3 is cross-sectional in nature and does not allow for determination of cause and effect. The committee, therefore, cannot definitively estimate the impact of substance use on STD transmission. The associations between drug and alcohol use and STD transmission, however, are substantial and have important implications for improving STD prevention. Substance use increases the risk of STDs on an individual level by making it more difficult for persons to take protective actions against STDs. In the case of crack cocaine, drug use not only increases personal risk for STDs, but also has an effect on the prevalence of STDs in certain communities by altering social structures. An increased emphasis on outreach services for substance users is indicated because health services for such persons are fragmented and often not accessible. STD prevention efforts need to include individuals who are at risk for substance use and specifically target venues where substance users can be effectively reached with tailored interventions.

The increasing number of persons in correctional facilities represents a growing pool of people at risk of STDs and a potential source of infection for others when inmates are released. Data cited in Chapter 3 indicate that screening and treatment of all prisoners and detainees is an important public health strategy for the following reasons: (a) the prevalence of STDs is extremely high in this population; (b) treatment may reduce the spread of STDs in the community once detainees are released; (c) detention represents an ideal opportunity to screen for health problems in a population that does not ordinarily have access to health care; and (d) treatment reduces spread of STDs within detention facilities and averts associated long-term health care costs. Rapid screening and treatment of persons in detention facilities represent an opportunity to effectively contain STDs in a high-risk group. Because of lags in obtaining laboratory results, rapid turnover of detainees, poor treatment compliance, drug contraindications during pregnancy, and other issues, the optimal screening and treatment program for detention facilities varies with the characteristics of the facility and population. At a minimum, all persons entering detention facilities should be screened and treated for STDs. As reviewed in Chapter 3, in addition to having high rates of STDs upon entry, some inmates continue to have high rates of unprotected sex and drug use while in prison. Therefore, diagnostic and treatment services, risk reduction, and other prevention programs for prisoners are needed. Prevention, early detection, and treatment are appropriate even for long-term prisoners because such a strategy is more cost-effective for the correctional system than treating the severe long-term complications of STDs.

Few correctional facilities currently provide access to condoms. Although condoms can be used as weapons or to conceal contraband, as cited in Chapter 3, the experience of correctional systems with condom availability programs indicates that such programs do not increase these problems. Given the circumstances under which sexual intercourse occurs among prisoners, research regarding the effectiveness of condom availability programs and other methods for reducing the prevalence of unprotected sexual intercourse within correctional facilities is indicated and should be supported by the Department of Justice and the Department of Health and Human Services.

Sex workers, runaways, and the homeless are at high risk of STDs and almost always lack health insurance and are difficult to reach. These populations, however, may be more accessible through nontraditional venues and mobile clinics. Examples of effective approaches to reach these groups are cited in Chapters 3 and 4. Migrant workers need access to STD-related services in an environment that minimizes cultural and language barriers. Because of the lack of education of most migrant workers, health education for STDs must begin at the most basic level. To address cultural and language barriers, peer educators may be effective in reaching many migrants and other groups.

Nontraditional venues for delivering STD-related services, such as detention facilities, drug treatment clinics, alcohol treatment facilities, and other sites where disenfranchised persons can be found, are appropriate sites for prevention activities. Most nontraditional venues for STD prevention have not been targeted by STD program staff, and there are many problems that may arise in implementing STD-related services in such settings. Appropriately trained staff and tools that are suitable for such situations are essential. For example, outreach workers commonly need multiple language and cultural sensitivity skills in order to effectively deliver services to these ethnically and culturally diverse groups. Despite the barriers that make delivery of services in these settings challenging, it is critical that STD-related services be provided in places where persons at high risk for STDs are frequently encountered. Such services may either be furnished by staff of these facilities or supplied through partnerships with local health departments, health plans, and other organizations. Given the evolving epidemiology of STDs, health officials need to continually monitor and reassess the most appropriate and effective community-based venues for prevention.

New biomedical, epidemiological, and behavioral tools are needed to contain persistent epidemics of STDs among disenfranchised populations. One of the major barriers to effective screening programs for disenfranchised populations is the relative lack of diagnostic tests that can be used outside of the health-care setting. Ideally, to maximize their usefulness in field situations, tests should be inexpensive and rapid and use noninvasive clinical specimens, such as urine or saliva. The ability to diagnose STDs using noninvasive clinical samples presents tremendous potential opportunities for innovative STD prevention programs. For example, this technology may enable more widespread clinician use of laboratory testing, allow for expansion of screening programs in venues not traditionally targeted by STD programs, and improve health-seeking behavior for STDs. In addition, improvements in the following areas would be beneficial in providing services to disenfranchised persons: rapid diagnostic tests for genital ulcer diseases; effective oral therapies that are suitable for use in community-based prevention campaigns; protocols for rapid assessments of community substance use patterns; and guidelines for STD screening in a variety of traditional and nontraditional health care settings. Innovative, effective, and rapid screening and treatment protocols for syphilis, such as that implemented in New York City's major facility for admission medical screening of female inmates (described in Chapter 3), should be considered.

Various government agencies have responsibility for delivering health services to disenfranchised persons but may not coordinate such services, thus gaps in services result. For example, a prisoner may be screened for an STD upon arrival but, unless the results are available before release, there is no assurance that the individual will be treated by a health care provider in the community. Given the variety of agencies that provide services to substance users, the Department of Health and Human Services, including the CDC and the Substance Abuse and Mental Health Services Administration, should work with other federal agencies to coordinate STD prevention programs for substance users. Providing STD-related services to disenfranchised persons requires innovative approaches, additional planning, and resource commitments because of the special considerations and staff skills that are needed to reach these populations.

Therefore, the committee makes the following recommendations:

• **Federal, state, and local agencies should focus on reducing STDs among disenfranchised populations (e.g., substance users, persons in detention facilities, sex workers, the homeless, migrant workers) by:**

1. coordinating their various health-related programs to ensure effective, comprehensive STD-related services for populations at high risk for STDs. Coordination of services and sharing of resources are especially important for federal agencies (e.g., the Department of Health and Human Services, the Department of Justice) and should be priorities both among and within agencies;

2. ensuring that STD prevention programs establish linkages with correctional facilities, substance use treatment programs, homeless and runaway programs, migrant health programs, and other facilities and programs that serve high-risk populations to ensure appropriate screening, diagnosis and treatment, and follow-up of infected persons and their partners. Such linkages should ensure that all adolescents and adults living in environments where the risk for STDs is high have access to confidential, comprehensive, high-quality STD-related services. In addition, the CDC, in collaboration with other appropriate agencies, should develop STD screening guidelines suitable for use in venues that have not been traditionally targeted by STD screening programs; and

3. developing and implementing interventions and services for STDs that are (a) focused, sustained, and culturally appropriate; (b) provided by a spectrum of health care professionals, including potential non-health-care professionals such as educators, peers, and community volunteers; (c) delivered through a variety of settings, including nontraditional settings such as substance use treatment centers, mobile clinics, and the streets; and (d) reinforced at multiple points and venues to sustain and maximize effectiveness.

- **Prisons and other detention facilities should provide comprehensive STD-related services, including STD prevention counseling and education, screening, diagnosis and treatment, partner notification and treatment, and methods for reducing unprotected sexual intercourse and drug use among prisoners.** Rapid screening and treatment programs for STDs should be developed and implemented. In addition to health agencies, prison administrators should seek assistance and guidance in developing and implementing the above services from correctional systems that have already implemented effective programs to prevent STDs.

- **The National Institutes of Health, the Food and Drug Administration, and the CDC should work with pharmaceutical and biotechnology companies to develop improved STD diagnostic tools (e.g., rapid saliva and urine tests) that are suitable for use in nontraditional health care settings (e.g., prisons, mobile clinics, the streets).** Pharmaceutical, biotechnology, and medical device companies should continue to invest in research to develop and improve vaccines, diagnostic tests, antiviral treatments, and mechanical and chemical barrier protection for women and assist in promoting public and health care provider awareness and knowledge of STDs. In addition, such companies should ensure that the cost of existing and new biomedical interventions for STDs are affordable to publicly sponsored STD programs.

STRATEGY 4: ENSURE ACCESS TO SERVICES

Strategy 4 is to ensure access to and quality of essential clinical services for STDs. As demonstrated in Chapter 5, both public and private sector clinical services for STDs are currently fragmented, inadequate, and sometimes of poor quality. Timely access to clinical services for STDs is vital to prevent further transmission. Access to clinical services is supported by the absence of financial barriers to obtaining health services, minimization of nonfinancial barriers, assurance that patients will not be stigmatized, and assurance that services are sensitive to sociocultural diversity. Assuring access, however, is not a sufficient method of ensuring that clinical services are effective. Providing access in both the public and private sectors allows those who need services to get them, while quality assurance improves the likelihood that services will be effective when delivered. Ensuring access to and quality of clinical services maximizes coverage and effectiveness of STD-related services. Therefore, universal and timely access to high-quality clinical services should be the goal of the clinical care system.

Under Strategy 4, the committee proposes to improve and expand clinical services for STDs by (a) ensuring access to services at the local level, (b) improving dedicated public STD clinics, (c) expanding the role of health plans and purchasers of health services, (d) improving the training of clinicians, and (e) improving clinical management of STDs.

Ensuring Access to Community Services

Access to services is facilitated by expanding availability of STD-related services through primary care clinicians and by coordinating services at the local level.

Incorporating STD-Related Services into Primary Care

Effective STD-related care encompasses biomedical interventions (e.g., diagnosis and treatment); behavioral interventions (e.g., patient counseling); and social interventions (e.g., substance use prevention and treatment). Primary care providers can be effective coordinators of these types of health and social services in the community (IOM, 1996b). This is especially important for disenfranchised persons who are at high risk for STDs and other infectious diseases and require multiple services. Because primary care treats the individual in the context of other physical and mental health problems and fosters ongoing relationships between the clinician and the individual, the likelihood of early STD detection and effective preventive interventions, such as regular clinician counseling, increases. In addition, incorporating STD-related services into primary care may improve access to services since primary care clinicians are much more numerous than public STD clinics. Primary care providers diagnose the majority of STDs in the United States, and it is likely that primary care health professionals in the private sector will play a greater role in STD prevention.

Another reason for incorporating STD-related clinical services into primary care is the wide variation in the quality, scope, accessibility, and availability of services currently provided by many public STD clinics. However, limited research has been performed regarding the quality and scope of STD-related services in primary care settings. While the committee is optimistic regarding the ability of primary care clinicians to improve STD-related services, it recognizes that barriers to their ability to provide comprehensive services, as outlined in this report, are substantial. Although many of these barriers need to be addressed before primary care clinicians are fully able to provide comprehensive STD-related services, the committee believes that the long-term process of incorporating STD-related services into primary care should begin as these barriers are addressed.

Whether in a fee-for-service or a managed care setting, privately insured patients usually receive STD-related services as part of comprehensive primary care or, for women, gynecological care. However, such services are isolated from public sector services and broader efforts to prevent STDs in the community. With very few exceptions, it appears that private health care professionals are unaware of both the prevalence of STDs among privately insured persons and the serious and expensive sequelae of undetected infections.

Therefore, the committee makes the following recommendation:

• **Comprehensive STD-related services should be incorporated into primary care, including reproductive health services.** Primary care should include the full range of STD-related services, including screening, diagnosis and treatment, partner notification and treatment, health education and counseling, and community outreach. Such services should be delivered by health care professionals with training in STD clinical management. These professionals may be STD specialists or primary care providers who have received STD-specific training. Regardless of the clinical setting, the provision of such services by poorly qualified health care professionals with no specific training in STDs is not recommended because it will result in inadequate diagnosis and treatment and poor coordination with other STD-related services.

Coordinating Services at the Community Level

Communities differ widely in their health needs and capacity to support a system of STD-related services. Therefore, the organization of community STD prevention services must be tailored to local needs and conditions. No single model will be appropriate for all communities. For example, only some communities will be able to depend on the teaching and research support of academic health centers that have established model STD prevention programs, including clinical capacity. Clinicians with training in STDs may be readily available in the private sector in urban areas, but difficult to find in rural areas. Communities with large numbers of high-risk persons and high STD rates may need a system of dedicated STD clinics, but communities with low STD rates may only require primary care providers trained in STD prevention, diagnosis, and treatment. In addition, dedicated public STD clinics are not likely to be cost-effective in some rural communities that have high rates of STDs but relatively small populations.

Each community, through the leadership of the local health department, should ensure universal access to high-quality, comprehensive STD-related services. At a minimum, public and private sector health services should be coordinated to increase coverage and ensure optimal use of resources. Depending on local conditions, public health departments should incorporate STD-related services into other public and private primary health care services. Depending on epidemiologic patterns, health insurance coverage, population density, and other community characteristics, communities may continue to support dedicated public STD clinics or may shift such services to community-based clinics or the private sector. Dedicated public STD clinics may be phased out in communities with relatively few uninsured high-risk persons if public-private contractual arrangements ensure that STD-related clinical services will be provided by community-based and private sector clinicians in a timely manner. However, communities with a high prevalence of STDs, a large number of uninsured residents, or difficulty forging public-private partnerships are likely to find that public STD clinics are necessary to ensure universal access to comprehensive STD-related services.

Public health agencies may consider one or a combination of alternative models for providing services, including provision of services through contracts or agreements with public sector health programs, community-based health programs, universities or teaching hospitals, or private health care professionals, including managed care organizations and other health plans. Contracts and partnerships may include agreements regarding patient referral for specific services, sharing of resources, or shared administration and management of programs. Regardless of how community services are organized, local health departments must provide leadership in the community to ensure universal access, promote preventive services, conduct disease surveillance, ensure confidentiality of services, assess the effectiveness of services, train clinicians, and implement policies to prevent STDs (IOM, 1988).

Therefore, the committee makes the following recommendation:

- **Local health departments, with the assistance of the state health department and in consultation with the community, should determine how to provide high-quality, comprehensive STD-related clinical services that meet federal and state quality standards most effectively in their communities.**

Improving Dedicated Public STD Clinics

Public STD clinics are the primary source of STD-related services for the uninsured and provide an important focus for STD prevention at the community level. The management and quality of services provided by dedicated public STD clinics, as described in Chapter 5, need significant improvement to ensure confidential, comprehensive, high-quality STD-related services for all persons. The committee has witnessed the wide variation in the quality, scope, accessibility, and availability of services provided by public STD clinics firsthand during their site visits and through their professional experience. Some public programs, usually university-affiliated, provide STD-related services that are personalized and efficient, and provide STD diagnostic and treatment services along with counseling and education, HIV testing and counseling, and family planning services. Many local health departments, especially in metropolitan areas, however, operate dedicated STD clinics that are isolated from other public health and personal health services, including HIV screening and counseling clinics. In many clinics, quality of care, monitoring, and assessment have not been a priority.

Ensuring Access and Quality

As discussed in Chapter 5, dedicated public STD clinics historically have emphasized serving large numbers of patients and their sex partners, who are identified through patient interviews. These clinics seldom emphasize the long-term disease management that chronic viral STDs require or effective long-term behavioral interventions that require multiple sessions. Examples of other appropriate long-term disease management activities include early management of HIV and hepatitis B virus infection, suppression of recurrent genital herpes, Pap smear screening and managing cervical dysplasia, administration of complete vaccination series for hepatitis B, and treatment of genital warts. In large cities, public STD clinics tend to be overwhelmed with patients, and provide impersonal care. Recruiting high-quality health care professionals to work in these settings is also difficult. In many small communities, dedicated STD clinics may be open for only several hours each week, relying on health personnel who may be inadequately trained in STDs and may have too many competing responsibilities. Moreover, these clinics often suffer from fragmentation and frequently are inefficiently managed.

Dedicated STD clinics help set community standards and train health professionals in STD prevention, including screening, risk assessment, diagnosis and treatment, partner notification, and education and counseling. In some areas, dedicated STD clinics serve as the focus for training of health professionals, performing clinical research in STDs, and setting standards for STD services in the public and private sectors. Although many small communities and communities with low STD rates do not require dedicated public STD clinics, nearly all states in the United States have one or more cities with such clinics. Again, local health officials need to assess the status of clinical services in their communities and determine the most appropriate model for delivering services. In all cases, health departments that operate dedicated public STD clinics should ensure that these clinics collaborate with community-based health clinics, including family planning clinics and school-based programs, university and hospital medical centers, and private sector health care professionals, to improve the scope and quality of care in dedicated public STD clinics.

As previously mentioned, the committee supports incorporating STD-related services into primary care. The committee believes that, in some communities and situations, dedicated public STD clinics should continue to be an important component of STD prevention because, in most areas, persons who use public STD clinics usually are uninsured. Data cited in Chapter 5 indicate that convenience, confidentiality, low cost, and perception of expert care at public STD clinics are important to clinic users. The populations at greatest risk for STDs—the young, disenfranchised groups, and certain ethnic and racial groups—tend to have the least access to health care. One of every four persons 15–29 years old is uninsured. Lack of private health insurance and dependence on Medicaid suggest why some ethnic groups and persons with lower incomes account for a disproportionately large share of public STD clinic visits in many urban areas. Therefore, without universal health care coverage in the United States or improved access to STD-related services in the public and private sector, effective STD prevention will continue to require public STD programs to ensure access to STD-related services for the uninsured.

The committee is particularly concerned regarding the potential adverse public health impact of the recently enacted welfare reform legislation, proposals to restrict social and health services to immigrants, and the proposed reductions in the rate of growth of Medicaid funds. It is likely that such legislation will increase the number of persons without health insurance coverage, and thus without financial access to health services. It is also possible that the above policies will indirectly promote certain behaviors that increase risk for STDs or inhibit prompt health-seeking behaviors. Adding to these public policies, the continuing decline in employer-provided health insurance also is likely to increase the number of uninsured. These developments raise grave concerns that even larger numbers of persons will be dependent on publicly financed STD clinics, increasing the importance of this safety net at the same time that such services are being curtailed in some places.

Therefore, the committee makes the following recommendations:

• **Based upon local conditions and health department determination, dedicated public STD clinics should continue to function as a "safety net" provider of STD-related services for uninsured and disenfranchised persons and for those who prefer to obtain care from such clinics.** Should universal health care coverage in the United States be achieved, or if proposed changes in the existing delivery system for STD-related clinical services, including incorporating STD-related clinical services into primary care and improved access to

STD-related services in the public and private sector, are realized, the role of public STD clinics should be assessed.

• **The CDC, in collaboration with state and local health departments, should ensure that services provided by dedicated public STD clinics are of high quality.** This involves initiating the development of quality indicators and implementing and monitoring performance measures that reflect quality of services and health outcomes rather than program operation. Quality standards are recommended in the following three general areas: (1) technical standards (e.g., diagnostic capability in STDs), (2) operational standards (e.g., hours of operation and convenience of services, staffing), and (3) program content standards (e.g., scope of services and referral networks). Quality standards for STD-related services should apply to services provided by both public and private sector health care professionals.

Collaborating with Academic Health Centers

Some of the most promising models for STD prevention in the United States have involved collaborative efforts between local public health departments and academic medical centers. Several such models (e.g., Albuquerque, Birmingham, Baltimore, Boston, Cincinnati, Raleigh (NC), Chicago, Indianapolis, Minneapolis, New Orleans, San Francisco, St. Louis, Seattle) have involved joint health department/medical center recruitment and appointments of medical staff and collaborative training of medical students and house staff. In some cases, the health department has contracted with the medical center for delivery of medical services while retaining direct control of outreach and laboratory support services. Less extensive collaboration models have been established in many other cities to provide medical staffing, training, research, and reference laboratory capabilities. These models most closely parallel the pattern of delivery of clinical services in other developed countries.

Although it is difficult to measure the impact of the academic health center/public health department collaboration model on community STD rates, the apparent success of these models in the United States is evidenced by their relatively greater effectiveness in obtaining local, state, and federal funding for programs; their role in training clinical and public health leaders in STD and HIV prevention; their roles as regional training centers for public and private sector clinicians; their development and early adoption of innovative methods for diagnosis, treatment, and behavioral intervention; and their role in surveillance and early recognition of emerging STDs. Although such models are effective in areas where they are implemented, the model is less feasible for rural areas and small communities with more limited access to academic health centers. Nevertheless, these partnerships have steadily increased and, in nearly every instance, have resulted in improved patient care and training for health care professionals and have increased the number of high-quality public STD programs. Such collaborations are particularly important not only in improving quality of dedicated STD clinics, but also in providing professional training required to expand STD-related services into the private sector.

Therefore, the committee makes the following recommendation:

*   **Health professional schools, including schools of medicine, nursing, and physician assistants, should partner with a local health department for purposes of STD clinic staffing, management, and professional training.** Support from federal and state governments should be provided as incentives for such collaboration.

Involving Managed Care Organizations and Other Health Plans

The committee believes that, if certain concerns are adequately addressed, there is substantial potential for managed care health plans to improve both the quality of and access to STD-related services. As summarized in Chapter 5, managed care organizations have several characteristics that represent important opportunities for enhancing STD-related services among persons enrolled in managed care health plans. Compared with other health plans, the structure and resources of many managed care organizations allow for improved coordination and integration of care, accountability of services, incentives to provide preventive services, and quality monitoring of services through information systems. Managed care organizations have the potential to provide higher quality, more comprehensive STD-related services than traditional indemnity health insurance plans and independent private practice clinicians, who may have little incentive to provide preventive services.

The committee identified some notable and impressive STD-related programs and activities among managed care organizations, as described in Appendix H. Some managed care organizations have developed and implemented STD or HIV prevention activities for both plan members and the community. Some large group- and staff-model managed care organizations are fully incorporating STD-related clinical services into routine practice. For example, Group Health Cooperative of Puget Sound, Harvard Pilgrim Health Care, and Kaiser-Permanente of Southern California offer a range of STD-related services, including education, screening, diagnosis, and treatment, relying on public health agencies for outreach, partner notification, and, often, counseling.

Although the committee believes that managed care health plans are capable of improving STD-related services, it recognizes that they have not yet fully demonstrated this capacity. Therefore, as managed care expands in the United States, the performance of such health plans in providing STD-related services should be carefully monitored and evaluated to determine the impact of such health plans on access and quality of services, especially among persons at high risk for STDs.

The potential concerns related to expanding the role of managed care organizations in STD prevention are summarized in Chapter 5. Practice constraints and financial incentives and methods for financing managed care and other health plans are potential barriers to health plans providing comprehensive STD-related services. As long as purchasers of health services are generally basing their decisions on premium costs rather than on enrollee health outcomes, many health plans are unlikely to fulfill their potential as providers of comprehensive STD-related care. It is important to note that there is great variation in the types of managed care plans and also variation within the types of managed care organizations. The extensive STD-related programs of a few group- and staff-model managed care organizations should not be assumed to reflect the interest or commitment of the less-structured health plans, which are far more numerous and cover a larger proportion of the population. In addition, the community outreach prevention programs of a few not-for-profit managed care organizations may not reflect the commitments or programs of investor-owned, for-profit managed care organizations. The committee is particularly concerned with the rapidly growing, less-structured health plans that do not have integrated delivery systems, lack health professionals with training in STDs, and have less-developed information systems. Some of these health plans do not fully participate in quality assurance activities or adequately monitor performance. Given the great variability in managed care organizations and other health plans, quality assurance and accrediting organizations, such as the National Committee for Quality Assurance, should promote measures that monitor the quality of STD-related services provided by health plans.

With very few exceptions, STDs are not yet high priorities among managed care organizations, and most are not involved in activities to prevent STDs in the general community. The committee's assessment is based on anecdotal information and was validated by a committee survey of managed care organizations that were considered to be likely providers of community health services (Appendix H). Given the limited data available regarding the scope and quality of STD-related services provided within the range of private sector health care settings, the CDC, in collaboration with the American Association of Health Plans, the National Committee for Quality Assurance, and the Health Insurance Association of America, should jointly sponsor or conduct a study to examine such services provided in private sector settings, including managed care organizations and other health plans.

There are several explanations for the general lack of involvement of managed care organizations and other health plans in STD prevention activities. STDs are not perceived as widespread problems among plan members or by purchasers and therefore are not a priority for many health plans. Second, the general lack of involvement in community-based prevention activities is consistent with market conditions. Driven by employers' and other purchasers' demands for lower premiums, virtually no health plan can afford to provide clinical services without payment. To do so would add to their cost base and increase their premiums, an undesirable action in a competitive market. It is in a plan's best interest to invest in preventive services if the member stays with the plan long enough to lower his or her use of more expensive treatment services, such as services required to treat late sequelae such as cervical cancer. It may be less expensive for health plans simply to treat STD infections than to invest in specialized training for clinicians and to support more comprehensive STD prevention programs. Plans that have a small market share or operate in a volatile market may be unlikely to invest significantly in disease prevention because of the high turnover rate of enrollees. Finally, many health plans have not supported STD prevention activities because they have traditionally relied on the availability of services in public STD clinics and, as a result, have not developed the capacity to deliver comprehensive STD-related care.

STD prevention services may be in the long-term interests of enrollees and of the community, but the plan itself may not realize the rewards of that investment in the short term. It is interesting to note that certain preventive services have been widely adopted by health plans. In the case of childhood immunizations, which are typically provided by health plans, the benefit of the intervention is likely to be realized within a span of a few years. In the case of cancer prevention services, such as tobacco cessation services, which are not as widely covered by health plans, the greatest benefit (averting lung cancer) usually occurs many years later, but some benefits (decrease in respiratory disease) may occur in a shorter time period. Similarly, some sequelae of STDs occur within a few years (e.g., pelvic inflammatory disease, infertility, ectopic pregnancy, preterm delivery), while others occur only after many years (e.g., cervical and liver cancer, AIDS). Further, coverage of childhood immunizations by health plans has been stimulated in part by consensus guidelines. The U.S. experience indicates that only with structural, enabling, societal changes (e.g., requiring immunizations for entrance to school) have major advances occurred in widespread support for childhood immunizations. This paradigm suggests that practice guidelines and structural pressures (e.g., Medicaid contract requirements to provide services) are necessary to strengthen STD prevention efforts.

The prevalence of STDs among health plan members is underrecognized. Managed care organizations and other health plans need to develop capacity and become more involved in STD prevention activities directed toward both plan members and the community in which they operate. Preventive services for STDs, such as risk assessment and screening, are likely to avert significant health care costs associated with serious complications of STDs, such as cancer, infertility, and perinatal problems. For example, a previously mentioned study conducted in a managed care organization showed that screening and treating women at increased risk for asymptomatic chlamydial infection dramatically reduced the rate of pelvic inflammatory disease in one year (Scholes et al., 1996). In addition, by aiding STD prevention efforts among persons in the community who are not plan members, health plans reduce the likelihood that their plan members will be exposed to infected partners. Health plans should also realize that screening and treating sex partners of plan members who are infected with an STD is in the interest of the health plan because such a strategy is likely to avert reinfections in the plan member. Finally, by participating in community-oriented activities and improving community health, health plans will help prevent long-term complications of STDs among persons who are not currently plan members, but may be in the future. Although the committee believes that health plans should develop capacity to provide comprehensive STD-related services, it recognizes that this will be a long process for many health plans. This is because some obstacles to full participation of health plans, such as assurance of confidentiality of services, coordination of services with public agencies, and legal considerations, must be addressed on several levels. In these cases, health plans, public health agencies, and purchasers of health services need to collaboratively address these issues.

It is important to note that, regardless of whether managed care and other health plans are successful in improving the scope and quality of STD-related care, private health plans are unlikely to provide services to uninsured persons in the near future. Therefore, this group of potentially high-risk individuals currently requires access to publicly sponsored services.

Therefore, the committee makes the following recommendation:

• **Health plans should provide for or cover comprehensive STD-related services, including screening, diagnosis and treatment, and counseling regarding high-risk behavior for plan members** *and their sex partners*, **regardless of the partners' insurance status.** The following actions should be taken to ensure that comprehensive STD-related services are available through health plans:

1. Federal, state, and local health agencies and health plan member associations should educate health plan executives regarding the need for, and benefits of, providing comprehensive STD-related services.

2. Employers and other purchasers of health services should require that STD-related services be provided as part of covered services in contracts with health plans.

3. State and local governments should require health plans participating in Medicaid contracts to provide or cover such services.

Involving Employers and Other Purchasers of Health Care

Employers, government agencies, and other purchasers of health care services have a potentially powerful influence on the scope and quality of STD-related services provided by health plans. Purchasers are the key to ensuring that managed care organizations and other health plans provide comprehensive, high-quality STD-related services. The committee believes that employers should be interested in the health of the general community because employers within a region are essentially drawing from the same employee pool. However, few managers who negotiate contracts with health plans are aware of the health and economic impact of STDs on their employees. Therefore, the public health community will need to encourage purchasers to consider STD prevention as a priority. Employers are interested in including preventive health services in their negotiated benefits packages, especially if the services are shown to be cost-saving for the company or organization. Some STD-related services are cost-effective, but may not be recognized as cost-saving; these services also need to be supported.

Therefore, the committee makes the following recommendation:

• **Federal, state, and local health agencies should educate employers, Medicaid programs, and other purchasers of health care regarding the broad scope and impact of STDs and the effectiveness of preventive services for STDs.**

Evaluating the Privatization of Services

In an effort to reduce costs, improve quality of services, or incorporate clinical services in primary care settings, many local governments are considering privatizing clinical services traditionally provided by local public health departments. Pressures on local health agencies, such as reduced funding for STD-related services and the enrollment of Medicaid beneficiaries into managed care health plans, are resulting in the shifting of services within the public sector and between the public and private sectors. Some agencies have begun to provide STD-related clinical services along with more comprehensive primary care services, and many are seeking ways to shift STD-related services to the private sector.

The costs, benefits, and sustainability of privatizing STD-related services should be carefully weighed. Several factors reduce the attractiveness of local health departments contracting out community-wide STD-related care to private health plans or private medical groups and clinics. First, health plans and private medical groups and clinics have generally shown little interest in providing clinical or other services to the entire community beyond their plan membership. Secondly, few health plans or private groups and clinics have experience providing comprehensive, high-quality STD-related services, especially to populations at high risk for STDs. Finally, and perhaps most important, many persons with STDs do not have health insurance and will not be served by any health plan. Although some private medical groups and clinics have offered to take over the role of public health clinics, they generally insist on receiving public funds to fulfill that responsibility. It is not clear that this approach would be cost-effective or would result in more effective STD prevention.

Further, there is concern among local health departments that, even if more health plans develop strong STD-related clinical services, some privately insured persons will continue to seek STD-related care from public programs. Some Medicaid enrollees and privately insured persons who may have an STD or have been exposed to an infected person may not feel confident in obtaining STD-related services from their health plan provider or in having their condition recorded in the medical records of their health plan. Effective prevention of STDs requires that all persons exposed to an STD and at risk of acquiring an STD, especially adolescents, have access to services in an environment that ensures confidentiality.

Proponents of contracting out STD-related clinical services argue that directly providing clinical services is not an essential role of public health departments and that these services are most efficiently and effectively provided by the private sector. The committee is aware of both successful and unsuccessful attempts to privatize STD-related clinical services. As discussed earlier, some partnerships with medical schools have improved the quality of services in dedicated public STD clinics. Current data are not sufficient to determine under what circumstances, if any, privatization is cost-effective or results in better clinical care for persons with STDs. Regardless of whether local health departments choose to privatize such services, it is essential that local health departments, with assistance from state health departments, ensure that access is available and quality of services is regularly monitored and evaluated. The monitoring and assessment role of public health agencies requires agencies to monitor the prevalence of STDs in the community, identify high-risk populations or communities, and assess the adequacy of treatment and prevention efforts. This role also requires that government agencies monitor and ensure compliance with minimum standards for quality and accessibility of services. Effective performance of these roles requires improved collaboration among local health departments and community-based health services, private sector health care professionals, health plans, and other community stakeholders.

The recent trend toward managed care in many states is increasing the proportion of Medicaid beneficiaries who will have to obtain their health care from managed care organizations. These changes could potentially improve their access to primary care services. Most health plans, however, will require beneficiaries to obtain STD-related services from specific providers, and thereby reduce access to STD-related services provided by out-of-plan providers. Therefore, standards for access and quality should be developed for STD-related services provided by managed care organizations, other health plans, and by public-private sector arrangements.

Medicaid could be an important source of reimbursement for STD clinics, but the rapid spread of Medicaid managed care requires STD clinics to obtain reimbursement for Medicaid patients from their health plans. To receive such payment, the clinics must become contract providers with the plans or receive payment for out-of-plan use of services, both of which could be encouraged or required by state Medicaid contracts. Agreements requiring managed care organizations and other health plans that participate in Medicaid contracts to reimburse public sector providers for STD-related services provided to plan beneficiaries, such as that developed by the Los Angeles County Department of Health Services, help ensure more equitable responsibility for supporting services (County of Los Angeles Department of Health Services, 1995). Local health departments should also consider incorporating performance requirements for STD-related services into any contracts with health plans. In addition, many federally supported STD clinics have provided free services to their patients. This has limited the ability of public STD clinics to obtain reimbursement from Medicaid for eligible patients. Public STD clinics should look to public health programs with a tradition of collecting patient fees and obtaining revenues from medical assistance programs, such as prenatal programs, community health centers, and family planning programs, as models. Health plans should provide enrollee access to public sector providers. As discussed in Chapter 5, some privately insured individuals may elect to go to a public STD clinic out of confidentiality or anonymity concerns or because of the perceived lack of quality or expertise in their health plan to provide STD-related services. Local health departments generally have not been prepared to bill private health plans for STD-related services, and since public sector providers are generally not in managed care organization networks, their services are considered "out of plan" and not reimbursed. This problem is made worse because health plans require enrollee permission for a provider to bill for services, thus threatening the very confidentiality sought by the enrollee.

Therefore, the committee makes the following recommendation:

- **Health plans, including managed care organizations, should develop collaborative agreements with local public health agencies to coordinate STD-related services, including payment for STD-related services provided to plan enrollees by public sector providers, including public STD clinics.** Local health departments should work with health plans to ensure fair reimbursement rates and confidentiality of services. State and local governments should require health plans that participate in Medicaid contracts to develop such agreements with local health departments. Collecting reimbursement for services will require health departments to develop billing capability for services, to seek permission from patients to bill, and, if this is denied, to require direct payment by the patient. In such cases, it is critical that patient confidentiality is not compromised. Given the current lack of data, federal health agencies such as the Health Care Financing Administration, the Health Resources and Services Administration, the CDC, and health plans should sponsor thorough evaluations of the impact of privatization of STD-related services on access and quality of such services in various communities before such privatization can be confidently endorsed.

Improving Training and Education of Health Care Professionals

Many factors, including availability of diagnostic and therapeutic resources, are important determinants of effective clinical management of STDs. However, more than any other factor, effective clinical management of STDs is dependent on adequate training and education of health care professionals. No matter how efficacious a clinical intervention may be under ideal conditions, it will not be effective unless the clinician delivering the intervention knows when and how to use it. The current system of clinical training for health care professionals, as outlined in Chapter 5, is inadequate in preparing clinicians to effectively manage patients with STDs. Studies examined by the committee suggest that many health care practitioners in both public or private settings are not sufficiently prepared to provide STD-related clinical services. Unless they are accompanied by appropriate training, changes in policy, increased funding, and implementation of clinical practice guidelines are not sufficient to ensure quality clinical care. Programs to train health professional students and practicing health care professionals in STD prevention are critical to increasing the capacity of the health care system to address STDs. The committee is encouraged by the apparent increase in clinical training in STDs in medical schools during the 1980s and urges all health professional schools to build upon this improvement and focus on the gaps in training identified in Chapter 5.

Inadequate professional training no doubt also contributes to the widespread tendency of clinicians to oversimplify and underestimate the importance of STDs. While STD diagnosis and management receives relatively little attention in health care training curricula, even less time is allocated to teaching STD risk assessment, patient counseling skills, methods of reducing risks for STDs, or treatment of sex partners. Training in diagnosis and treatment of sex partners is particularly important for health professionals who primarily treat persons of one gender. Discussion of risk and personal responsibility for sexual behavior is often awkward and uncomfortable for both the patient and health professional. As mentioned in Chapters 4 and 5, widespread misconceptions are shared by health professionals and their patients regarding STD risks, the signs and symptoms of STDs, and the importance of treating STDs promptly. These misconceptions contribute to the failure of many individuals with STDs, or at risk for STDs, to seek care and the failure of many health professionals to improve their own abilities to provide such services. There are limited data regarding the knowledge, skills, and training needs of specific types of health care professionals, and an assessment of these issues is necessary.

Familiarity with population-based health promotion and disease prevention techniques, skills in evidence-based clinical decision-making, and patient communication skills are essential for every clinician. Many clinicians, however, do not have these skills or are not being consistently trained to use them to effectively prevent disease or diagnose and treat patients with STDs. Given the limited amount of time that is available in educational curricula, it may be most appropriate to focus primary care training on a core set of clinical competencies. The clinical skills needed to effectively manage patients with STDs are consistent with those identified as essential for primary care providers (IOM, 1996b).

Expanded training programs are urgently needed to ensure expertise in STD case management at the primary care level. In areas with university-affiliated public STD clinics, it is most efficient for primary care clinicians to develop expertise in STD case management given the high volume and range of STDs seen in these facilities. Thus, courses specifically designed for primary care providers should present the management of STDs within a primary care context, where patient care issues and other clinical resources are different from those of dedicated STD clinics. Continuing medical education courses should include STD practice management in settings without the specific diagnostic testing resources of an STD clinic and should emphasize patient management and partner treatment issues appropriate for a primary care setting.

Given evidence that health information provided by primary care clinicians has resulted in positive individual behavior change, the committee believes that communicating effectively with patients regarding sexuality issues and STDs is a critical skill for primary care professionals. Training in this area can be conducted in a number of ways and environments. Training modules should be modified to ensure that primary care providers will be able to fully incorporate this type of training into their practice situation.

The committee believes that training and education of health care professionals are paramount, but also recognizes the need to address other major factors that influence a clinician's ability to provide comprehensive services. These factors include practice format constraints such as inadequate time for risk assessment and counseling, especially within managed care environments that emphasize high productivity levels, and lack of systematically promulgated and institutionally supported approaches for risk assessment, screening, diagnostic testing, and counseling for STDs. In some situations, these factors may be problems of equal or greater importance than training.

New computer and telecommunications technology should be applied to improve training of health care professionals. Awareness and clinical knowledge of STDs among health care professionals should be improved by distance learning activities such as televised courses, developing interactive software modules for teaching clinical skills, and increasing electronic access to clinical information such as clinical practice guidelines. For example, medical and other health professional students may be able to practice STD-related diagnostic and patient communication skills with interactive computer software. In addition, primary care practitioners in rural areas or areas where specialized training in STDs in not available may be able to access training modules or courses sponsored by the CDC, professional societies, or other organizations through distance learning programs. Staff in academic infectious disease clinics, dedicated STD clinics, federal, state, and local health departments, and primary care providers can develop shared information networks to exchange new information and epidemiologic data regarding STDs in order to improve clinical and public health practice. In addition, through telemedicine, infectious disease specialists may be able to assist in diagnosis and treatment of patients with STDs.

Therefore, the committee makes the following recommendation:

- **The training of primary care providers in STD prevention should be improved by:**

1. training based on a core set of clinical competencies, including population-based health promotion and disease prevention techniques, evidence-based clinical decision-making skills, and patient communication skills. The training experience should include experience in both dedicated STD clinics and primary care settings and instruction regarding techniques to promote individual behavior change and improve disease reporting;

2. improving medical student training in STDs by encouraging medical schools to provide clinical instruction in STD clinics to ensure that students see a sufficient variety of STDs;

3. conducting an annual survey of medical schools through the Liaison Committee on Medical Education of the Association of American Medical Colleges and the American Medical Association to determine the extent to which medical schools are providing appropriate instruction in STD diagnosis and treatment;

4. expanding collaborations among federal, state, and local STD programs; health professional organizations; graduate medical education; and other health professional training programs to include STD diagnosis and treatment as part of continuing medical education for all primary care providers;

5. providing additional federal support to academic health centers to establish clinical expertise and clinic-based training opportunities for STDs; and

6. encouraging state and local public health departments to identify primary care clinicians and clinics serving populations with high rates of STDs and provide STD-related education materials, training modules, and other technical assistance to them. The CDC should work with STD clinical training centers to develop training programs specifically designed for primary care providers.

Improving Clinical Management of STDs

The major components of effective clinical management for STDs include appropriate screening, diagnosis and treatment, risk reduction counseling and education, and identification and treatment of sex partners. Each of these components represents essential responsibilities of every clinician and needs to be improved and expanded. Appropriate clinical management of STDs also requires access to quality laboratory services for screening and evaluation of potential STDs.

Improving and Expanding Screening Programs

Screening allows for the detection of infected persons who would otherwise remain undetected, develop complications of STDs, and potentially transmit the infection to their partners. Screening is only effective, however, if appropriate treatment and counseling are provided to identified persons. As summarized in Chapter 4, the U.S. Preventive Services Task Force has identified effective clinical preventive services for STDs, and several agencies and health professional organizations have published similar recommendations. These guidelines are important in establishing preventive services for STDs as standard clinical practice for all clinicians. The full implementation of clinical guidelines will require additional investment of resources, but, as discussed earlier, many of these preventive services are cost-effective and some are cost-saving.

Although the recommendations of various health professional groups regarding clinician screening are generally very similar, many of these organizations' recommendations differ in their definition of appropriate populations for screening. These and other differences in clinical guidelines can lead to confusion among clinicians and make it more difficult to ensure a consistent standard for STD-related clinical care.

There is considerable need to expand screening programs for STDs, especially for chlamydial infection and certain other STDs.[5] Studies cited in Chapter 4 (e.g., Scholes et al., 1996), clearly show that associated serious health complications of STDs such as pelvic inflammatory disease and other reproductive health problems can be prevented by treatment of infections identified through screening. Expanded screening for STDs, particularly for chlamydial infection and in regions or population groups with inadequate access to health services, will have a significant impact in preventing health consequences of STDs among women. The committee does not recommend diagnostic screening for those viral STDs for which curative treatment or a clinically important intervention is not available. Given the association between HIV infection and other STDs and the impact of STDs on transmission of HIV, persons who utilize HIV testing and counseling services should also be screened for STDs as appropriate for the clinical setting.

Screening programs should be appropriately focused and should be based on

---

[5]The guidelines of the U.S. Preventive Services Task Force and the CDC should be consulted regarding recommended indications for individual- and population-based screening for STDs.

surveillance data and knowledge of the populations or geographic prevalence of STDs. These expanded programs should utilize diagnostic tests that are appropriate for screening persons in a variety of settings. Family planning clinics, prenatal clinics, facilities that provide pregnancy termination services, and other settings where obstetric or gynecological care is available should screen and treat women and their partners for sexually transmitted infections.

Premarital testing for syphilis, as a requirement for marriage licenses, is unnecessary and contributes little to containing syphilis because persons applying for marriage licenses are generally at lower risk for syphilis compared with the general population. Although these tests represent a source of revenue for some states, studies cited in Chapter 4 indicate that the number of previously undetected cases identified through premarital testing is extremely low; the tests are not cost-effective; and they have little public health impact. In addition, unnecessary testing may undermine public support for more appropriate screening programs, such as syphilis screening of women during early pregnancy.

Therefore, the committee makes the following recommendations:

• **All primary care providers, including managed care organizations and other health plans, should implement the recommendations of the U.S. Preventive Services Task Force and the CDC regarding clinical screening and management of STDs.** The CDC, the Agency for Health Care Policy and Research, the National Institutes of Health, and other federal agencies should collaborate with health professional organizations and representatives of health plans to develop comprehensive, consensus clinical practice guidelines for primary care clinicians for STD-related services including screening, risk assessment, and counseling and other clinical interventions to promote healthy sexual behaviors. These guidelines should build on the work of the U.S. Preventive Services Task Force and the CDC STD treatment guidelines. These agencies and organizations should also work together to minimize any differences in current recommendations regarding clinical screening and management of STDs and to promote consistent clinical guidelines.

• **States that still have laws requiring premarital syphilis testing as a condition for marriage licenses should repeal these laws.** Resources devoted to such testing would be more effective if used in other ways. States that rely heavily on revenue generated by such testing should consider alternative sources of revenue.

Improving Diagnosis and Treatment

The CDC's STD Treatment Guidelines are a valuable resource that represent the standard for treatment of STDs. Such treatment guidelines help to promote appropriate therapy for STDs on a national basis. Compliance with treatment guidelines is important because it helps ensure that patients receive the most effective therapy. However, as documented in Chapter 5, there is limited awareness of, and compliance with, these guidelines, especially among private sector health care professionals in some regions. Appropriate diagnosis and treatment of STDs is most effectively accomplished by improving awareness and training of clinicians. Clinicians are ultimately responsible for ensuring that patients and their sex partners who are diagnosed with STDs are appropriately followed up and treated. When the diagnosis of an STD is laboratory-based, a mechanism for communicating results and following up on treatment should be established between the patient and the clinician.

Single-dose therapy for bacterial STDs is important in preventing complications and further transmission of STDs because it averts the problems of ineffective treatment associated with the failure of infected individuals to return for subsequent treatment or to take multiple doses of drugs. This attribute is especially valuable when treating disenfranchised persons. Single-dose therapy is most effective when it is directly provided and observed by the clinician, thereby ensuring patient compliance. Although single-dose therapy is more expensive than multidose therapy, it may be more cost-effective from a public health perspective for those populations in which compliance or follow-up are problematic.

Therefore, the committee makes the following recommendations:

• **All clinicians should follow STD treatment guidelines recommended by the CDC and national medical professional organizations.** The CDC should continue to publish and update the STD Treatment Guidelines. All health plans and national and state professional organizations, such as the American Medical Association, the American Academy of Pediatrics, the American College of Obstetrics and Gynecology, and the American Academy of Family Practitioners, should assist in the dissemination of these guidelines to their members and clinical staff.

• **Single-dose therapy for bacterial and other curable STDs should be available and reimbursable in all clinical settings where STD-related clinical care is routinely provided to populations in which treatment compliance or follow-up are problems.** Such therapy should be reimbursed by Medicaid programs and private health insurance plans. Although the pharmaceutical industry has been willing to provide single-dose therapies to public STD clinics at reduced contract prices, some public STD clinics and other public programs still lack sufficient funds to offer single-dose therapy in all situations where it is clinically indicated. Therefore, the pharmaceutical industry should consider further price reductions for public providers of STD treatment.

Improving Counseling and Education

Risk reduction counseling and education of patients during routine clinical encounters and during evaluations for potential STDs are important components of STD clinical management. The U.S. Preventive Services Task Force and other professional organizations have recommended that all primary care providers counsel patients regarding the avoidance of high-risk sexual behaviors as part of the periodic health examination. The committee believes that although the ability of clinician counseling in primary care settings to change behavior is unproven, focused counseling in both specialized and general clinical settings has great potential for changing behaviors related to the transmission of STDs. The effectiveness of client-centered counseling for STD prevention in a randomized behavioral intervention trial (Project RESPECT) was mentioned in Chapter 4. Thus, counseling is most likely to be highly effective when it is tailored to the individual and is provided in the context of, and reinforced by, other individual-focused and community-based interventions. The experience of STD infection presents an important opportunity to motivate behavior change.

Counseling and education are especially important for adolescents and other groups at high risk of STDs. Major barriers described in Chapters 4 and 5 that hinder clinicians from providing counseling are primarily lack of training and skills in counseling, lack of time allocated for counseling, and lack of reimbursement for such services. To maximize the time available for individualized counseling, new methods of providing information, such as interactive computer software programs and use of other clinic-based counseling staff, should be used to supplement person-to-person counseling by time-constrained clinicians. It is important to develop and evaluate such innovative approaches to counseling and education because some clinicians may be unable, for various reasons, to provide comprehensive preventive services in all the primary care areas that are expected from them. These approaches not only reinforce prevention messages delivered directly by clinicians, but also allow clinicians an opportunity to provide more effective, individually tailored prevention messages.

Therefore, the committee makes the following recommendation:

• **All health care professionals should counsel their patients during routine and other appropriate clinical encounters regarding the risk of STDs and methods for preventing high-risk behaviors. Counseling for STDs, including HIV infection, should be reimbursed without copayments or other financial disincentives by Medicaid programs, managed care organizations, and other health plans.** The recommendations of the U.S. Preventive Services Task Force regarding counseling for high-risk sexual behaviors should be implemented. Clinical encounters, such as the new diagnosis of an STD or unintended pregnancy, evaluation for HIV infection, or the prescribing of contraceptives, present unique teaching opportunities, when patients may be particularly receptive to health education and counseling; these opportunities should be utilized.

Improving Partner Notification and Treatment

As discussed in Chapter 4, identification and treatment of partners is an essential component of STD clinical management because it reduces further transmission of STDs, prevents reinfection, and reduces risk of long-term complications of STDs in the infected partner. The case-finding activities of STD disease intervention specialists have been effective in containing outbreaks of bacterial STDs in discrete communities by promptly identifying and treating infected partners. In some countries, such as Sweden, partner notification for gonorrhea, syphilis, and chlamydial infection has been highly effective. However, the current methods of partner notification utilized by public STD clinics in the United States are extremely resource-intensive, inefficient, and in need of redesign. This is especially important given the high incidence of STDs among persons whose partners are unidentifiable, not easily reached, or uncooperative (and often participate in extended sexual networks).

No single model for partner notification is appropriate for all communities. One approach is to identify sex-partner networks in high morbidity areas and screen and treat members of the network. Another option is to replace the current method of notification with a combination of outreach efforts to identify partners and other individuals at high risk for STDs. The optimal combination of activities that are most effective at reaching persons at risk for STDs will vary depending on the local epidemiology of STDs, available resources, and the spectrum of local public and private health care professionals treating STDs.

STD programs need to develop new strategies and techniques for community outreach in partnership with other health care professionals rather than relying solely on health department or public STD clinic staff. It is essential that disease intervention specialists be sensitive to the local community. Other approaches include involving community-based organizations, designing and implementing outreach and screening activities, motivating private health care professionals to assist in partner notification, and assisting and motivating index patients to notify and assist their partners in seeking treatment. Limited data are available regarding the effectiveness and potential benefits of different approaches to partner notification, and further research is urgently needed to identify innovative and more cost-effective strategies for partner outreach at the individual and community levels.

As reflected in the committee's model, notifying partners of potential exposure to an STD should be a major responsibility of those persons who are infected. Community norms regarding the roles of groups or individuals in patient and partner referral need to be changed. However, health professionals need to recognize that certain individuals, especially adolescents and women, may experience difficulty notifying their partners and will require assistance in doing so. Few efforts have been made to explore the factors that affect the willingness or ability of individuals to participate in patient referral, and research in this area is important to improve the overall effectiveness of patient referral.

Partner treatment should be addressed as part of the comprehensive STD care of anyone with an STD, whether managed in the private or public sector. A comprehensive strategy for partner outreach needs to include private sector health care professionals, because they treat a large proportion of STDs. Health care professionals who primarily treat patients of one gender (e.g., obstetricians and gynecologists) should be given appropriate training to improve clinical management of sex partners. Managers of clinical settings need to identify and address other potential clinic-specific barriers to effective partner diagnosis and treatment.

The concept that partner treatment is part of standard STD clinical management should be reinforced among private sector clinicians as well as among health plans. The committee believes that health care professionals and health plans have an ethical and public health obligation to ensure that the sexual contacts of their patients with STDs are notified promptly of potential exposures, counseled regarding risk factors for infection, and offered diagnostic testing and treatment. The responsibility for these activities in private health care settings historically has been relegated to public health agencies. This is often an inappropriate or ineffective method of ensuring prompt notification, counseling, testing, and treatment. The committee also believes that this obligation extends beyond health plan members because health plans have a responsibility to improve the health of the communities from which they draw their revenue (Showstack et al., 1996). As previously mentioned, treating partners in the community is in the long-term interest of both the health plan and health plan members.

Therefore, the committee makes the following recommendations:

• **State and local health departments, with the assistance of the CDC, should redesign current partner notification activities for curable STDs in public health clinics to improve outreach, mobilize public health staff in new ways, and enlist support from community groups or other programs that provide services to high-risk populations.** Changes in the system should be driven by results of cost-effectiveness research and formal prevention intervention trials on innovative approaches to partner notification. Communities and clients should also be involved in designing partner notification approaches to improve effectiveness and acceptability. Identifying sex-partner networks in high morbidity areas, with screening and outreach activities occurring within high-risk networks, should be one component of refocused partner notification activities. The CDC should support research to identify and evaluate innovative and cost-effective strategies for partner outreach and to determine those factors that may influence personal behavior or responsibility related to patient referral. In addition, local health departments should promote the coordination of partner notification activities by establishing linkages with other public agencies and private health plans.

- **All health plans and clinicians should take responsibility for partner treatment and provide STD diagnosis and treatment to sex partners of plan members or others under their care as part of standard clinical practice. Diagnosis and treatment of partners should be reimbursable by third-party payers, including Medicaid, or by the partner's health plan if he or she is insured.** All health plans and appropriate private health care professionals should participate, and develop capacity, in partner notification. Health professional organizations should educate their members regarding the importance of partner diagnosis and treatment.

Improving Availability and Capability of Laboratory Services

As reviewed in Chapter 4, access to appropriate laboratory testing is critical for accurate diagnosis of STDs and STD screening programs. Clinicians may have limited access to materials for diagnosis or laboratories with appropriate diagnostic tests. Therefore, qualified laboratories need to be available on a regional basis and do not need to be located in every clinical facility. Quality control and standardization of diagnostic tests are essential and should be systematically performed. Qualified public sector laboratories are available in many areas, but long-term availability of these laboratories may be jeopardized if health plans do not provide reimbursement for services or if competition with established commercial or hospital-based laboratories increases. Clinicians need to be aware that specimen adequacy and proper handling and transport of diagnostic specimens are needed to ensure accurate test results. Even with access to diagnostic testing, clinicians must have adequate training to appropriately select and interpret such tests. Use of nucleic acid detection rather than culture and sensitivity analysis, and syndromic diagnosis rather than laboratory-based diagnosis, may reduce the capability of public sector laboratories to perform certain public health functions such as the monitoring of antibiotic resistance of sexually transmitted pathogens. Public STD laboratory expertise should be maintained at the federal, state, and local levels to support clinical care of patients, monitor microbial resistance, and support surveillance of emerging STDs.

Therefore, the committee makes the following recommendation:

- **Public sector laboratories should be reimbursed for STD-related laboratory tests performed on persons who have private health insurance coverage.** Such laboratories should develop mechanisms to bill health plans for laboratory services. State and local health departments should negotiate adequate reimbursement for such services from health plans. In addition, public sector laboratories should ensure that the quality and cost of their services are competitive with those in the private sector. Qualified STD reference laboratories should be preserved at the regional level and strengthened where regional capabilities are lacking. Outsourcing and collaboration with private or university-based STD reference laboratories should be considered in sustaining and developing public sector reference laboratory capabilities.

COLLABORATING TO IMPROVE SERVICES

In this section, the committee describes potential models for how the various providers of clinical services can work together to improve access to, and quality of, clinical services. In examining potential models for delivering services, the committee considered the many ongoing programs that they visited and heard about during the course of the study. The committee believes that the programs summarized in Appendix I serve as valuable models for agencies and organizations that are planning to develop collaborative activities. Because most of these programs have not been systematically evaluated for effectiveness, the committee does not necessarily endorse these specific programs, but rather encourages agencies and organizations to use these examples as the basis for developing collaborations to improve services.

Collaborating with Other Public Sector Health Programs

As in the case of community-based and private sector clinics, local health departments that provide STD-related clinical services should ensure that such services are provided in primary care settings, including reproductive health programs. The DeKalb County health department in Georgia, for example, has integrated STD and HIV screening and counseling services and is beginning to provide both services in family planning and primary care clinics. Some of the most promising efforts to provide STD-related services along with other public health services are focused on high-risk populations. For example, the Teen Services Program, sponsored by Emory University at Grady Memorial Hospital in Atlanta, and the Young Adult Clinic, operated by the Chicago Health Department with Vida/Sida, a community outreach program, target high-risk adolescents and young adults in inner-city communities. These projects focus on the comprehensive health and social needs of populations and individuals within the community, not just STDs. They bring together high-priority services for adolescents and young adults, such as STD screening and treatment, HIV testing and counseling, and contraceptive services and pregnancy testing, in a comprehensive health care setting. Although the Chicago project focuses on STDs, including HIV infection, and the Atlanta project focuses on pregnancy prevention, both emphasize education and behavior change related to sexuality. They are also both closely linked to schools; the Grady program is closely aligned with the Atlanta middle-school curriculum. Both programs also utilize "peer experts" who provide outreach and education to other adolescents.

These various models reflect many of the characteristics of the Youth Clinics implemented in Sweden in 1972. There are 187 such clinics in existence in Sweden—a country with a population under nine million. These clinics provide comprehensive services to adolescents and are credited with a major positive impact on prevention of STDs and unintended pregnancy.

Collaborating with Community-Based Health Programs

Community-based health providers such as community health centers, family planning programs, and school-based health clinics are potentially important sources of STD-related services because they serve a patient population with a high prevalence of STDs. Although many community-based health programs currently provide STD-related clinical services, most have not made STD prevention a priority, despite its high prevalence in their patient population, and some do not have expertise in providing such services. There are, however, some notable exceptions to this observation.

Programs that provide family planning services, for example, have long recognized the importance of integrating STD clinical and educational services into family planning services, although not all programs provide STD-related services. In Chicago, Planned Parenthood provides STD- and HIV-related services in the context of comprehensive primary care for women and adolescents, while focusing on reproductive health. Using a population-based public health approach, the Chicago Planned Parenthood program provides outreach and education services directly to several high schools and through its clinics. The West End Community Health Center in Atlanta has developed a substantial STD program and provides STD-related services along with extensive primary care services. In this comprehensive model, clients receive STD screening, diagnosis, and treatment through their primary care provider of choice. Outreach, follow-up, and special counseling and education are available through clinic-based staff in collaboration with the local health department STD program staff. Most important, services are centered on the patient, coordinated by a primary care provider, documented in a single medical record, and monitored by relevant public health agencies.

In addition, local health departments in several cities (e.g., Baltimore, Boston, Denver, Minneapolis, and Portland) have developed collaborative pilot programs linking school-based health centers sponsored by the health department with local managed care organizations (Schlitt et al., 1995; Zimmerman and Reif, 1995). These programs provide comprehensive primary care, easily accessed at school, and multidisciplinary health education, health promotion, and mental health and social services. All routine STD- and reproductive-health-related care is provided through these centers. Agreements with the participating managed care organizations have enabled the providers in the school-based health center to act as primary care providers, referring plan enrollees to other plan services as needed.

An example of an effort to promote collaboration at the national level is the CDC's National Partnership to Prevent STD-Related Infertility, which is intended to prevent infertility and other serious complications of chlamydial and gonococcal infections. The partnership seeks to prevent these infections through collaborations with a variety of traditional and nontraditional stakeholders in STD prevention. The action plan for the partnership focuses on coordination and integration of STD-related services, public education, health professional education, quality assurance for diagnosis and treatment, community-level behavior change, and surveillance and program evaluation (CDC, DSTD/HIVP, 1995). In addition, the demonstration projects cosponsored by the CDC and the Office of Population Affairs are increasing collaboration among dedicated public STD clinics, family planning clinics, and public laboratories. The committee believes that these types of collaborative approaches should be expanded to all STDs.

CONCLUDING STATEMENT

STDs are hidden epidemics of tremendous health and economic consequence in the United States. They are hidden because many Americans are reluctant to address sexual health issues in an open way and because of the biologic and social characteristics of these diseases. STDs are diseases of national and global importance that have a dramatic impact on local communities. All Americans have an interest in STD prevention because all communities are impacted by STDs, and all individuals directly or indirectly pay for the costs of these diseases. STDs are public health problems that lack easy solutions because they are rooted in human behavior and fundamental societal problems. Indeed, there are many obstacles to effective prevention efforts. The first hurdle will be to confront the reluctance of American society to openly address issues surrounding sexuality and STDs. Despite the barriers, there are existing individual- and community-based interventions that are effective and can be implemented immediately. Although these interventions are not perfect, they can have a synergistic, positive impact in reducing the risk of STDs in the population. That is why a multifaceted approach is necessary at both the individual and community levels. Populations at high risk, such as adolescents and disenfranchised persons, will need special attention.

An effective system of STD prevention in the United States will have to be developed at the local, state, and national levels, with full participation of both the public and private sectors. Many of the essential components of an effective system already exist, but they need to be integrated or coordinated, particularly at the local level. Many of these components also need to be improved and redesigned in order to maximize effectiveness and optimize resources. This means that many stakeholders need to redefine their mission, refocus their efforts, modify how they deliver services, and accept new responsibilities. In this process, strong leadership, innovative thinking, partnerships, and adequate resources will be required. The additional investment required to effectively prevent STDs may be considerable, but it is negligible when compared with the likely return on the investment. The process of preventing STDs must be a collaborative one. No one agency, organization, or sector can effectively do it alone; all members of the community must do their part. A successful national initiative to confront and prevent STDs requires widespread public awareness and participation and bold national leadership from the highest levels.

REFERENCES

AGI (Alan Guttmacher Institute). Lawmakers grapple with parents' role in teen access to reproductive health care. Issues in Brief. New York and Washington, D.C.: AGI, 1995.

AMA (American Medical Association). Policy compendium on reproductive health issues affecting adolescents. Gans Epner JE, ed. Chicago: AMA, 1996.

Aral SO, Holmes KK, Padian N, Cates W. Overview: individual and population level approaches to the epidemiology and prevention of sexually transmitted diseases and human immunodeficiency virus infection. J Infect Dis 1996;174(Suppl 2):S127-33.

ASTHO (Association of State and Territorial Health Officials). Access and managed care: oxymoron or reality? Washington, D.C.: ASTHO, Managed Care Monograph Series, November, 1995a.

ASTHO. Communicable disease control in a managed care environment. Washington, D.C.: ASTHO, Managed Care Monograph Series, November, 1995b.

ASTHO. Ensuring and improving the quality of care in a managed care environment. Washington, D.C.: ASTHO, Managed Care Monograph Series, November, 1995c.

Cates W Jr. Contraception, unintended pregnancies, and sexually transmitted diseases: why isn't a simple solution possible? Am J Epidemiol 1996;143:311-8.

CDC (Centers for Disease Control and Prevention). Trends in sexual risk behavior among high school students—United States, 1990, 1991, and 1993. MMWR 1995;44:124-5, 131-2.

CDC, DSTD/HIVP (Division of STD/HIV Prevention). Plan for a national partnership to prevent STD-related infertility. Draft internal document, January 10, 1995.

County of Los Angeles Department of Health Services. Draft agreement between the County of Los Angeles and plan. March 29, 1995.

Grosskurth H, Mosha F, Todd J, Mwijarubi E, Klokke A, Senkoro K, et al. Impact of improved treatment of sexually transmitted diseases on HIV infection in rural Tanzania: randomized controlled trial [see comments]. Lancet 1995;346:530-6.

Halpern CT, Udry JR, Suchindran C. Effects of repeated questionnaire administration in longitudinal studies of adolescent males' sexual behavior. Arch Sex Behav 1994;23:41-57.

IOM (Institute of Medicine). The future of public health. Washington, D.C.: National Academy Press, 1988.

IOM. Healthy communities: new partnerships for the future of public health. Stoto MA, Dievler A, Abel C, eds. Washington, D.C.: National Academy Press, 1996a.

IOM. Primary care: America's health in a new era. Donaldson MS, Yordy KD, Lohr KN, Vanselow NA, eds. Washington, D.C.: National Academy Press, 1996b.

IOM. Improving health in the community: a role for performance monitoring. Durch JS, Bailey LA, Stoto MA, eds. Washington, D.C.: National Academy Press, 1977.

NACCHO (National Association of County and City Health Officials). Blueprint for a healthy community: a guide for local health departments. Washington, D.C.: NACCHO, July 1994.

NCASH (National Commission on Adolescent Sexual Health). Facing facts: sexual health for America's adolescents. New York: SIECUS, 1995.

NIH (National Institutes of Health). NIH AIDS Research Program Evaluation. Behavioral, social science, and prevention research area review panel. Findings and recommendations. Bethesda, MD: National Institutes of Health, 1996.

NRC (National Research Council). Assessment of performance measures in public health. Phase 1 report. Washington, D.C.: National Academy Press, in press.

Russell LB. Educated guesses. Making policy about medical screening tests. Berkeley, CA: University of California Press, 1994.

SAM (Society for Adolescent Medicine). Special issue on guidelines for adolescent health research. J Adolesc Health 1995;17:259-332.

Schlitt JJ, Rickett KD, Montgomery LL, Lear JG. State initiatives to support school-based health centers: a national survey. J Adolesc Health 1995;17:68-76.

Scholes D, Stergachis A, Heidrich FE, Andrilla H, Holmes KK, Stamm WE. Prevention of pelvic inflammatory disease by screening for cervical chlamydial infection. New Engl J Med 1996;334:1362-6.

Showstack J, Luire N, Leatherman S, Fisher E, Inui T. Health of the public. The private-sector challenge. JAMA 1996;276:1071-4.

Sparling PF, Aral SO. The importance of an interdisciplinary approach to prevention of sexually transmitted diseases. In: Wasserheit JN, Aral SO, Holmes KK, Hitchcock PJ, eds. Research issues in human behavior and sexually transmitted diseases in the AIDS era. Washington, D.C.: American Society for Microbiology, 1991:1-8.

Stryker J, Coates TJ, DeCarlo P, Haynes-Sanstad K, Shriver M, Makadon HJ. Prevention of HIV infection. Looking back, looking ahead. JAMA 1995;273:1143-8.

Wasserheit JN. Effect of changes in human ecology and behavior on patterns of sexually transmitted diseases, including human immunodeficiency virus infection. Proc Natl Acad Sci 1994;91:2430-5.

Wasserheit JN, Aral SO. The dynamic topology of sexually transmitted disease epidemics: implications for prevention strategies. J Infect Dis 1996; 174 (Suppl 2):S201-13.

Wasserheit JN, Hitchcock PJ. Future directions in sexually transmitted disease research. In: Quinn TC, ed. Sexually transmitted diseases. New York: Raven Press Ltd., 1992:291-325.

Zimmerman DJ, Reif CJ. School-based health centers and managed care health plans: partners in primary care. J Public Health Manage Prac 1995;1:33-9.

APPENDIXES

A
Sexually Transmitted Pathogens and Associated Diseases, Syndromes, and Complications

TWENTY-FIVE SEXUALLY TRANSMITTED PATHOGENS AND ASSOCIATED DISEASES OR SYNDROMES

Pathogen	Associated Disease or Syndrome
BACTERIA	
Neisseria gonorrhoeae	Urethritis, epididymitis, proctitis, cervicitis, endometritis, salpingitis, perihepatitis, bartholinitis, pharyngitis, conjunctivitis, prepubertal vaginitis, prostatitis (?), accessory gland infection, disseminated gonococcal infection (DGI), chorio-amnionitis, premature rupture of membranes, premature delivery, amniotic infection syndrome
Chlamydia trachomatis	All of the above except DGI, plus otitis media, rhinitis, and pneumonia in infants and Reiter's syndrome
Mycoplasma hominis	Postpartum fever, salpingitis (?)
Ureaplasma urealyticum	Nongonococcal urethritis

Treponema pallidum	Syphilis
Gardnerella vaginalis	Bacterial ("nonspecific") vaginosis (in conjunction with *Mycoplasma hominis* and vaginal anaerobes, such as *Mobiluncus spp*)
Haemophilus ducreyi	Chancroid
Calymmatobacterium granulomatis	Donovanosis (granuloma inguinale)
Shigella spp	Shigellosis in homosexual men
Campylobacter spp	Enteritis, proctocolitis

VIRUSES

Human immunodeficiency virus, types 1 and 2	AIDS
Herpes simplex virus	Initial and recurrent genital herpes, aseptic meningitis, neonatal herpes
Human papillomavirus (more than 70 types identified)	Condyloma acuminata, laryngeal papilloma, cervical intraepithelial neoplasia and carcinoma, vaginal carcinoma, anal carcinoma, vulvar carcinoma, penile carcinoma
Hepatitis B virus	Acute hepatitis B virus infection, chronic active hepatitis, persistent (unresolved) hepatitis, polyarteritis nodosa, chronic membranous glomerulonephritis, mixed cryoglobulinemia (?), polymyalgia rheumatica (?), hepatocellular carcinoma
Hepatitis A virus	Acute hepatitis A
Cytomegalovirus	Heterophil-negative infectious mononucleosis; congenital CMV infection with gross birth defects and infant mortality, cognitive impairment (e.g., mental retardation, sensorineural deafness); protean manifestations in the immunosuppressed host

Molluscum contagiosum virus	Genital molluscum contagiosum
Human T-cell lymphotrophic virus, types I and II	Human T-cell leukemia or lymphoma
Human herpes virus type 8	Kaposi's sarcoma (?), body cavity lymphoma

PROTOZOA

Trichomonas vaginalis	Trichomonal vaginitis
Entamoeba histolytica	Amebiasis in men who have sex with men
Giardia lamblia	Giardiasis in men who have sex with men

FUNGI

Candida albicans	Vulvovaginitis, balanitis

ECTOPARASITES

Phthirus pubis	Pubic lice infestation
Sarcoptes scabiei	Scabies

SELECTED SYNDROMES AND COMPLICATIONS OF SEXUALLY TRANSMITTED PATHOGENS

Syndrome or Complication	Associated Sexually Transmitted Pathogen

IN MEN

AIDS	Human immunodeficiency virus, types 1 and 2
Urethritis	*Neisseria gonorrhoeae, Chlamydia trachomatis*, herpes simplex virus, *Ureaplasma urealyticum*
Epididymitis	*C. trachomatis, N. gonorrhoeae*

Intestinal infections

Proctitis	*N. gonorrhoeae*, herpes simplex virus, *C. trachomatis*
Proctocolitis or enterocolitis	*Campylobacter spp, Shigella spp, Entamoeba histolytica*
Enteritis	*Giardia lamblia*
Hepatitis	Hepatitis A and B viruses, cytomegalovirus, *Treponema pallidum*

IN WOMEN

AIDS	Human immunodeficiency virus, types 1 and 2

Lower genitourinary tract infection

Vulvitis	*Candida albicans*, herpes simplex virus
Vaginitis	*Trichomonas vaginalis*, *C. albicans*
Vaginosis	*Gardnerella vaginalis, Mobiluncus spp*, other anaerobes, *Mycoplasma hominis*
Cervicitis	*N. gonorrhoeae, C. trachomatis*, herpes simplex virus
Urethritis	*N. gonorrhoeae, C. trachomatis*, herpes simplex virus
Pelvic inflammatory disease	*N. gonorrhoeae, C. trachomatis, M. hominis*, anaerobes, Group B streptococcus

Infertility

Postsalpingitis, postobstetrical, postabortion	*N. gonorrhoeae, C. trachomatis, M. hominis* (?)
Pregnancy morbidity Chorioamnionitis, amniotic fluid infection, prematurity, premature rupture of membranes, preterm delivery, postpartum endometritis, ectopic pregnancy	Several STDs have been implicated in one or more of these conditions.

IN MEN AND WOMEN

Neoplasia Cervical, vulvar, vaginal, anal, and penile; intraepithelial neoplasia, carcinoma	Human papillomavirus

Hepatocellular carcinoma	Hepatitis B virus
Kaposi's sarcoma, non-Hodgkin's lymphoma	Human immunodeficiency virus, types 1 and 2
Genital ulceration	Herpes simplex virus, *T. palladium, Haemophilus ducreyi, Calymmatobacterium granulomatis, C. trachomatis* (LGV strains)
Acute arthritis with urogenital or intestinal infection	*N. gonorrhoeae, C. trachomatis, Shigella spp, Campylobacter spp*
Genital warts	Human papillomavirus
Molluscum contagiosum	Molluscum contagiosum virus
Ectoparasite infestations	*Sarcoptes scabiei, Phthirus pubis*
Heterophil-negative mononucleosis	Cytomegalovirus, Epstein-Barr virus (some evidence for sexual transmission)
Tropical spastic paraparesis	Human T-cell lymphotrophic virus, type I

IN NEONATES AND INFANTS

TORCHES syndrome[a]	Cytomegalovirus, herpes simplex virus, *T. pallidum*
Conjunctivitis	*C. trachomatis, N. gonorrhoeae*
Pneumonia	*C. trachomatis, U. urealyticum* (?)
Otitis media	*C. trachomatis*
Sepsis, meningitis	Group B streptococcus
Cognitive impairment, deafness	Cytomegalovirus, herpes simplex virus, *T. pallidum*

NOTE: For each of the above syndromes, some cases cannot yet be ascribed to any cause and must currently be considered idiopathic. An "?" indicates a possible associated syndrome.

[a] TORCHES is an acronym for toxoplasmosis, rubella, cytomegalovirus, herpes, and syphilis. The syndrome consists of various combinations of encephalitis, hepatitis, dermatitis, and disseminated intravascular coagulation (DIC).

SOURCES: Cates W Jr, Holmes KK. Sexually transmitted diseases. In: Last JM, Wallace RB, eds. Maxcy-Rosenau-Last public health and preventive medicine. 13th ed. Norwalk, CT: Appleton & Lange, 1992:99–114; 121–3. Holmes KK, Handsfield HH. Sexually transmitted diseases. In: Isselbacher KJ, Braunwald E, Wilson JD, Martin JB, Fauci AS, Kasper DL, eds. Harrison's principles of internal medicine. 13th ed. New York: McGraw Hill, 1994:534–43.

APPENDIX
B
Characteristics of Major STDs in the United States

STD (etiologic agent)	Estimated Annual Incidence, 1994[a]	Estimated Prevalence, 1994[b]	Estimated Annual Total Costs (millions of 1994$)[c]	Routes of Transmission[d]	Frequency of Asymptomatic Infections[e]
Chlamydial infection (*Chlamydia trachomatis*)	4,000,000	NA	2,013	Vaginal, anal, and oral sex. Mother-to-infant transmission.	Women: very common. Men: common.
Gonorrhea (*Neisseria gonorrhoeae*)	800,000	NA	1,051	Vaginal, anal, and oral sex. Mother-to-infant transmission.	Women: common. Men: uncommon.
Syphilis (all stages) (*Treponema pallidum*)	101,000	NA	106	Vaginal, anal, and oral sex. Mother-to-infant transmission. Very rarely by direct nonsexual contact with infectious lesions. Rarely through blood transfusion if donor is in early stages of disease.	Women: common. Men: common or less common.
Human papillomavirus infection (human papillomavirus)	500,000– 1,000,000	24,000,000	3,827	Vaginal, anal, and probably oral sex. Occasional mother-to-infant transmission.	Women and men: very common.
Genital herpes (herpes simplex virus types 1 and 2)	200,000– 500,000	31,000,000	237	Vaginal, anal, and oral sex. Direct nonsexual contact with infectious lesions. Mother-to-infant transmission.	Women and men: common.

Major Long-Term Health Consequences:[f]		Increases Risk for Acquisition or Transmission of HIV Infection? [g]	Effective Curative Treatment Available/ Vaccine Available? [h]
Adults	Pregnant Women and Infants		
Women: pelvic inflammatory disease, infertility, ectopic pregnancy, chronic pelvic pain. Men: epididymitis, urethral stricture. Women and men: Reiter's syndrome (arthritis), complications of septicemia.	Infants: neonatal eye disease, pneumonia. Pregnant women: prematurity and other complications.	Yes	Yes/No
Women: pelvic inflammatory disease, infertility, ectopic pregnancy, chronic pelvic pain. Men: epididymitis, urethral stricture. Women and men: complications of septicemia.	Infants: eye infections (conjunctivitis), blindness. Pregnant women: prematurity and other complications.	Yes	Yes (but antibiotic-resistant strains exist)/No
Women and men: cardiovascular problems, neurological disorders, damage to other organ systems, often years after the initial infection.	Infants: congenital syphilis. Pregnant women: stillborn fetus, premature delivery.	Yes	Yes/No
Women: genital cancer (vulvar, cervical, vaginal). Men: penile cancer. Women and men: anal cancer.	Infants: wart-like tumors of larynx.	No evidence	Yes/No
Women and men: recurrent lesions.	Infants: fetal malformations, severe mental retardation, brain damage. Pregnant women: spontaneous abortion, premature delivery.	Possible	No/No

STD (etiologic agent)	Estimated Annual Incidence, 1994[a]	Estimated Prevalence, 1994[b]	Estimated Annual Total Costs (millions of 1994$)[c]	Routes of Transmission[d]	Frequency of Asymptomatic Infections[e]
Hepatitis B virus infection (hepatitis B virus)	53,000 (sexually transmitted cases)	NA	156 (sexually transmitted cases)	Vaginal, anal, and oral sex. Parenterally, through exposure to infectious blood, especially intravenous drug use. Mother-to-infant transmission. Close direct contact with infectious body fluids, especially in health care settings, including blood, saliva, semen, and vaginal fluids.	Women and men: common.
Chancroid (*Haemophilus ducreyi*)	3,500	NA	1	Vaginal and anal sex.	Women: common. Men: uncommon.
Trichomoniasis (*Trichomonas vaginalis*)	3,000,000	NA	NA	Vaginal sex.	Women: common. Men: very common.
HIV-1 infection (human immuno-deficiency virus)	NA	630,000–897,000 (estimate for January 1993)	6,683 (sexually transmitted cases)	Vaginal, anal, and oral sex. Parenterally, through exposure to infectious blood, especially through intravenous drug use. Mother-to-infant transmission.	Women and men: common.

NOTE: NA = not available.

[a] CDC, DSTD/HIVP (Division of STD/HIV Prevention). Annual report, 1994. U.S. Department of Health and Human Services, Public Health Service. Atlanta: Centers for Disease Control and Prevention, 1995. CDC, DSTDP (Division of STD Prevention). Sexually transmitted disease surveillance, 1994. U.S. Department of Health and Human Services, Public Health Service. Atlanta: Centers for Disease Control and Prevention, 1995.
[b] CDC, DSTD/HIVP, 1995 (see above). Rosenberg PS. Scope of the AIDS epidemic in the United States. Science 1995;270:1372-5.
[c] IOM Committee on Prevention and Control of STDs, Chapter 2 of this volume.
[d] Benenson AS, ed. Control of communicable disease manual. 16th ed. Washington, D.C.: American Public Health Association, 1995. Wasserheit JN, Aral SO, Holmes KK, Hitchcock PJ, eds. Research

Major Long-Term Health Consequences:[f]		Increases Risk for Acquisition or Transmission of HIV Infection? [g]	Effective Curative Treatment Available/ Vaccine Available? [h]
Adults	Pregnant Women and Infants		
Women and men: chronic liver disease, cirrhosis, liver cancer, death.	Infants: same as adults, chronic infection more likely.	No evidence	No/Yes
Long-term consequences uncommon.	Unknown.	Yes	Yes/No
Women: chronic vaginal discharge.	Infants: possible low birth weight. Pregnant women: possible preterm delivery.	Possible	Yes/No
Women and men: AIDS.	Infants: pediatric AIDS.		No/No

issues in human behavior and sexually transmitted diseases in the AIDS era. Washington, D.C.: American Society for Microbiology, 1991. Donovan P. Testing positive: sexually transmitted disease and the public health response. New York: Alan Guttmacher Institute, 1993.
[e] Categories are (a) very common: > 75 percent of infections; (b) common: > 25 to 75 percent of infections; (c) less common: 5 to 25 percent of infections; and (d) uncommon: < 5 percent of infections are asymptomatic. SOURCE: Wasserheit et al., 1991 (see above).
[f] Wasserheit et al., 1991 (see above). Donovan, 1993 (see above).
[g] Wasserheit et al., 1991 (see above).
[h] CDC. 1993 Sexually transmitted diseases treatment guidelines. MMWR 1993;42(No. RR-14).

C
Transmission Dynamics of Coexisting Chlamydial and HIV Infections in the United States

Marie-Claude Boily[1]

INTRODUCTION

Predicting HIV prevalence and incidence trends in the United States is hazardous because the mechanisms of heterosexual HIV transmission, the interrelationships between classical STDs and HIV infection, and sexual behavior among the U.S. population are not fully understood. These factors are particularly important when determining the rate of spread of HIV in different risk groups and the potential impact of STDs on heterosexual HIV transmission. Nevertheless, mathematical models of disease transmission can be used to investigate whether HIV, once introduced in the general heterosexual population, is able to establish and persist solely by heterosexual transmission, without the contribution of high-risk groups such as intravenous drug users or bisexuals. If so, how fast will HIV spread and to what extent will new HIV infections be attributable to curable STDs? A deterministic mathematical model has been developed to represent the natural course of STD and HIV infection in the general, sexually active, heterosexual population of the United States. Chlamydial infection is specifically modeled because it affects a large proportion of individuals not usually at risk for STDs and could therefore play an important role in heterosexually transmitted HIV infections, not only from high-risk to low-risk groups but also within low-risk groups. Results of the model will be discussed in relation to all curable STDs.

---

[1]Centre de Recherche Hôpital du St-Sacrément and Département de Médecine Sociale et Préventive, Université Laval (Center for Research, Hospital of St. Sacrement and Department of Social and Preventive Medicine, University of Laval, Quebec City, Canada).

MODEL AND PARAMETER ASSUMPTIONS

The deterministic mathematical model used, which is compartmental in structure, describes dynamically the course of both chlamydial and HIV infections in an active heterosexual population stratified by sex and sexual activity. The different stages of HIV and chlamydial infections are represented by six compartments. In the model, an individual can be susceptible to HIV, be infected with HIV but asymptomatic, or have full-blown AIDS. Each of these groups could be infected with an STD or not. Individuals can pass from one disease state to another at different rates, depending on the demographic and behavioral characteristics of the population as well as the natural history of the STD and HIV infections. The details of the model, including information on the system of nonlinear differential equations describing changes in the size of the population with time for the different disease states, are described by Boily and others (in press) in an upcoming paper.

The numerical studies of the model are based upon an initial population size of 171,481,800 individuals corresponding to the general, sexually active, heterosexual population of the United States in 1995 (Leigh et al., 1993; CIA, 1995; U.S. Census Bureau, 1996). The population growth rate is assumed to be 1.1 percent in absence of HIV infection, with a 1.01:1.00 female-to-male ratio (CIA, 1995; U.S. Census Bureau, 1996). It is assumed that an individual remains sexually active for a period of 55 years from age 15 to 70 (Anderson and Dahlberg, 1992; Leigh et al., 1993; Seidman and Rieder, 1994). Each gender is divided into six sexual activity classes to represent people with different rates of partner acquisition.

The most important assumptions when evaluating the potential impact of STDs on heterosexual HIV transmission center around HIV transmission probabilities in the absence of STDs, the sexual network and the distribution of sexual activity in the general population, the prevalence of STDs, and the nature and the magnitude of the interrelationships between STDs and HIV infection. These parameters determine whether HIV, in the presence or absence of STDs, can establish in the population and what the rate of spread of HIV in different risk groups will be. In the absence of the enhancing STD, the male-to-female per partner transmission probability for HIV is assumed to be two times that of female-to-male transmission (European Study Group on Heterosexual Transmission of HIV, 1992; Garnett and Anderson, 1993b; de Vincenzi and European Study Group on Heterosexual Transmission of HIV, 1994; Mastro et al., 1994;). In addition, HIV transmission probabilities are reduced when partnerships are formed with individuals from the high-activity classes (Jewell and Shiboski, 1990; Brookmeyer and Gail, 1994; Downs and de Vincenzi, 1996) to reflect the fact that very active individuals perform fewer acts per partnership than those with fewer partners (Garnett and Anderson, 1995; Boily and Anderson, 1996; Boily et al., in press). Lastly, different mechanisms have been postulated about the way STDs interact with HIV infection (Pepin et al., 1989; Piot and Tezzo, 1990; Laga et al., 1991, 1993; Wasserheit, 1992; Wald et al., 1993; Laga, Diallo, et al., 1994; Grosskurth et al., 1995).

The interrelationship between HIV infection and chlamydial infection is defined strictly as an increase in HIV transmission probability (the relative risk) due to increased HIV susceptibility and infectivity in presence of the cofactor chlamydia (May and Anderson, 1989; Boily and Anderson, 1996). To account for the variability in the estimates from different studies (Plummer et al., 1991; Wasserheit, 1992; Laga et al., 1993; Wald et al., 1993), it was assumed that chlamydia increases HIV transmission probability by 3.6- and 5-fold. In this model, the epidemic is seeded by introducing one HIV infected person in the female activity class 6 in 1980. The annual rates of new partner acquisition of the six sexual activity classes for the model (Table C-1) were derived from different national sex surveys of the general population (Anderson and Dahlberg, 1992; Leigh et al., 1993; Laumann et al., 1994; Seidman and Rieder, 1994) that report approximately 10 percent of the general population had more than two partners in the previous year (Table C-2). The problems with such data, as with most data on sexual behavior in the general population (ACSF Investigators, 1992; Anderson and Dahlberg, 1992; Johnson et al., 1992; Leigh et al., 1993; Seidman and Reider, 1994; Laumann et al., 1994; Turner et al., 1995), are that for a variety of reasons (Morris, 1993; Wadsworth et al., 1996), men usually report more female partners than females do male partners. This is inconsistent with the fact that men and women are having sex with each other (Blower and McLean, 1991; Boily and Anderson, 1991; Morris, 1993; Wadsworth et al., 1996). Thus, for simplicity and to ensure that the mean number of sex partners between the male and female population is balanced (Blower and McLean, 1991; Boily and Anderson, 1991; Lepont and Blower, 1991), we assumed that males and females have a similar distribution in sexual activity. The simulations have been performed under an assortative mixing scenario (Garnett and Anderson, 1993b; Garnett et al., 1996) or, in other words, one where the individual prefers to choose his or her partners within the same activity class (a minimum of 44 percent of partner formation occurs within members of the same activity class). The fact that, under proportionate mixing (individuals choose their sexual partners at random, depending on availability only) (Haralosottir et al., 1992; Boily and Brunham, 1993), chlamydial and HIV infections cannot establish in the population even with a relative risk of 5 further supports this hypothesis.

The predicted HIV and AIDS trends and estimates of the fraction of cases attributable to cofactor chlamydia were produced using different sets of realistic parameter assumptions in which HIV transmission probabilities were varied depending on the magnitude of association used. The various biological and demographic parameter values used for chlamydial and HIV infection are summarized in Table C-3, and those on sexual behavior and initial chlamydia prevalence are

TABLE C-1 Equilibrium Prevalence of Chlamydia (the STD "Cofactor") by Sex and Sexual Activity Classes

Set 1

Sexual Activity Classes, i	Females			Males		
	Mean Rate of Sex Partner Change at $t = 0$ (per year)	Proportion in Class at $t = 0$ (%)	Initial Prevalence of Chlamydia (%)	Mean Rate of Sex Partner Change at $t = 0$ (per year)	Proportion in Class at $t = 0$ (%)	Initial Prevalence of Chlamydia (%)
1	0.1	86.600	0.10	0.1	88.600	0.10
2	1.1	5.500	1.59	1.1	5.500	1.48
3	2.1	3.250	3.50	2.1	3.250	3.27
4	3.2	2.425	6.58	3.2	2.425	6.16
5	6.9	1.800	7.55	6.9	1.800	7.09
6	22.0	0.355	39.27	22.0	0.355	37.53
Overall mean/ prevalence	0.5		0.73	0.5		0.68

TABLE C-2 Distribution of General U.S. Population by Reported Number of Sex Partners in Past Year

Reported Number of Sex Partners in Past Year	Total (%)	Male (%)	Female (%)
0	18.3	13.2	22.6
1	69.0	69.1	68.9
2	5.2	5.3	5.2
3	3.1	4.6	1.8
4	1.7	2.8	0.7
5–10	2.0	3.6	0.6
11–20	0.3	0.6	0.1
21–100	0.3	0.7	0.0
>100	0.0	0.1	0.0
Total	100.0	100.0	100.0

SOURCE: Anderson JE, Dahlberg LL. High-risk sexual behavior in the general population. Results from a national survey, 1988-1990. Sex Transm Dis 1992;19:320-5.

TABLE C-3 Epidemiological and Demographic Parameters Used in the Simulations

Parameters	Symbols	Values
Sexually active population size in 1995	$Pop_{female}=1.01Pop_{male}$	171,481,800
Population growth rate in absence of HIV	Λ	1.1%
Age at sexual maturation	τ	15 yrs
Average duration of sexual activity (taking account of background mortality) in the absence of HIV-1 infection	D_{sa}	55 yrs
Perinatal transmission {probability}	ε	30%
Life expectancy of AIDS patient	D_{AIDS}	1 yr
Average time from infection to the development of AIDS (incubation period) in STD-negative and -positive individuals	D_{HIV}	10 yrs
Average duration of chlamydial (Ct) infection in absence of treatment in HIV-negative and -positive individuals	D_{Ct}	10.2 mths

TABLE C-3 Continued

Parameters	Symbols	Values
Probability of HIV-1 transmission per partnership (varied)		Fast scenario
from female class <5 to male class <5	β_{1ij}	0.020
from female class ≥5 to male class ≥5	β_{1ij}	0.008
from male class <5 to female class <5	β_{2ij}	0.040
from male class ≥5 to female class ≥5	β_{2ij}	0.016
Probability of chlamydia transmission per partnership		
from female class <5 to male class <5	ξ_{1ij}	0.450
from female class ≥5 to male class ≥5	ξ_{1ij}	0.145
from male class <5 to female class <5	ξ_{2ij}	0.550
from male class ≥5 to female class ≥5	ξ_{2ij}	0.175
Magnitude of association between chlamydia and HIV	RR	3.6 or 5
Sexual network structure or mixing pattern	ρ_{kij}	Assortative
Initial number of HIV infections in 1980	Female class 6	1

NOTE:
Probability of HIV-1 transmission per partnership (varied):
β_{1ij} = Probability of HIV-1 transmission per partnership from a female of activity class i to her male partner in sexual activity class j.
β_{2ij} = Probability of HIV-1 transmission per partnership from a male of class i to his female partner of sexual activity class j.
(1) = female; (2) = male; (i) = sexual activity class of the HIV-infected partner; (j) = sexual activity class of the HIV-susceptible partner.
Probability of chlamydia transmission per partnership:
ξ_{1ij} = Probability of chlamydia transmission per partnership from a female of activity class i to her male partner in sexual activity class j.
ξ_{2ij} = Probability of chlamydia transmission per partnership from a male of class i to his female partner of sexual activity class j.
(1) = female; (2) = male; (i) = sexual activity class of the chlamydia-infected partner; (j) = sexual activity class of the chlamydia-susceptible partner.
RR = relative risk of HIV transmission due to chlamydia.
ρ_{kij} = Probability that an individual from sex k and activity class i will choose his/her partner of the opposite sex in activity class j.

presented in Table C-1. Additional details can be found in an upcoming paper by Boily and others (in press).

RESULTS

The predicted prevalence and incidence trends of HIV infection from 1980 to the year 2005 in the sexually active heterosexual population are depicted in (a) the general population (both sexes and all sexual activity classes), (b) the low-risk group (annual rate of partner change less than one per year), and (c) the high-risk group (annual rate of partner change greater than one per year) in Figure C-1. Fast and slow spread scenarios are represented. Both are based on the parameters described in Table C-3 with a relative risk of 5 except that, for the slow scenario, HIV transmission probabilities are reduced by 25 percent.

HIV trends predicted by the model suggest that the establishment of HIV in the heterosexual population is possible and may affect a considerable proportion of the general population and different risk groups. The rate at which HIV will propagate and the maximum fraction of the population afflicted by HIV infection are highly dependent on the degree to which chlamydial infection enhances HIV transmission and on the prevalence of chlamydial infection. At the time of introduction of HIV in the population in 1980, chlamydial infection affected 0.72 percent and 0.68 percent of the general female and male population (weighted average of the different activity classes), but rates were higher in the most sexually active individuals (Table C-1), thus emphasizing their contribution to HIV transmission. Under the set of conditions investigated, HIV infection cannot establish in the absence of chlamydial infection, without a minimum degree of within-group mixing between high-activity classes or in the absence of the highest-activity class (class 6). Under the latter two conditions, chlamydial infection cannot persist either. Thus, a large fraction of HIV infections will, even over a short time period, be attributable to the cofactor chlamydia and the core group population.

The predicted fraction of the total incident heterosexual HIV and AIDS cases attributable to chlamydial infection for the periods 1980–1994 inclusive, 1995–1999, and 1995–2004 are presented in Table C-4 for the slow and fast scenarios with a relative risk of 3.6 and 5.

For all scenarios investigated, a large fraction of HIV infections can, even over a short time period, be attributed to cofactor chlamydia. For example, the model predicts that during 1990–1994, more than 86 percent and 95 percent of the heterosexual AIDS and HIV cases, respectively, could have been prevented by treating chlamydial infections.

DISCUSSION

Despite limitations of the model due to major uncertainties concerning parameter assumptions, mathematical modeling can be used to evaluate the magnitude of the HIV/AIDS epidemic and the role of STDs in heterosexual HIV transmission. The real impact of STDs on the pattern of HIV incidence and prevalence in the United States remains uncertain because it mainly depends on the prevalence of STDs in different risk groups, the interrelationships between STD and HIV infection, the real magnitude of association, and the estimates of HIV trans-

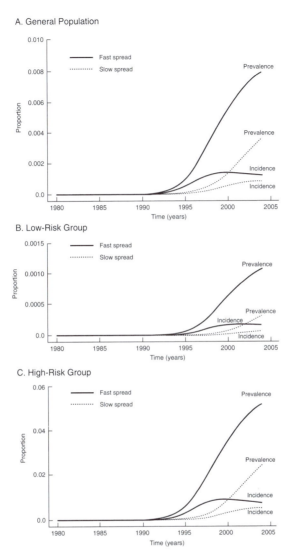

FIGURE C-1   Predicted prevalence and incidence trends of HIV infection, 1980 to 2005, in the sexually active U.S. heterosexual population. Graph A represents the general population (both sexes and all sexual activity classes), with initial prevalence of chlamydial infection = 0.70 percent; Graph B depicts the low-risk group (annual rate of partner change less than one per year), with initial prevalence of chlamydial infection = 0.01 percent; and Graph C represents the high-risk group (annual rate of partner change greater than one per year), with initial prevalence of chlamydial infection = 4.63 percent. Fast and slow spread scenarios also are represented. Both are based on the parameters described in Table C-3 with a relative risk of 5 except that, for the slow scenario, HIV transmission probabilities are reduced by 25 percent.

TABLE C-4 Fraction of Total New HIV and AIDS Cases in the General Heterosexual Population Attributable to Cofactor Chlamydia, 1980–1994, 1995–1999, and 1995–2004

Scenarios	Slow		Fast	
Parameters Relative risk (RR):	RR = 3.6	RR = 5	RR = 3.6	RR = 5
HIV transmission probabilities:				
fem. cl. <5 to male cl. <5	$\beta_{1ij} = 0.025$	$\beta_{1ij} = 0.015$	$\beta_{1ij} = 0.030$	$\beta_{1ij} = 0.020$
fem. cl. ≥5 to male cl. ≥5	$\beta_{1ij} = 0.010$	$\beta_{1ij} = 0.006$	$\beta_{1ij} = 0.012$	$\beta_{1ij} = 0.008$
male cl. <5 to fem. cl. <5	$\beta_{1ij} = 0.050$	$\beta_{1ij} = 0.030$	$\beta_{1ij} = 0.060$	$\beta_{1ij} = 0.040$
male cl. ≥5 to fem. cl. ≥5	$\beta_{1ij} = 0.020$	$\beta_{1ij} = 0.012$	$\beta_{1ij} = 0.024$	$\beta_{1ij} = 0.016$
	Population Attributable Risk (%)			
1980–1994:				
AIDS	99	99	99	99
HIV	99	99	99	99
1995–1999:				
AIDS	76	80	68	58
HIV	92	96	88	80
1995–2004:				
AIDS	93	95	78	67
HIV	97	98	88	80

NOTE: See Table C-1 and C-3 for parameters and symbols.

mission probability in the absence of STDs. Additional data are needed for all these factors.

From the different scenarios considered, there are a variety of reasons to conclude that a self-sustaining HIV epidemic in the general heterosexual population is possible. First, the behavioral parameter values used underestimate the variability in sexual activity of the general population because the most sexually active individuals, who constitute a small fraction of the population, are most probably undersampled in a random sample of the general population. Greater heterogeneity in sexual activity and higher activity levels of the most active individuals are conditions that favor the establishment of an STD. Second, previous results (Garnett et al., 1992; Whitaker and Renton, 1992; Garnett and Anderson, 1993a; Boily et al., in press) show that a more assortative mixing or a majority of individuals having a low rate of partner change accentuate partner formation between high-activity classes. Thus, even with a lower level of sexual activity, a more assortative mixing would favor STD establishment and transmission. Third, chlamydial infection prevalence rates produced in the different risk groups before the introduction of HIV are lower than the rates currently reported (prevalence of chlamydial infection in young adult women and sexually active adolescents greater than 5 percent and 10 percent, men from STD clinics up to 15 to 20 percent, young asymptomatic men seen in more general medical settings greater than 3 to 5 percent). Fourth, by considering the general heterosexual population exclusively, the model does not account for the fact that many heterosexual contacts and transmissions occur with high-risk individuals such as intravenous drug users and bisexuals, for whom HIV and STD rates are higher. Fifth, if a causal relationship exists between chlamydial and HIV infections, then the magnitude of association is very likely to be underestimated (Hayes et al., 1995; Boily and Anderson, 1996). Thus, the real increase in HIV transmission probabilities per partnership or per contact due to the cofactor chlamydia could be higher than what has been reported, a relative risk of 3.6, in the best study (Laga, Alary, et al., 1994).

Two elements that have the potential to modify the global picture of HIV spread and that were not included in the model are spatial heterogeneity and the heterogeneity in HIV transmission probabilities during the long incubation period. It was assumed that the U.S. population was homogeneously distributed geographically. This implies that the rate of spread of HIV predicted may be faster than in reality, as HIV might be introduced at different times in different agglomerations. Thus, on the one hand, spatial heterogeneity could retard diffusion of HIV from one agglomeration to another and display great variability in the rate of spread between regions or districts, but it should not compromise the reproductive success of HIV infection, which was shown to be viable in a spatially homogeneous population. On the other hand, if heterogeneity in HIV transmission probabilities (with high transmission probabilities in the first and last phase of the incubation period) were included in the model, then, in its initial phase, the epidemic could develop at a faster rate than predicted by the model (Blythe and Anderson, 1988).

Given a fixed trend, the effect of STD treatment on future HIV trends and the maximum proportion of HIV infections prevented are highly dependent on the degree to which STDs enhance HIV transmission, on the prevalence of STDs, and on the combination between the pattern of sexual behavior in the general population and the estimates of HIV transmission probability in the absence of STDs. The strongest assumption of this analysis is the extent to which HIV spread depends on chlamydia, since HIV cannot establish in the absence of enhancing chlamydia. This assumption is not totally unrealistic if we consider (despite other dissimilarities) that in many Northern European countries, where STDs are better controlled compared to the United States, there is little evidence of an indigenous heterosexual HIV epidemic (King K. Holmes, University of Washington, personal communication, August 1996). Thus, the model and parameters used may portray an overly optimistic scenario of the impact of chlamydia treatment on HIV incidence trends, because the model suggests that heterosexually transmitted HIV could in theory be eradicated if chlamydia were eliminated. Note that even if HIV could establish in the absence of chlamydia, a considerable fraction of HIV cases could still be attributed to cofactor chlamydia. HIV spread would slow down, but would not be eradicated by effective STD treatment alone. In addition, in the United States, the continued force of heterosexual transmission from intravenous drug use would remain. Note also that even if chlamydial infection accounts for a large fraction of new HIV cases in this model, this does not preclude the possibility that other STDs have also contributed to the spread of HIV once it has become established. The model with chlamydia is equivalent to assuming that all STDs are required for HIV to establish. Under this assumption, the eradication of heterosexually transmitted HIV is possible by eliminating only one curable STD or by reducing the prevalence of all curable STDs below a certain threshold. Another way the same HIV epidemic could be established is by assuming that it requires the presence of only one STD, such as chlamydia. This scenario is more conservative regarding the impact of STD treatment on HIV incidence trends, since the elimination of HIV would require the eradication of all STDs or the reduction of the prevalence of all curable STDs below a threshold much lower that that for the first scenario.

Despite the depressing forecast of the model on the potential impact of chlamydial infection and other STDs on HIV spread in the general U.S. heterosexual population, one optimistic point emerges from this study. This is the important fraction of heterosexually transmitted HIV infections that can be prevented by treating chlamydial infection and other curable STDs. Simulation work confirms previous results (Hethcote and Yorke, 1984) showing that screening high-risk individuals or core groups can be much more efficient than the screening of the more general population (Hethcote and Yorke, 1984; Brunham and

Plummer, 1990; Garnett and Anderson, 1995), because the noncore population contributes relatively little to the reproductive success of STDs and HIV infection. Thus, a 50 percent reduction in chlamydia (from 10 to 5 percent), such as observed in Region X of the United States (DeLisle et al., 1993) following the implementation of a chlamydia screening program in family planning clinics, could play an important role in slowing HIV transmission in the area. Moreover, treating STDs offers a complementary approach to interventions to change sexual behavior (such as reduction of sexual activity). Furthermore, changes in sexual behavior can produce pernicious effects by modifying the structure of social networks (Boily and Anderson, 1990; Thompson Fullilove, 1995).

Considering the great heterogeneity in seroprevalence rates of infection between regions (CDC, 1994, 1995), it can be assumed that the HIV epidemic in the heterosexual population in most U.S. states and cities might still be in its early stages (i.e., anywhere between 1980 and 2000 on our time scale). Results indicate that improved efforts to contain and prevent STDs should be made immediately and that such efforts could prevent, if initiated early enough, many new HIV infections, even over a relatively short time period. However, since exposure of the general heterosexual population to HIV via high-risk individuals such as intravenous drug users or bisexuals has not been included in the model (deliberately done in order to remain conservative), one should bear in mind that constant introduction of the virus in the general heterosexual population by these high-risk groups can always occur despite excellent STD control. Therefore, it is important when designing prevention strategies for the general heterosexual population not to ignore these remaining reservoirs of STDs, including HIV infection.

REFERENCES

ACSF (Analyse des Comportements Sexuels en France) Investigators. AIDS and sexual behaviour in France. Nature 1992;360:407-9.

Anderson JE, Dahlberg LL. High-risk sexual behavior in the general population. Results from a national survey, 1988-1990. Sex Transm Dis 1992;19:320-5.

Blower SM, McLean AR. Mixing ecology and epidemiology. Proc R Soc Lond B 1991;245:187-92.

Blythe SP, Anderson RM. Variable infectiousness in HIV transmission models. IMA J Math App Med Biol 1988;5:181-200.

Boily M-C, Anderson RM. Assessing change in sexual behaviour using mathematical models: the impact of sexual mixing (Part A). Proceedings of the International Conference on Assessing AIDS Prevention, October 29-November 1, 1990; Montreux, Switzerland [abstract no. C2.4].

Boily M-C, Anderson RM. Sexual contact patterns between men and women and the spread of HIV-1 in urban centres in Africa. IMA J Math App Med Biol 1991;8:221-47.

Boily M-C, Anderson RM. Human immunodeficiency virus transmission and the role of other sexually transmitted diseases: measures of association and study design. Sex Transm Dis 1996;23:312-30.

Boily M-C, Brunham RC. The impact of HIV and other STDs on human populations. Are predictions possible? Inf Dis Clin North Am 1993;7:771-91.

Boily M-C, Desai KN, Garnett GP. Transmission dynamics of co-existing chlamydia and HIV infections in the heterosexual population of the United States. IMA J Math Appl Med Biol, in press.

Brookmeyer R, Gail MH. Risk factors for infection and the probability of HIV transmission. In: AIDS epidemiology—a quantitative approach. New York: Oxford University Press, 1994:19-50.

Brunham RC, Plummer AA. A general model of sexually transmitted disease epidemiology and its implications for control. Sex Transm Dis 1990;74:1339-52.

CDC (Centers for Disease Control and Prevention). National HIV serosurveillance summary: results through 1992. Atlanta: U.S. Department of Health and Human Services, 1994:3:51.

CDC. HIV/AIDS surveillance report, U.S. HIV and AIDS cases reported through December 1995. Atlanta: U.S. Department of Health and Human Services, 1995;5:38.

CIA (Central Intelligence Agency). CIA World Factbook. http://www.odci.gov/cia/publications/95fact/us.html, 1995.

DeLisle S, Fine D, Kaetz S, Johnson RE, Schrader M, Lee V, et al. A multi-site model for the prevention and control of sexually transmitted chlamydia infections. Tenth International Meeting of the International Society for STD Research, August 29-September 1, 1993, Helsinki [abstract no. 162].

de Vincenzi I, European Study Group on Heterosexual Transmission of HIV. A longitudinal study of human immunodeficiency virus transmission by heterosexual partners. N Engl J Med 1994;331:341-6.

Downs AM, de Vincenzi I. Probability of heterosexual transmission of HIV: relationship to the number of unprotected sexual contacts. European Study Group in Heterosexual Transmission of HIV [see comments]. J Acquir Immune Defic Syndr Hum Retrovir 1996;11:388-95.

European Study Group on Heterosexual Transmission of HIV. Comparison of female to male and male to female transmission of HIV in 563 stable couples. Br Med J 1992;304:809-13.

Garnett GP, Anderson RM. Contact tracing and the estimation of sexual mixing patterns: the epidemiology of gonococcal infection. Sex Transm Dis 1993a;20:181-91.

Garnett GP, Anderson RM. Factors controlling the spread of HIV in heterosexual communities in developing countries: patterns of mixing between different age and sexual activity classes. Phil Trans R Soc Lond B 1993b;342:137-59.

Garnett GP, Anderson RM. Strategies for limiting the spread of HIV in developing countries: conclusions based on studies of the transmission dynamics of the virus. J Acquir Immune Defic Syndr Hum Retrovirol 1995;9:500-13.

Garnett GP, Hughes JP, Anderson RM, Stoner BP, Aral SO, Whittingham WL, et al. Sexual mixing patterns of patients attending sexually transmitted disease clinics. Sex Transm Dis 1996;23:248-57.

Garnett GP, Swinton J, Brunham C, Anderson RM. Gonococcal infection, infertility, and population growth: the influence of heterogeneity in sexual behaviour. IMA J Math Appl Med Biol 1992;9:127-44.

Grosskurth H, Mosha F, Todd J, Mwijarubi E, Klokke A, Senkoro K, et al. Impact of improved treatment of sexually transmitted diseases on HIV infection in rural Tanzania: randomized controlled trial [see comments]. Lancet 1995;346:530-6.

Haralosottir S, Gupta S, Anderson RM. Preliminary studies of sexual networks in a male homosexual community in Iceland. J Acquir Immune Defic Syndr 1992;5:374-81.

Hayes RJ, Schulz KF, Plummer FA. The cofactor effect of genital ulcers on the per-exposure risk of HIV transmission in sub-Saharan Africa. J Trop Med Hyg 1995;98:1-8.

Hethcote HW, Yorke JA. Gonorrhea transmission dynamics and control. In: Levin S, ed. Lecture notes in biomathematics. New York: Springer-Verlag, 1984:56:99.

Jewell NP, Shiboski SC. Statistical analysis of HIV infectivity based on partner studies. Biometrics 1990;46:1133-50.

Johnson AM, Wadsworth J, Wellings K, Bradshaw S, Field J. Sexual lifestyles and HIV risk. Nature 1992;360:410-2.

Laga M, Alary M, Nzilambi N, Manoka AT, Tuliza M, Behets F, et al. Condom promotion, sexually transmitted treatment, and declining incidence of HIV-1 infection in female Zairian sex workers. Lancet 1994;344:246-8.

Laga M, Diallo MO, Buv A. Inter-relationship of sexually transmitted diseases and HIV: where are we now? AIDS 1994;8[1 Suppl]:S119-S124.

Laga M, Manoka A, Kivuvu M, Malele B, Tuliza M, Nzila N, et al. Non-ulcerative sexually transmitted diseases as risk factors for HIV-1 transmission in women: results from a cohort study. AIDS 1993;7:95-102.

Laga M, Nzilambi N, Goeman J. The interrelationships of sexually transmitted diseases and HIV infection: implication for the control of both epidemics in Africa. AIDS 1991;5[1 Suppl]:S55-S65.

Laumann EO, Gagnon JH, Michael RT, Michaels S. The social organization of sexuality: sexual practices in the United States. Chicago: University of Chicago Press, 1994:718.

Leigh BC, Temple MT, Trocki KF. The sexual behavior of U.S. adults: results from a national survey. Am J Public Health 1993;83:1400-8.

Lepont F, Blower SM. The supply and demand dynamics of sexual behaviour: implications of heterosexual HIV epidemics. J Acquir Immune Defic Syndr 1991;4:987-99.

Mastro TD, Satten GA, Nopkesorn T, Sangkharomya S, Logini IM Jr. Probability of female-to-male transmission of HIV-1 in Thailand [see comments]. Lancet 1994;343:204-7.

May RM, Anderson RM. Heterogeneities, cofactors and other aspects of the transmission dynamics of HIV/AIDS. J Acquir Immune Defic Syndr 1989;2:33-67.

Morris M. Telling tails explain the discrepancy in sexual partner reports. Nature 1993;365:437-40.

Pepin J, Plummer FA, Brunham RC, Piot P, Cameron CW, Ronald AR. The interaction of HIV infection and other sexually transmitted diseases. AIDS 1989;3:3-9.

Piot P, Tezzo R. The epidemiology of HIV and other sexually transmitted infections in the developing world. Scan J Inf Dis Suppl 1990;69:89-97.

Plummer FA, Simonsen JN, Cameron DW, Ndinya-Achola JO, Kreiss JK, Gakinya MN, et al. Co-factors in male-female transmission of human immunodeficiency virus type 1. J Infect Dis 1991;163:233-9.

Seidman SN, Rieder RO. A review of sexual behavior in the United States. Am J Psychiatry 1994;151:330-41.

Thompson Fullilove M. Risk behaviors and STD/HIV transmission. Paper presented at the Institute of Medicine workshop "Understanding the relationship of STD control to HIV prevention in the United States." Committee on Prevention and Control of Sexually Transmitted Diseases, National Academy of Sciences, Washington, D.C., July 10, 1995.

Turner CF, Danella RD, Rogers SM. Sexual behavior in the United States, 1930-1990: trends and methodological problems. Sex Transm Dis 1995;22:173-90.

U.S. Census Bureau. http://www.census.gov/, 1996.

Wadsworth J, Johnson AM, Wellings K, Field J. What's in a mean? An examination of the inconsistency between men and women in reporting sexual partnerships. J R Statist Soc A 1996; 59[Part 1]:111-23.

Wald A, Corey L, Handsfield HH, Holmes KK. Influence of HIV infection on manifestations and natural history of other sexually transmitted diseases. Ann Rev Public Health 1993;14:19-42.

Wasserheit JN. Interrelationships between immunodeficiency virus infection and other sexually transmitted diseases. Sex Transm Dis 1992;19:61-5.

Whitaker L, Renton AM. A theoretical problem of interpreting the recently reported increase in homosexual gonorrhoea. Eur J Epidemiol 1992;8:187-91.

Estimates of the Economic Burden of STDs: Review of the Literature with Updates

Joanna E. Siegel[1]

INTRODUCTION

STDs impose a significant burden of morbidity and mortality in the United States. They range from diseases that, for the most part, cause temporary discomfort and inconvenience to illnesses that impair fertility, result in long-term morbidity, or shorten life.

This paper summarizes information in the literature to provide estimates of the economic impact of seven sexually transmitted diseases. These are gonorrhea, chlamydial infection, syphilis, genital herpes, human papillomavirus (HPV), chancroid, and hepatitis B virus infection. This list of STDs is far from comprehensive, but it includes most of the reportable STDs, with the exception of HIV infection, and some additional STDs that potentially impose a large burden of illness. Estimates are presented for the annual costs of these illnesses for the year 1994.

ECONOMIC BURDEN OF ILLNESS

The economic burden of an illness reflects the opportunity cost of all resources used as a result of the illness, that is, the value of these resources in their

---

[1]Department of Maternal and Child Health, Harvard School of Public Health, Boston, MA.
Acknowledgments: Thanks are due to the following individuals for their assistance with this project: James Ida (research assistant), Melinda Flock, Alan Friedlob, Mike St. Louis, Tom Eng, and Gene Washington.

preferred alternative use, assuming the illness had not arisen. A measure of the economic burden of STDs thus indicates the quantity of resources that would be available for other purposes if they were not used to address STDs. The actual source of funds may be the government, individuals, or other parties such as insurers. In some cases, resources may be used with no accompanying transfer of money.

The costs associated with STDs and other illnesses include "direct" costs, both medical and nonmedical, for services and materials. Major categories of direct costs incurred because of illness include the costs of health care workers' services (those of physicians, nurses, technicians, and others), costs associated with hospital admissions, costs of pharmaceuticals, and costs of medical equipment. The costs of transportation, home care, special schooling, and other such resources are also direct costs.

Productivity costs are also incurred by illness. These costs, often termed "indirect" costs, reflect the opportunity cost of the productive time the affected individual (and society) lose because of illness. Productivity costs include both time spent sick, when an individual is unable to engage in the activities he or she otherwise would, and premature mortality. The time an individual invests in treatment—traveling to obtain care, waiting in the clinic waiting room, filling a prescription, undergoing a procedure—could be categorized either as a direct cost or a productivity cost. Regardless of how it is categorized, it entails an opportunity cost.

The economic burden of a disease can be demonstrated by calculating either its prevalent costs (the annual costs of cases prevalent during a given year) or the lifetime costs of individual cases (incident costs). This review focuses on the former measure of economic burden, often termed the "cost-of-illness." This approach seeks to capture the costs associated with the cross-section of existing cases—including current costs for cases that occurred previously—but does not reflect future costs associated with a disease. Prevalent costs provide an estimate of economic burden that is useful for comparisons in an annual context, such as for federal, state, or institutional budgets. Incident costs, in contrast, demonstrate the full impact of an illness over time on a cost-per-case basis. They include the present value of future costs associated with the cases occurring during a given year.

For some illnesses, the distinction between prevalent and incident costs is of minimal importance, as the primary costs of the disease relate to the acute infection and occur during the first year of the disease. For most illnesses, however, costs occur over a longer period of time. This is clearly true for debilitating congenital illnesses, for which costs of care may extend over a lifetime. It is also true for STDs that have long-term consequences, such as pelvic inflammatory disease (PID) and infertility. For this reason, the prevalent costs of STDs cannot be assumed to reflect the full costs per case of these diseases.

This effort focuses on the collection and adjustment of existing estimates. It estimates prevalent costs (costs-of-illness) for the year 1994, reflecting the most current data available at the time of this research. The emphasis is on direct costs, although productivity loss estimates are reported where they exist.

WHY THE COST OF ILLNESS IS ASSESSED

Policymakers solicit and researchers undertake cost-of-illness studies to demonstrate the impact of an illness on society. As noted earlier, these studies place the burden of illness in the context of annual spending related to a specific cause. Consumers of this information then can more accurately assess the priority of a problem or the appropriateness of the level of spending. For example, the Senate Appropriations Committee recently requested that the National Institutes of Health compile a table of annual costs of illness for leading causes of mortality. The request specified that a column indicating the fiscal year research funding for each cause of death should be included in the table (NIH, 1995).

Annual spending may reflect a minor or a major proportion of the total expenditures related to an illness. In the early 1980s, for example, annual costs for HIV infection represented only a very small part of the costs eventually attributable to existing infection. In addition, the annual burden of an illness gives no indication of the effectiveness of dollars invested in alleviating it. Nonetheless, the annual figure gives an indication of the importance of the problem at a point in time. As a result, federal offices and congressional committees have demonstrated interest in clarifying the methodology for these studies, in conducting them, and in assembling their results (Rice et al., 1985).

CHALLENGES TO ASSESSING ECONOMIC IMPACT

There are numerous obstacles to accurately accounting for resource use associated with disease and to the assignment of dollar values to these resources. Some problems are specific to assessing the cost of STDs, while other problems apply equally to the assessment of cost of both STDs and other illnesses.

A basic problem in assessing the cost of STDs is the difficulty in establishing incidence and prevalence. Counts of cases are critical when estimates are based on an annual cost per case that is multiplied by the estimated total number of cases. Because the United States has no integrated and comprehensive medical data system, incidence of illnesses must be estimated. The reporting of many STDs is required, and therefore their incidence should be easier to ascertain than the incidence of nonreportable diseases. However, the government does not require the reporting of some important (particularly viral) STDs, and even reportable STDs are commonly underreported. The extent of underreporting is not well understood. Surveys completed over two decades ago demonstrated that private physicians reported only 25–50 percent of the gonorrhea cases they treated (IOM, 1985; Moran et al., 1995). Updated information on reporting is currently being gathered. Meanwhile, the CDC assumes that only half of all gonorrhea cases are reported. Reported syphilis cases, in contrast, are believed to provide a good indicator of the incidence of that disease (Moran et al., 1995).

Other factors complicating the determination of STD counts are errors in the communication of reported statistics, obstacles to clinical diagnosis, and error in laboratory testing (Schmid et al., 1987; Corey, 1994). In addition, some afflicted individuals never seek treatment and therefore are not counted in data systems. This is true, for example, for genital herpes, where primary infection is asymp-tomatic (or at least unrecognized) in more than half of cases (Johnson et al., 1989; Corey, 1994). Alternatively, patients may seek treatment long after the initial infection is acquired. Sequelae of STDs that motivate treatment, such as PID, may occur years later.

The valuation of resources used in the identification and treatment of illness, which links counts of events and medical interventions to final estimates of cost, can also be problematic. In most analyses, opportunity costs are approximated by market prices, which is generally the most tractable method of estimation. According to economic theory, prices are an adequate reflection of the opportunity cost of resources in competitive markets. However, health care markets are gen-erally acknowledged not to meet the standard criteria for competitive markets, so prices may deviate significantly from resource costs. For example, hospital costs for most patients have long been covered by health insurance, creating a situation in which the buyers and sellers of hospital services have had no direct contact. As a result, the consumers have exhibited little price sensitivity. Health care markets have become dramatically more competitive in recent years, owing principally to the buying power of managed care organizations and other large purchasers. However, it is unclear whether these changes have caused "prices"—i.e., fees and charges—to become more reflective of costs.

Many of the prices used to estimate costs in the literature are administrative and are likely to be only rough surrogates for cost. It is difficult to obtain full information with which to compute administrative prices. In addition, these prices inevitably lag behind technological changes in the delivery of care. A particular problem affecting the estimation of STD-related costs is that a large proportion of patients are treated in public STD clinics. Little is known about the units of service provided and their costs in these settings because the clinics are allocated budgets and do not generate case-by-case claims records for purposes of reim-bursement. A problem common to cost estimates of a range of diseases is that treatment patterns and costs vary geographically and by care setting. Studies using a variety of data sets would be required to accurately assess the distribution of costs.

The estimation of the economic burden of illness suffers further from the virtual lack of information on certain categories of resource use. In general, there are few data available describing the "out-of-pocket costs" paid by patients and family members. The units of time lost in pursuing treatment of, and recovery from, a particular disease often are not available. The valuation of productive time lost, once it is identified, is complicated both by practical and ethical issues. For example, the wage rates most frequently used to value time lost to illness generally do not reflect the replacement of labor by unemployed workers, and they do not apply readily to some categories of individuals affected by illness, such as the unemployed, children, homemakers, and the retired.

The obstacles to obtaining adequate measures of cost are reflected in the estimates of economic impact presented in this literature review. In some cases, the estimates are carefully developed, subject to the broader constraints of the field. In other instances, estimates are rough; these are usually intended to provide policymakers and the research community with a general gauge of costs.

METHODS

Literature on the Economic Impact of STDs

This paper reviews the existing literature to identify estimates of the economic impact of STDs in the United States. The MEDLINE and Health databases produced by the National Library of Medicine were the primary means of identifying literature. MEDLINE covers the international biomedical literature, including the allied health fields, the biological and physical sciences, selected humanities, and information services as they relate to medicine and health care. The database from 1966 through December 1995, which includes some 3,600 journals and selected monographs of scientific congresses and symposia, was searched. In addition, the Health database from 1975 through December 1995 was searched. This database contains references from the Hospital Literature Index and other selected journals in addition to MEDLINE information.

The following headings were used as keywords in both titles and abstracts: cervical cancer, cost and cost analysis, chlamydia, chancroid, economics, genital herpes, gonorrhea, health expenditures, herpes simplex, hepatitis B, human papillomavirus, pregnancy, sexually transmitted diseases, and syphilis. These headings were used separately and in selected combinations to search for materials to be reviewed for their relevance to the present study. Additional information was obtained from the Centers for Disease Control and Prevention (CDC), from members of the Institute of Medicine (IOM) Committee on Prevention and Control of Sexually Transmitted Diseases, and through citations in journals and textbooks.

Adjustments

Two primary adjustments are made to cost estimates from the literature in order to present annual costs for 1994. The first is an adjustment for inflation: All cost estimates are converted to 1994 dollars. This adjustment is made using the general medical component of the Consumer Price Index (CPI), except in a few cases where another conversion factor is more specific to the cost being considered. In those cases, the specific category is identified (e.g., the hospitals component of the CPI). In most of the literature containing cost estimates, the year of costs is given in the study. When it is not, it is assumed that costs in the original literature were collected for the year prior to the year of publication.

The second major adjustment to estimates in the literature is for changes in the incidence or prevalence of illness. Many of the estimates in the literature reflect incidence rates from the early 1980s, which were higher in many cases than 1994 STD incidence rates. In adjusting overall cost estimates for current trends, the assumption is made that the cost per case has remained constant. Therefore, if estimated 1994 incidence was 60 percent as high as an earlier year, the overall cost estimate was adjusted to 60 percent of the original figure.

In some cases, estimates for STD treatment costs for an STD are calculated. The recommended treatment regimens are obtained from the CDC STD Treatment Guidelines (CDC, 1993). Costs for a physician visit are estimated at $61, based on a survey of physician fees charged to privately insured patients (AMA, 1994). This is the estimated charge for a new patient office visit for a general/family practice physician. New patient visits for other types of physicians can be much higher (e.g., the comparable fee for an internist is $122). However, fees for established patients are in this range for most relevant physician specialties (general/family: $44; internal medicine: $62; all physician average: $56). In addition, Medicaid fees and costs of physicians at public clinics are likely to be lower. Thus, the $61 fee seems a reasonable approximation for a majority of visits. Costs of drug treatments are obtained from the Drug Topics Red Book (1995).

To estimate costs consistently for STDs, a standard set of expenditures should be utilized. Many categorizations would be reasonable. For example, Bowie (1995) divides resource use associated with STDs into the following categories:

- Routine STD laboratory testing for screening or diagnosis (diagnostics, specimen collection and transport, laboratory resources, reporting)
- Nonroutine diagnostic testing
- Physician costs (counseling, acute management, follow-up evaluations, complications)
- Other health care providers
- Medication-associated costs for treatment (drug costs, prescribing fees, equipment for packaging)
- Hospitalization
- Costs to affected individuals
- Preventive medications/ barrier methods
- Administration (collection of statistical data, control programs, accounting)

Ideally, costs should be counted for all STDs in all relevant categories. In this review and in the estimates presented, this type of consistency is not attempted. For example, in some cases, an estimate of treatment costs was conducted that included costs of personnel, laboratory testing, and contact tracing. In other estimates, some of these costs were purposely excluded. In far more cases, there was simply no detailed assessment of many categories of the relevant costs in the literature. In this review, all available information is presented, and the limited number of adjustments listed above are used. Because many components of cost are missing, the totals calculated should be considered a lower bound for estimates of the economic burden of most STDs individually, and STDs as a group.

RESULTS

Types of Studies

There are several types of studies in the literature that bear on economic impact. The first, and most relevant for the purpose of this review, are studies evaluating the overall, or global, annual cost of an illness. In the area of STDs, there are studies on the overall costs of gonorrhea, chlamydial infection, and herpes simplex virus. A second type of study assesses costs for a component of an illness—that is, for some subset of the resource use associated with the broad category of the STD. The articles reviewed here focus either on relatively narrow subsets, such as treatment of an STD, or on larger subsets, such as the costs of congenital syphilis or PID. These studies are useful building blocks for estimates of overall economic burden.

Finally, there are cost-effectiveness and cost-benefit studies, often termed "economic evaluations." These studies are of limited use in assessing economic burden, although they may contain information relevant to calculating annual costs. They are often prescriptive, assessing costs for medical technologies that are not yet used or only partially implemented. Their assessment of economic impact is almost always based on an analysis of lifetime costs of an illness.

Studies containing cost estimates or data used in the estimates presented in Table D-1 and Table D-2 are reviewed below. This review seeks to be comprehensive in its discussion of overall cost-of-illness estimates. However, only cost-effectiveness analyses from which specific data have been obtained for estimates are reviewed. There are many others in the literature.

Studies of Overall Costs of STDs

A study on the overall costs of gonorrhea was conducted as part of the IOM report *New Vaccine Development: Establishing Priorities* (IOM, 1985). The study sought to demonstrate the cost of vaccine-preventable gonorrhea, which required, in part, development of an estimate of the total economic burden of disease.

The authors of the IOM study estimate annual cases of gonorrhea, adjusting for underreporting and misdiagnosis. They divide symptomatic cases into morbidity categories, assigning costs based on treatment profiles for each of these categories. Costs attributable to sequelae of gonorrhea (PID and ectopic pregnancy) are included, based on estimates of the annual occurrence of these conditions. Costs of infertility resulting from PID are also included; these appear to be calculated using an incident cost-of-illness approach, rather than the annual estimates otherwise used in their calculations. Incidence of epididymitis, ophthalmia neonatorum, and disseminated infection are assumed to be negligible and are not included.

The IOM estimates exclude productivity costs. In addition, they exclude the costs of public health measures to prevent further spread of gonorrhea, such as contact tracing. The advantages of these estimates are related to their comprehensiveness: all major components of cost attributable to the illness, from acute infection to sequelae, are included. The disadvantages stem from the lack of detail in cost calculations and lack of data to verify treatment protocols and cost estimates used in the calculations. The IOM estimate is clearly intended to provide a "ballpark" figure rather than a precise estimate.

In the same report and using the same general procedures, the IOM estimates costs for herpes simplex viruses (HSV) types 1 and 2. The same basic strengths and weaknesses apply. Due to a striking lack of information on such components of cost as the number of annual recurrent cases of herpes and the frequency and extent of treatment of these cases, important aspects of these costs estimates are based on relatively crude estimates. Similarly, the judgment of experts is used to categorize cases in terms of severity (and likely treatment) and treatment protocols. However, the estimates are ambitious, broad, and comprehensive—and often cited in the literature (Cates, 1988; CDC, DSTD/HIVP, 1995). It should be noted in using the IOM's unadjusted estimate that it is for both HSV-1 and HSV-2.

Costs of herpes in the IOM document are estimated separately for primary and recurrent cases of genital and labial herpes as well as for herpes keratitis. A substantial proportion (40 percent) of the total costs calculated for herpes are associated with herpes keratitis, reflecting costs of corneal transplants, blindness, and treatment. Costs for other sequelae reflect encephalitis, immunocompromised and disseminated HSV, and long-term costs associated with central nervous system (CNS) impairment. Neonatal herpes and its prevention are also included, although costs associated with HSV cultures during pregnancy are now outdated as a result of changes in obstetrical practice. Annual costs are cited, with the exception of those associated with CNS impairment, which are available in the report. However, the cost estimates for CNS impairment use total costs per case rather use costs on an annualized basis.

Washington and others (1987) provide an overall cost estimate for chlamydial infection. Their estimates of chlamydia incidence are based on gonorrhea incidence, using ratios of diagnosed gonorrhea to chlamydial infection among men and women at sentinel sites and in published reports. They obtained estimates of epididymitis from national data sets, and from this information estimated a proportion of physician visits and hospital admissions attributable to chlamydial epididymitis. Similarly, costs of uncomplicated infection among women and of PID are estimated nationally and a proportion assigned to chlamydia. Incidence of conjunctivitis among infants is based on a CDC estimate of births to chlamydia-infected women and an attack rate estimated from published sources (A. Eugene Washington, University of California, San Francisco, personal communication, 1996).

Cost data are based on national average physician fees, a survey of bills from two hospitals (for epididymitis), and published estimates. The authors base their estimates for conjunctivitis on assumptions about hospitalization rates, Diagnosis-Related Group rates, and physician fees. Indirect costs are based on assumptions about work loss and loss of homemaking services resulting from illness. Indirect costs for infants are included as the cost of lost work for parents. This is an unusual interpretation of the indirect cost for infants, which ordinarily seeks to capture the value of the infant's time; the parent's care-taking time would be included additionally.

The authors note exclusion of a number of cost sources, such as adverse pregnancy outcomes and some sequelae of infection. However, probably the most important sources of uncertainty relate to disease incidence. Cost data, because they reflect only private practice physicians and exclude clinics, may also pose a source of error. In addition, PID costs comprise a substantial proportion of the costs attributed to chlamydia. These estimates are taken from the literature (Washington et al., 1986); their limitations are discussed above.

Component Studies

De Lissovoy and others (1995) constructed a model to estimate direct medical costs of congenital syphilis cases during 1990. The study generated a case-severity distribution for true and presumptive cases and estimated costs for five treatment protocols, assuming treatment was based on severity. The cost of hospital care was obtained from Maryland hospital per diems; Resource-Based Relative Value Scale rates (using a Maryland conversion factor) were used for outpatient visits and procedures. The estimate included direct, first-year medical costs only. It accounted for neither costs of stillbirths resulting from congenital syphilis nor annual costs associated with long-term disability after the first year of life. The authors tested their model for sensitivity to the assumptions contained in the model, reporting that the cost estimates were significantly sensitive to the assumed severity of cases.

Hibbs and Gunn (1991) examined an on-site syphilis control intervention conducted during a cocaine-related syphilis outbreak in Chester, Pennsylvania. The program involved screening and treatment, targeting cocaine users and sex workers. The study reports costs and cases identified by the program, as compared to routine syphilis identification and treatment activities at public STD clinics. Its purpose was to assess the viability of this type of targeted intervention, and it does not address issues of generalizability to other populations, situations, or intervention strategies.

Washington and others (1986), Washington and Katz (1991), and Curran (1980) have conducted studies of costs of pelvic inflammatory disease. The Curran study is not reviewed here, because it is based on data from the early 1970s, now quite dated. However, estimates from this study appear in Table D-1.

The other two studies, Washington and colleagues (1986) and Washington and Katz (1991), used similar methodologies. Incidence and cost data were updated in the 1991 study. Both studies calculate indirect as well as direct costs. Costs were estimated separately for hospitalized cases of PID, outpatient visits, ectopic pregnancies, and infertility.

Data on hospitalized cases of PID and ectopic pregnancy are from the Hospital Discharge Survey for both studies. Data for outpatient visits were obtained from the National Ambulatory Medical Care Survey for the earlier study and from the National Disease Therapeutic Index for the later study. Both studies used the National Health Survey of Physician Visits to estimate costs of clinic and emergency room visits.

Data were collected to estimate costs of PID hospitalization for both studies. The later study is more detailed, including a longer time period and statewide discharge data as well as individual hospital data. Costs for outpatient physician visits are more approximate. The number of physician visits per case (2.5) does not appear to be based on data. Outpatient expenses included an estimate of lab tests and medications in addition to physician charges, but these estimates were derived from national average private practice data on physician costs and, in the case of the 1991 study, from information on a specific hospital physician group. The alternative to these approximations would have been to survey these costs, as no obviously better sources of data were available.

Indirect cost calculations were based on assumptions regarding work loss and assumptions regarding the distribution of occupation for affected women. There are few data available to perform this type of calculation.

These studies confronted problems of inadequate data regarding outpatient services, including those for treatment of PID, ectopic pregnancy, and infertility. The extent of bias introduced by the assumptions used is not clear. For example, the ratio of initial physician visits to office-based practices versus clinics or emergency departments is 2.27 to 1 in the 1986 study, while in the 1991 study this ratio was assumed to be the reverse (1:2 physician offices to clinics and emergency departments). As no explanation is given for this difference, the data

TABLE D-1 Estimates of Overall Cost of Illness in the Literature (millions of dollars)

STD[a]	Original Estimate (direct costs)	Original Estimate (indirect costs)	Original Year	Source	Estimate in 1994 Dollars
Gonorrhea[b]	$937		1984	IOM, 1985	$1,980
Chlamydial infection[b]	$727	$687	1985	Washington et al., 1987	$1,350 (direct) $1,280 (indirect)
PID[c]	$2,730	$1,510	1990	Washington and Katz, 1991	$3,540 (direct) $1,950 (indirect)
PID[c]	$699	$557	1980	Curran, 1980	$2,230 (direct) $1,780 (indirect)
Congenital syphilis	$12.4 (first-year costs only)		1990	de Lissovoy et al., 1995	$16.1
Herpes simplex[d] (genital)	$84.5		1984	IOM, 1985	$178

NOTE: Cost estimates are reported using 3 significant digits.
[a]There are no published overall estimates of costs for syphilis, human papillomavirus, chancroid, and hepatitis B virus infection.
[b]The estimates of costs for chlamydial infection and gonorrhea contain costs for PID.
[c]The estimates of costs for PID include cases resulting from chlamydial infection or gonorrhea.
[d]The IOM estimate for all types and sequelae of herpes simplex virus is $452.20 (1984$) or $954.56 (1994$).

SOURCES:
Curran JW. Economic consequences of pelvic inflammatory disease in the United States. Am J Obstet Gynecol 1980;138:848-51.
de Lissovoy G, Zenilman J, Nelson KE, Ahmed F, Celentano DD. The cost of a preventable disease: estimated U.S. national medical expenditures for congenital syphilis, 1990. Public Health Rep 1995;110:403-9.
IOM (Institute of Medicine). New vaccine development: establishing priorities; vol. I, Diseases of importance in the United States. Washington, D.C.: National Academy Press, 1985.
Washington AE, Johnson RE, Sanders LL. *Chlamydia trachomatis* infections in the United States: what are they costing us? JAMA 1987;257:2070-2.
Washington AE, Katz P. Cost of and payment source for pelvic inflammatory disease: trends and projections 1983 through 2000 [see comments]. JAMA 1991;266:2565-9.

available and the authors' interpretation of them (rather than changes in utilization of medical services) may be responsible for the discrepancy. All data on ectopic pregnancy pertain to hospitalization. These data are likely to exclude an increasing number of cases, since more than half of all ectopic pregnancies are now treated on an outpatient basis rather than requiring hospital admission (CDC, DSTDP, 1995).

For infertility, both studies used estimates of numbers of cases of PID as the basis for estimating the number of cases of infertility due to PID treated annually. This method is approximate; it assumes that cases of infertility originate in the same year they are treated (or, alternatively, that the annual incidence of PID is constant). Because of the delay between occurrence of PID and desired childbearing, it is conceivable that the current costs of infertility are more closely related to the higher incidence of PID in the 1980s. Costs of infertility treatment are based on a 1989 study, and, owing to the rapid change in technology and insurance coverage in that field, those costs may have changed significantly in the past five years.

Cost-Effectiveness Analyses and Related Studies

Randolph and others (1993) conducted a cost-effectiveness analysis examining the practice of cesarean delivery for women presenting with genital herpes lesions. The analysis estimates the cost per case averted and cost per Quality-Adjusted Life-Year of this practice. It was conducted for the purpose of demonstrating the excess cost associated with cesarean sections, given evidence of a low attack rate for women with recurrent HSV, who comprise the majority of women undergoing cesarean sections for genital herpes. The analysis is model-based. It considers a cohort of one million pregnant women. No national figures are presented. Some cost data are included, but no aggregate costs are calculated.

Cost Estimates of STDs

Gonorrhea

During 1994, a total of 418,738 cases of gonorrhea were reported to the CDC. Assuming a stable incidence in the state of Georgia, which did not report cases that year, an estimated 450,221 cases occurred in the United States and outlying areas. This total reflects a significant decrease in gonorrhea incidence since the 1980s. The peak numbers of reported cases occurred earlier, but since 1990 the number of cases has decreased by about 35 percent. The decreasing trend has been less marked in the last few years, and the number of cases in 1993 and 1994 was similar.

As noted earlier, reported cases are likely to underestimate the actual number of cases, although the true extent of current underreporting is not well docu-

TABLE D-2 Derived and Adjusted Estimates of Direct Costs of STDs (1994$)

STD	Original Overall Estimate (1994$)[a]	Adjusted Overall Estimate (1994$)[b]	Components (1994$) Treatment	Other
Gonorrhea[c]	1,980	791–1,050	72.9–96.4	
Chlamydial infection[c]	1,350	668–1,510		
PID[c]	3,560	3,120		
Syphilis			35.8–67.0	
Congenital	16.1	10.1–12.4		
Herpes Simplex	178			20.9–31.3[d] (induced cesarean)
Neonatal HSV			10.5 (first year treatment)	2.47 (care for existing cases)
HPV				(see cervical cancer)
Chancroid			0.066 (drug treatment)	
Hepatitis B virus infection			111 (acute infection)	
Cervical cancer[e]	791	396–712		

NOTE: Cost estimates are reported using 3 significant digits.
[a]See Table D-1 for original estimate adjusted to 1994 dollars.
[b]Overall estimate recalculated to account for data on incidence changes and other changes.
[c]The estimates of costs for chlamydial infection and gonorrhea contain costs for PID.
[d]Lower estimate based on Randolph et al., 1993; higher estimate based on IOM, 1985.
[e]It is questionable to which STD costs should be ascribed, but generally cervical cancer is assumed to be caused by sexually transmitted agents. Estimate assumes cervical cancer attributable to STDs is responsible for 50–90 percent of total cervical cancer costs.

SOURCES:
IOM. New vaccine development: establishing priorities; vol. I, Diseases of importance in the United States. Washington, D.C.: National Academy Press, 1985.
Randolph AG, Washington AE, Prober CG. Cesarean delivery for women presenting with genital herpes lesions: efficacy, risks, and costs. JAMA 1993;270:77-82.

mented. Assuming, as the CDC does, that only half of all cases are reported, the 1994 reported cases represent an actual number of cases is closer to 900,442. In a recent publication, however, the CDC estimated an incidence of 800,000 (CDC, DSTD/HIVP, 1995).

Global Cost Estimates.   The 1985 IOM study estimated the total direct cost of gonorrhea at $936.68 million (1984$) (IOM, 1985). This estimate was based on 960,933 *reported* cases. The 238,730 cases reported in private physicians' offices were assumed to represent only 25 percent of the caseload, so that after adjustment for both underreporting and misdiagnosis, the total cases were estimated to number two million. A subset of these cases—those estimated to be symptomatic—were assumed to receive care according to a treatment profile. The estimate includes costs for primary infection, PID, ectopic pregnancies, and infertility.

If the 1994 estimate of 900,442 cases is adjusted for misdiagnosis in the same manner, the true figure is closer to 1,059,345 total cases. Keeping all other aspects of the cost estimate constant, the IOM estimates would imply a current cost of $496.13 million (in 1984 dollars) or $1,046.84 million (in 1994 dollars). Alternatively, using the CDC estimated incidence of 800,000, the 1994 annual cost is estimated at $790.56 million.

Although a more recent detailed review of the cost of gonorrhea is not available in the literature, there are more recent estimates of some of the major components of its cost.

Treatment.   Begley and others (1989) reviewed the costs of gonorrhea treatment in a family planning clinic serving high-risk adults. For symptomatic patients, they estimated a cost of $46 in 1987 for diagnosis, treatment, and contact-tracing activities. This cost, adjusted for inflation and to reflect changes in the current treatment of gonorrhea (Table D-3), is $81 (1994$). The majority of the STDs treated in this study were identified through the screening of family planning patients. While the marginal cost was lower for each of these cases, total costs reflect the screening of negative patients. The cost per case of gonorrhea or chlamydial infection found was $66 in 1987, or $107 in 1994, dollars. (More than twice as many patients had chlamydial infection than gonorrhea, so the cost per case found of gonorrhea alone is higher than this estimate.)

Based on these estimates and current incidence, and assuming these costs apply to all reported cases, the cost of treatment of primary infection with gonorrhea is an estimated $72.94 million to $96.35 million annually (1994$).

Pelvic Inflammatory Disease (PID).   PID is an important complication of both gonorrhea and chlamydial infection, resulting from the spread of these or other microorganisms to the fallopian tubes and other reproductive organs. PID can cause chronic pelvic pain and recurrent infection. The resultant scarring can cause ectopic pregnancy and/or impaired fertility. In a long-term study of preg-

TABLE D-3 Treatment Costs for Gonorrhea in a
Family Planning Clinic and Adjustment for Current
Recommended Treatment (dollars)

Type of Visit	Cost per Case ($)
Screening visit	9.74
Treatment-related costs	
Contact letters	3.32
Treatment visit	6.64
Test of cure (includes lab)	12.84
Medications (ampicillin+probencid)	1.92
Pharmacist ($100.08/85 cases)	1.19
Total = 35.65 (1987$)	
Subtotal without medication	33.73
Adjustment to $1994	54.70 (1994$)
Adjustment for medication[a]	64.42[a] (1994$)
Diagnostic Visit	
Drop-in visit	19.92
Treatment-related costs	
Contact letters	3.32
Treatment visit	6.64
Test of cure (includes lab)	12.84
Medications (ampicillin+probencid)	1.92
Pharmacist ($100.08/85 cases)	1.19
Total = 45.83 (1987$)	
Subtotal without medication	43.91
Adjustment to $1994	71.21 (1994$)
Adjustment for medication[a]	80.93[a] (1994$)

Cost per Case Found: $65.82 (1987$) for 96 cases of gonorrhea and
chlamydial infection ($106.75 in 1994 dollars). (No adjustment for changes
in treatment.)

[a]Adjustment: Current recommended treatment for gonorrhea is ceftri-
axone 125 mg plus doxycycline (for chlamydial infection) 1400 mg. Estimated cost: $5.22 (ceftriaxone) + $4.50 (doxycycline 1400 mg) = $9.72.

SOURCE: Begley CE, McGill L, Smith PB. The incremental cost of
screening, diagnosis, and treatment of gonorrhea and chlamydia in a family planning clinic. Sex Transm Dis 1989;16:63-7.

nancy rates, about 20 percent of women were unable to conceive following PID
(Weström and Mårdh, 1990). STDs appear to be responsible for up to 80 percent
of all cases of PID (Weström and Mårdh, 1990).

In their study of the costs of PID, Washington and Katz (1991) estimated
annual direct medical costs of this infection and its sequelae at $2.73 billion
(1990$) or $3.54 billion in 1994 dollars. This figure is based on an estimated

TABLE D-4 Original and Adjusted Direct Costs of Pelvic Inflammatory Disease (dollars)

Item	Original Estimate in Millions (1991)	Adjusted to 1994[a]
Hospitalized PID[b]	1,850.40	1,476.64
Outpatient PID[c]	249.15	734.07
Ectopic pregnancy (PID-related)[d]	392.18	317.82 (hospitalized)
		312.01 (outpatient)
Infertility (PID-related)[e]	236.34	278.25
Total direct costs	2,728.07	3,118.79

[a]1991 estimates adjusted for incidence and inflation.

[b]Original: $1,850.40 million (200,000 admissions x $9,252 [1990$]); adjusted: $1,476.6 million (115,670 admissions × $12,766 [1994$]) (Hosp CPI).

[c]Original: $249.15 million (1,277,000 × $195 [1990$]); adjusted: $734.07 million (1994$) (1,160,580 initial visits × 2.5 visits/case = 2,901,450 visits) (2,901,450 × $253 [1994$]).

[d]*Hospitalized:* Original: $392.18 million (44,000 x 8913 [1990$]) (Assumes 0.5 of total ectopic pregnancies related to PID); adjusted: $317.82 million (1994$) (0.5 × 51,687 × $12,298 [1994$] (Hosp CPI)). *Outpatient:* Original: (no estimate); estimate: $312.02 million (1994$) (0.5 × 57,000 × $10,948 [1994$]); costs estimated to be $1,350 less than hospitalized costs.

[e]Original: $236.34 (255,000 cases × $3700 [1990$] × 0.25) (assumes 25 percent of cases of PID-related infertility seek treatment); adjusted: $278.25 (232,116 × $4795 [1994$] × 0.25).

SOURCE: Washington AE, Katz P. Cost of and payment source for pelvic inflammatory disease: trends and projections 1983 through 2000 [see comments]. JAMA 1991;266:2565-9.

200,000 hospitalizations (average of 1987–1988), 1,277,000 outpatient cases (average of 1985–1989), 44,000 ectopic pregnancies, and 25,500 new cases of infertility annually.

Table D-4 revises this cost calculation based on 1994 incidence data, reflecting a decreasing trend in hospitalization but a relatively constant rate of initial visits for PID. In 1993, the number of PID hospitalizations was 115,670 (including admissions for both acute and chronic PID) (CDC, DSTDP, 1995), and there were 386,860 initial visits to physicians' offices for PID (CDC, DSTDP, 1995). Assuming, as Washington and Katz did, that initial visits occur in clinics and hospital emergency rooms twice as often as in private offices, these data suggest 1,160,580 total initial visits for PID. There were 51,687 hospitalizations for ectopic pregnancy in 1993 (CDC, DSTDP, 1995), half of which may be attributed to PID (Washington and Katz, 1991). However, these cases do not reflect the estimated half of all cases that are treated on an outpatient basis. The CDC estimates that a total of 108,800 ectopic pregnancies occurred in 1992 (CDC, 1995), implying an estimated 57,000 women were treated as outpatients. Costs for these individuals are an estimated $1,200–$1,500 lower per case (Creinin and

Washington, 1993) (Table D-4). Assuming that 20 percent of women with PID become infertile each year and that 25 percent of those seek treatment (Washington and Katz, 1991), the incidence of infertility would have been an estimated 232,116 cases in 1993, with 928,464 seeking treatment. Adjusting the 1991 estimates for inflation and for current incidence, the 1994 estimate of the total cost of PID is $3,118.79 million (Table D-4).

Chlamydial Infection

Reporting of *Chlamydia trachomatis* is not consistently mandated across the United States. The 451,752 cases reported to the CDC in 1994 therefore understate the incidence of chlamydial infection (CDC, DSTD, 1995). In an article estimating the impact of chlamydial infection, Washington and colleagues (1987) used case ratios from sentinel sites to estimate the incidence of chlamydial infection relative to gonorrhea. If those 1983–1985 rates applied today (1.4 chlamydia cases for each case of gonorrhea for men, and 2.6 for women), the annual incidence would be closer to 1,765,539 adult cases (Table D-5).

This annual incidence is about one-half of the 3,570,000 adult cases estimated for 1985 (Washington et al., 1987), which was the basis for an overall cost estimate for chlamydia of $727 million in direct costs (1985$). This estimate includes costs for an estimated 73,800 cases of conjunctivitis and 37,100 cases of

TABLE D-5 Calculation of 1,765,539 Cases of Chlamydial Infection Using Estimates of Gonorrhea Incidence

1. Estimate of total gonorrhea
   CDC total reported cases of gonorrhea: 450,221
   (Adds 1993 state estimate for Georgia (31,483) to total (418,738).
   Total estimated cases of gonorrhea accounting for underreporting: 900,442
2. Estimate of ratio of chlamydial infections in men and women
   Ratio of men to women cases of gonorrhea: 1.14[a]
   Ratio of 1.14 applied to total gonorrhea cases gives:
      479,675 cases of gonorrhea among men
      420,767 cases of gonorrhea among women
   Using chlamydia/gonorrhea case ratio[b]
      Men: 479,675 × 1.4 = 671,545 cases of chlamydia
      Women: 420,767 × 2.6 = 1,093,994 cases of chlamydia
3. Estimate of total chlamydia cases: 1,765,539

[a]CDC/DSTDP (Division of STD Prevention). Sexually transmitted disease surveillance 1994. U.S. Department of Health and Human Services, Public Health Service. Atlanta: Centers for Disease Control and Prevention, September 1995. Tables 12, 13: 1994 men (222,718); 1994 women (195,576).

[b]Washington AE, Johnson RE, Sanders LL. *Chlamydia trachomatis* infections in the United States: what are they costing us? JAMA 1987;257:2070-2.

pneumonia among infants. Without accounting for changes in costs associated with treatment of chlamydial infection and its complications, but accounting for inflation, the change in incidence would imply that 1994 costs should have been in the range of $668.39 million (1994$). A recent CDC estimate of chlamydia incidence, however, is much higher—4,000,000 cases (CDC, DSTD/HIVP, 1995)—implying 1994 costs of $1,513.87 million (1994$).

Syphilis

The recent incidence of primary and secondary syphilis peaked in 1990 and has declined consistently since then. In 1994, the CDC reported a total of 83,751 cases of syphilis (all stages). This included 20,947 cases of primary and secondary syphilis; 32,970 cases of early latent syphilis; and 27,597 cases of late and late latent cases. An estimate of incidence from a CDC report is higher: 101,000 cases (CDC, DSTD/HIVP, 1995). No reports of the overall cost of syphilis are available in the literature.

Treatment. Hibbs and Gunn (1991) estimated costs for the identification and treatment of patients at STD clinics at $469 per case treated in 1989 dollars ($663 per case in 1994 dollars). This estimate, from an area of high incidence (Chester, Pennsylvania), includes investigator hours, practitioner wages, and diagnostic and treatment costs. If applied to the 1994 incident cases of primary, secondary, and early latent syphilis (53,917 cases), this estimate would amount to some $35.75 million (1994$) in treatment costs. The implied treatment costs would be $66.96 million (1994$) using the higher CDC incidence estimate.

Congenital Syphilis. Mirroring the incidence of primary and secondary syphilis, the incidence of congenital syphilis rose during the late 1980s, peaked in 1991, and has since declined. Some 2,224 U.S. cases were reported in 1994 (CDC, DSTDP, 1995).

In a model of congenital syphilis costs, de Lissovoy and others (1995) assigned a treatment protocol to patients as a function of the estimated level of the severity of illness. According to their estimates, some 75 percent of patients required hospitalization for treatment, for a median charge of $3,171 (1990$). They estimate direct, first-year medical costs (charges) of $12.4 million in 1990 dollars, based on 3,484 reported cases and an assumed 916 (20 percent) unreported cases.

Using the estimates of de Lissovoy and others, and adjusting for current incidence, the current estimated cost of congenital syphilis is $7.8 million in 1990 dollars or $10.1 million in 1994 dollars. This assumes, as did de Lissovoy and his colleagues (1995), that 20 percent of current cases go unreported. Using a higher CDC estimate of 3,400 cases (CDC, DSTD/HIVP, 1995), this figure is $12.4

million (1994$). These figures do not reflect nonmedical costs and do not reflect annual costs for infants who were infected in earlier years.

Genital Herpes

Although nationwide statistics for the incidence and prevalence of genital herpes are not available, studies from the early and mid-1980s indicated that an estimated 200,000 to 500,000 primary episodes of genital herpes occur each year (USPSTF, 1996). The IOM (1985) estimate was higher: 724,000 new cases annually. As a result of high annual incidence, HSV prevalence has continued to increase (Corey, 1994). A national study found that the prevalence of HSV-2 (the predominant causative agent for genital herpes) was 16.4 percent among U.S. adults in the late 1970s (Johnson et al., 1989); a decade later, prevalence is estimated to be 23 percent (Corey, 1994). The national survey cited above estimated the number of cases of HSV-2 to be 25.4 million in the late 1970s (Johnson et al., 1989), and the number of all genital herpes cases has been estimated to be 26 million to 31 million (Johnson et al., 1989; CDC, DSTD/HIVP, 1995). Some concurrent estimates are as high as 35 million (Fish, 1992).

Recent counts of initial physician visits demonstrate a general upward trend in incidence since the 1970s. In 1993, estimates based on data from the National Disease and Therapeutic Index (NDTI) indicated that there were 171,565 initial visits to private physicians' offices for genital herpes (IMS America, 1993; CDC, DSTDP, 1995). This estimate does not reflect visits to STD clinics and other types of practices. The incidence of herpes simplex is clearly much higher than this figure, because the infection is often asymptomatic; even when symptoms are present, patients may not seek medical treatment.

The IOM estimates (IOM, 1985) of the costs of herpes simplex include $84.5 million (1984$) attributable to genital herpes. This figure, adjusted for inflation, is $178.3 million in 1994 dollars. The calculation incorporates costs in the following categories: primary genital herpes, recurrent genital herpes, neonatal HSV, costs associated with culturing during pregnancy, and cesarean section (Table D-6). It does not include costs for keratitis or encephalitis, some cases of which may be due to HSV-2. This IOM cost calculation is based on the estimated 724,000 new infections, plus an estimated 4,826,667 annual recurrences. A simple (proportional) adjustment for incidence is not attempted here.

Induced Cesarean Sections.   An important cost generated by genital herpes is that of cesarean deliveries performed to reduce the risk of viral transmission from the mother to the newborn. Studies have questioned the necessity and wisdom of the aggressive approach (Chang and O'Keefe, 1977; Randolph et al., 1993); however, cesarean delivery in the presence of herpetic lesions during labor is currently standard practice (USPSTF, 1996).

In their study of the cost-effectiveness of cesarean section to prevent neona-

TABLE D-6   Costs of Genital Herpes (dollars)

Category	Costs (1984$)
Primary genital	
Severity A	5,680,000
Severity B	5,287,000
Recurrent genital	25,581,000
Neonatal HSV	7,156,000
Neonatal HSV	
Mild CNS impairment	702,000
Serious CNS impairment	1,495,000
Very severe CNS impairment	15,982,000
Cultures during pregnancy	5,391,000
Cesarean sections	17,250,000
Total 84,524,000 (1984$) (178.3 million [1994$])	

NOTE: This estimate does not include costs of encephalitis or herpes keratitis. Some cases of these complications are due to genital herpes and should be included. It includes present value of future costs attributable to central nervous system (CNS) impairment.

SOURCE: IOM. New vaccine development: establishing priorities; vol. I, Diseases of importance in the United States. Washington, D.C.: National Academy Press, 1985.

tal herpes, Randolph and colleagues (1993) estimated the cost of excess cesarean sections in hypothetical cohorts of pregnant women with and without a history of HSV infection. Costs for cesarean among women with recurrent HSV were $22.3 million (1992$) ($24.7 million in 1994$) *per million pregnant women*, and costs for women with a negative history were $341,000 (1992$) ($378,000 in 1994$) *per million pregnant women*. These calculations are based on the assumption that the incremental cost of a cesarean section instead of a vaginal delivery is $3,725 in 1992 dollars ($4,135 in 1994$). The estimate of 20 percent prevalence of HSV-2 infection among pregnant women (Randolph et al., 1993) implies that current costs for excess cesareans are about $20.9 million (1994$) annually.

The IOM (1985) estimated the total costs of cesareans at a higher value of $17.3 million (1984$) or $36.4 million in 1994 dollars. This total cost estimate would be somewhat lower if Randolph and others' (1993) estimate of the incremental cost of a cesarean were used: $31.3 million (1994$). However, the IOM estimate is still higher than the $20.9 million figure, despite a lower assumed prevalence of HSV-2 of 5 percent. This difference may reflect the number of cesarean sections attributed to herpes infection. Under the current policy, it is no longer recommended to perform a cesarean section based on a series of prenatal viral cultures, but only if a herpetic lesion is present.

TABLE D-7   Calculation of Annual Costs for Central Nervous System (CNS) Impairment Secondary to Neonatal HSV Infection (dollars)

IOM (1985) estimates:[a]
- 7 percent of cases mild CNS impairment, $2,000 per year (1984$), for 20 years ($4,220 in 1994$)
- 6 percent of cases serious CNS impairment, $5,000 per year (1984$) for 20 years ($10,550 in 1994$)
- 16 percent of cases very severe CNS impairment, 20,000 per year (1984$) for 20 years ($42,200 in 1994$)

Assume average incidence of 322 per year (between the IOM's estimate [380] and current estimates [265]).

Total: $2.47 million (1994$)

---

[a]SOURCE: IOM. New vaccine development: establishing priorities; vol. I, Diseases of importance in the United States. Washington, D.C.: National Academy Press, 1985.

Neonatal HSV.   Neonatal herpes infection is not reported to the CDC, so most estimates of incidence depend on surveys. Based on a review of surveys, Chuang (1988) estimated incidence to be between 1/7,500 births and 1/30,000 births, depending on the geographic location and the population included in the survey. Chuang gives 1/15,000 as the most likely incidence. With 3.979 million births in 1994 (Singh et al., 1995), this estimate suggests a 1994 incidence of 265 cases.

The 1985 IOM study estimated first-year treatment costs for neonatal herpes to be $7.156 million (1984$). If adjusted to reflect 265 cases, this figure would suggest costs of $10.530 million (1994$). The IOM estimates were computed by determining the present value of future spending for cases involving CNS impairment. Using the IOM estimates of mild, severe, and very severe impairment and their corresponding costs of annual care, the cost for 1994 cases would be an estimated $2.47 million (1994$) (Table D-7). Thus, in 1994, total annual costs of neonatal HSV would have been an estimated $13.00 million (1994$).

Human Papillomavirus (HPV) Infection

Like many STDs, the incidence of HPV infection rose through the 1970s and 1980s, but appears to have decreased since 1987. In that year, there were 351,370 initial visits to physicians' offices to seek care for HPV, in contrast to 166,796 initial visits to physicians' offices in 1993 (CDC, DSTDP, 1995). However, some estimates of HPV incidence are several times higher than these figures suggest. The CDC estimates an annual incidence of 500,000 to 1,000,000 cases (CDC, DSTD/HIVP, 1995). Prevalence estimates range from 10 million to 40 million (Fish, 1992); the CDC's estimate is 24 million (CDC, DSTD/HIVP, 1995).

Treatment.   An estimated 20 percent to 30 percent of genital wart infections resolve without treatment (CDC, 1993). The CDC does not recommend a particular treatment for other patients, although some expensive regimens are specifically not recommended. Treatment of HPV often entails multiple office visits, adding to its cost. No estimates of treatment costs or the number of patients treated are available in the literature.

Cancer.   HPV infection is associated with the risk of genital and anal cancers. Genital warts become precancerous in about 20 percent of affected women, and about 1 percent of these develop into invasive cervical cancer (Fish, 1992). The extent to which HPV infection is responsible for specific cancers, however, is unclear. One recent study found HPV to be responsible for about three-fourths of invasive cervical cancer (Schiffman et al., 1993). Some reviews are more cautious in their assessment of the causative role of this specific agent, noting that epidemiologic evidence does not yet support the theoretical link between HPV and cervical cancer (Reeves et al., 1989; Oriel, 1990; Paavonen et al., 1990). However, there is less reservation about the link between sexually transmitted diseases generally and cervical cancer.

The National Institutes of Health estimated the direct cost of cervical cancer to be $610 million in 1990 (1990$) (NIH, 1995) or $791 million in 1994 dollars. Assuming that 50 percent to 90 percent of this cost is attributable to STDs, if not to HPV alone, this would imply an annual cost burden of $396 to $712 million (1994$).

Chancroid

A total of 773 cases of chancroid were reported to the CDC in 1994 (CDC, DSTDP, 1995). This number represents a decrease from the mid-1980s, when the occurrence of chancroid reached its highest levels since the 1950s (Schmid et al., 1987). Chancroid is difficult to diagnose because of the complexity of laboratory testing procedures. Reliance on clinical diagnosis may result in either underreporting or overreporting (Schmid et al., 1987).

The treatment recommended by CDC is azithromycin 1g (CDC, 1993). The current cost for this drug is $24 per treatment regimen. The cost of this treatment, with physician visit, for all cases would be $66,000 (1994$).

Hepatitis B Virus Infection

Some 200,000 to 300,000 cases of hepatitis B virus infection are estimated to occur annually in the United States, and approximately one million individuals are chronic carriers (Margolis et al., 1991; Hall and Halsey, 1992). Most (90 percent) cases occur among adults. Although drug abuse and occupational exposure are important modes of transmission, sexual intercourse appears to be responsible for the more cases than any other mode of transmission—34 percent of cases, according to one source (Margolis et al., 1991), 38 percent according to another (USPSTF, 1996). In at least an additional 30 percent of cases, the mode of transmission is unknown (Margolis et al., 1991). In 1994, the CDC estimated an incidence of 53,000 cases of sexually transmitted hepatitis B virus infection (CDC, DSTD/HIVP, 1995).

The cost of hepatitis B virus infection has been a subject of relatively strong interest in the literature; however, no estimates that can reasonably be considered to reflect overall costs are available. Cost estimates for hepatitis B virus infection prepared by the IOM attribute $146.22 million (1984$) to acute infection (IOM, 1985). Using 36 percent (the median of the above estimates) as the proportion attributable to sexual activity, this would imply $111.07 (1994$) in annual costs for acute hepatitis.

The sequelae of hepatitis B virus infection (chronic persistent hepatitis, chronic active hepatitis, cirrhosis, and primary hepatocellular carcinoma) are clearly responsible for a large proportion of the costs of this disease. The IOM attributes an additional $138.38 (1984$) to these sequelae. However, this estimate reflects the discounted present value of treatment for these conditions and thus is not an annual cost. More recent studies have focused on the calculation of lifetime costs of hepatitis B virus infection for the purpose of assessing the cost-effectiveness of hepatitis B vaccine (Arevalo and Washington, 1988; Bloom et al., 1993; Margolis et al., 1995). These studies do not present annual costs for sequelae.

INDIRECT COSTS

Although the estimation of indirect costs was not undertaken for this review, morbidity and mortality are clearly an important part of the burden of STDs. In a recent study, Ebrahim and others (1995) estimated the number of STD-related deaths occurring among women related to STDs to be 9,179 in 1992. This total represents a relatively stable number of STD-related deaths (around 6,500 per year) from non-HIV-related causes and a rapidly increasing annual number of deaths from HIV/AIDS. Cervical cancer is by far the most common cause of STD-related death, representing 5,210 deaths in 1992 (57 percent of the total). (This estimate assumes that sexually transmitted agents are responsible for all deaths from cervical cancer.) The next most common causes of death are HIV/AIDS (2,665 cases, 29 percent of the total), hepatitis B and C virus infection (960 deaths; 10 percent of the total), and PID (220 deaths, 2 percent of the total). An earlier study estimated that STDs were responsible for 20 percent of reproductive mortality among women in 1975. However, this estimate precedes HIV infection and does not include cervical cancer (Grimes, 1986).

Indirect costs reflect the quantification of health effects—both morbidity and mortality—in terms of their monetary value. Few studies have examined indirect costs of STDs. Those that have done so *assumed* quantities of work loss due to STD morbidity, including both formal employment and household management (Curran, 1980; Washington et al., 1986, 1987; Washington and Katz, 1991). These assumptions are particularly important in the computation of indirect costs of STDs, because productivity costs related to morbidity appear to dwarf those related to mortality for most STDs (Washington et al., 1986). A preferable option would be to obtain survey data describing the work time lost to STDs, as has been done for other illnesses (Rice et al., 1985); however, this has not yet been attempted. It should also be noted that the value of leisure time is not included in these estimates.

The studies assessing indirect costs use gender-specific average wages to place a value on morbidity time. Because many STDs disproportionately affect people earning below average wages—i.e., the poor, certain racial and ethnic groups, and younger people (CDC, DSTDP, 1995)—it can be argued that a lower wage should be used. However, it can also be argued that the use of gender-specific wages for women, because they are lower than those of men, undervalues the economic burden (Curran, 1980).

CONCLUSIONS

The cost estimates reviewed here demonstrate the limited amount of research that has been conducted to quantify the current annual economic burden imposed on society by sexually transmitted diseases. The primary sources of information in this area are the IOM (1985) study, conducted a decade ago, and a series of studies conducted by the Institute for Policy Studies at the University of California at San Francisco (Washington et al., 1986, 1987; Washington and Katz, 1991). Far more research has assessed the cost-effectiveness of specific policies—both proposed and realized—related to sexually transmitted disease. This review also demonstrates the shortage of literature describing the national incidence and prevalence of sexually transmitted diseases and of data documenting the validity of the reporting system for diseases that are reported.

Despite the limits of the present review, it is clear that STDs exact a substantial direct cost. Conservatively, the subset of STDs examined here costs the nation *at least* 4 billion annually.

The costs of national STD prevention efforts, including surveillance and education programs, are not included in any studies reviewed in this report. Whether these should be considered part of the burden of disease is not clear. What is clear, however, is that current prevention outlays should not be weighed against current costs of illness. The size of a prevention effort should relate to the benefit of that effort, not to the remaining burden of illness. In fact, the benefit of many preventive measures—those targeting the risky sexual behaviors responsible for the transmission of STDs—includes not only a reduction in the burden of STDs, but also reductions in abortions and other consequences of unwanted pregnancy.

As described earlier, the estimates compiled in this report must be viewed as only partially describing the economic burden of STDs. Many costs associated with these diseases are not documented in the literature, often because collection of the data necessary to accurately describe these categories of resource use would require large and new research efforts. It should also be noted that this report reviews costs only for a subset of STDs. There are many other STDs, some of which clearly impose a large economic burden. AIDS, for example, was estimated to cost $45,700 (1994$) per patient in one report, a figure that implies an annual cost of $8.4 billion (Hellinger, 1992). Others, such as lymphogranuloma venereum (LGV), are relatively rare and likely to incur low costs. This report thus does not provide a comprehensive estimate of the burden of STDs but summarizes the available information relevant to assessing this burden for a specific subset of sexually transmitted illness.

REFERENCES

AMA (American Medical Association). Physician marketplace statistics 1994. Chicago: Center for Health Policy Research, 1994.

Arevalo JA, Washington AE. Cost-effectiveness of prenatal screening and immunization for hepatitis B virus. JAMA 1988;259:3:365-9.

Begley CE, McGill L, Smith PB. The incremental cost of screening, diagnosis, and treatment of gonorrhea and chlamydia in a family planning clinic. Sex Transm Dis 1989;16:63-7.

Bloom BS, Hillman AL, Fendrick M, Schwartz JS. A reappraisal of hepatitis B virus vaccination strategies using cost-effectiveness analysis. Ann Internal Med 1993;118:298-306.

Bowie WR. Drug therapies for sexually transmitted diseases: clinical and economic considerations. Drugs 1995;4:496-515.

Cates Jr W. The "other STDs": do they really matter? JAMA 1988;259:24:3606-8.

CDC (Centers for Disease Control and Prevention). 1993 Sexually transmitted diseases treatment guidelines. MMWR 1993;42(No. RR-14):56-66.

CDC. Ectopic pregnancy—United States, 1990-1992. MMWR 1995;44:46-8.

CDC, DSTD/HIVP (Division of STD/HIV Prevention). Annual report 1994. U.S. Department of Health and Human Services, Public Health Service. Atlanta: Centers for Disease Control and Prevention, 1995.

CDC, DSTDP (Division of STD Prevention). Sexually transmitted disease surveillance 1994. U.S. Department of Health and Human Services, Public Health Service. Atlanta: Centers for Disease Control and Prevention, September 1995.

Chang TW, O'Keefe P. Cesarean section and genital herpes. N Engl J Med. 1977;296:573.

Chuang TY. Neonatal herpes: incidence, prevention, and consequences. Am J Prev Med 1988;4:47-53.

Corey L. The current trend in genital herpes: progress in prevention. Sex Transm Dis 1994;21[2 Suppl]:S38-S44.

Creinin MD, Washington AE. Cost of ectopic pregnancy management: surgery versus methotrexate. Fertil Steril 1993;60:963-9.

Curran JW. Economic consequences of pelvic inflammatory disease in the United States. Am J Obstet Gynecol 1980;138:848-51.

de Lissovoy G, Zenilman J, Nelson KE, Ahmed F, Celentano DD. The cost of a preventable disease: estimated U.S. national medical expenditures for congenital syphilis, 1990. Public Health Rep 1995;110:403-9.

Drug Topics Red Book. Montvale, NJ: Medical Economics Company, Inc., 1995.

Ebrahim SH, Peterman TA, Zaidi AA, Kamb ML. Mortality related to sexually transmitted diseases in women, U.S., 1973-1992. Eleventh Meeting of the International Society for STD Research, August 27-30, 1995, New Orleans, LA [abstract no. 343].

Fish RM. Herpes simplex. In: Fish RM, Campbell ET, Trupin SR, eds. Sexually transmitted diseases: problems in primary care. Los Angeles: Practice Management Information Corporation, 1992.

Grimes DA. Deaths due to sexually transmitted diseases: the forgotten component of reproductive mortality. JAMA 1986;255:1727-9.

Hall CB, Halsey NA. Control of hepatitis B: to be or not to be? Pediatrics 1992;90 [2 Pt. 1] 274-7.

Hellinger FJ. Forecasts of the costs of medical care for persons with HIV: 1992-1995. Inquiry 1992;29:356-65.

Hibbs JR, Gunn RA. Public health intervention in a cocaine-related syphilis outbreak. Am J Public Health 1991;81:1259-62.

IMS America. National disease and therapeutic index (NDTI). Plymouth Meeting, PA: IMS America, 1993.

IOM (Institute of Medicine). New vaccine development: establishing priorities; vol. I, Diseases of importance in the United States. Washington, D.C.: National Academy Press, 1985.

Johnson RE, Nahmias AJ, Magder LS, Lee FK, Broods CA, Snowden CB. A seroepidemiologic survey of the prevalence of herpes simplex virus type 2 infection in the United States. N Engl J Med 1989;321:7-12.

Margolis HS, Alter MJ, Hadler SC. Hepatitis B: evolving epidemiology and implications for control. Semin Liver Dis 1991;11:84-92.

Margolis HS, Coleman PJ, Brown RE, Mast EE, Sheingold SH, Arevalo JA. Prevention of hepatitis B virus transmission by immunization. An economic analysis of current recommendations. JAMA 1995;274:1201-8.

Moran JS, Kaufman JA, Felsenstein D. Survey of health care providers: who sees patients needing STD services, and what services do they provide? Sex Transm Dis 1995;22:67-9.

NIH (National Institutes of Health). Disease-specific estimates of direct and indirect costs of illness and NIH support. Draft document, February 1995.

Oriel D. Genital human papillomavirus infection. In: Holmes KK, Mårdh P-A, Sparling PF, Wiesner PJ, Cates W Jr, Lemon SM, Stamm WE, eds. Sexually transmitted diseases. 2nd ed. New York: McGraw-Hill, 1990.

Paavonen J, Koutsky LA, Kiviat N. Cervical neoplasia and other STD-related genital and anal neoplasms. In: Holmes KK, Mårdh P-A, Sparling PF, Wiesner PJ, Cates W Jr, Lemon SM, et al., eds. Sexually transmitted diseases. 2nd ed. New York: McGraw-Hill, 1990.

Randolph AG, Washington AE, Prober CG. Cesarean delivery for women presenting with genital herpes lesions: efficacy, risks, and costs. JAMA 1993;270:77-82.

Reeves WC, Rawls WE, Brinton LA. Epidemiology of genital papillomaviruses and cervical cancer. Rev Infect Dis 1989;11:426-39.

Rice DP, Hodgson TA, Kopstein AN. The economic costs of illness: a replication and update. Health Care Financ Rev 1985;7:61-80.

Schiffman MH, Bauer HM, Hoover RN, Glass AG, Cadell DM, Rush BB, et al. Epidemiologic evidence showing that human papillomavirus infection causes most cervical intraepithelial neoplasia. J Natl Cancer Inst 1993;85:958-64.

Schmid GP, Sanders LL, Blount JH, Alexander ER. Chancroid in the United States: re-establishment of an old disease. JAMA 1987;258:3265-8.

Singh GK, Mathews MS, Clarke SC, Yannicos T, Smith BL. Annual summary of births, marriages, divorces, and deaths: United States, 1994. Centers for Disease Control and Prevention, National Center for Health Statistics, Monthly Vital Statistics Report, October 23, 1995.

USPSTF (U.S. Preventive Services Task Force). Guide to clinical preventive services. 2nd ed. Washington, D.C.: U.S. Department of Health and Human Services, 1996.

Washington AE, Arno PS, Brooks MA. The economic cost of pelvic inflammatory disease. JAMA 1986;255:1735-8.

Washington AE, Johnson RE, Sanders LL. *Chlamydia trachomatis* infections in the United States: what are they costing us? JAMA 1987;257:2070-2.

Washington AE, Katz P. Cost of and payment source for pelvic inflammatory disease: trends and projections 1983 through 2000 [see comments]. JAMA 1991;266:2565-9.

Weström L, Mårdh P-A. Acute pelvic inflammatory disease (PID). In: Holmes KK, Mårdh P-A, Sparling PF, Wiesner PJ, Cates W Jr, Lemon SM, et al., eds. Sexually transmitted diseases. 2nd ed. New York: McGraw-Hill, 1990.

APPENDIX
E
Summary of Empirical Studies of HIV Prevention Mass Media Campaigns

SUMMARY OF EMPIRICAL STUDIES OF HIV PREVENTION MASS MEDIA CAMPAIGNS

Country	Study	Population[a]	Primary Channel	Outcome Measure[b] Knowledge	Attitude	Behavior	Other
U.S.	Woods et al., 1991	General	TV, radio				Dollar value of donated airtime
	Keiser, 1991	General	TV, radio				Media Coverage
	Gerbert and Maguire, 1989	General	Mailing				Recall of exposure to ANM
	Snyder, 1991	General	Mailing	+/o			Perceived risk
	Caron et al., 1992	College students	TV, radio		o	o	
	Gentry and Jorgensen, 1991	General	TV, radio		+	+	Dollar value of donated airtime
	Bryce et al., 1990	General, Injecting drug users	Mass media			+	Seek information, obtain services
Australia	Rigby et al., 1989	General	TV	o	o		
	Bray et al., 1991	General	TV	o	o		Anxiety
	Ross et al., 1990	General	TV		+		
	Ross and Carson, 988	General	Mass media		+		
Brazil	Fox and Cortes, 1992	Urban adults		+			Awareness, concern, perceived risk

Country	Reference	Population	Media				Outcome
Bulgaria	Chileva and Metodieff, 1994	General	Print			+	Media coverage
France	Moatti et al., 1992	General adults	General media	+	+/o	+	Perceived risk
The Gambia	Sekou et al., 1989	General	General media			+	
Italy	Bortolotti et al., 1992	Drug users	Print		+	+	HIV seroconversion
Japan	Maeda et al., 1994	Young adults	Mass media	+	+	+	
Mexico	Izazola et al., 1988					+	Social response
	Helguera et al., 1990	General	Multiple		+		
	Sepulveda et al., 1989	General	Press, mass media	+	+	o	
Philippines	Margo et al., 1991	General	Multiple	+	+	+	Perceived risk
Switzerland	Wasserfallen et al., 1993	General	TV, print			+	
	Dubois-Arber et al., 1992	General	General media			+	
	Stutz Steiger et al., 1992	Clients of prostitutes	Print			o	
	Lehmann et al., 1987	General	Print	+			
	Hausser et al., 1988	General	TV, print			+	

continued on next page

Country	Study	Population[a]	Primary Channel	Outcome Measure[b] Knowledge	Attitude	Behavior	Other
U.K.	Beck et al., 1990	General	TV, print			+	
	Weller et al., 1984	Men	TV, print				Decrease in gonorrhea rate
	Wober, 1988	General	TV, print, radio	+			
	Mills et al., 1986	General	Print, TV	o			
	Sherr, 1987	General		o		+	Anxiety
Zaire	Kaseka et al., 1992	General	TV, radio	+			
	Rukarangira et al., 1990	General	Mass media	+		+	
	Kyungu et al., 1990	General	TV	+		+/o	HIV seroincidence

[a]Reach of program is national unless otherwise specified.
[b]A "+" indicates a favorable outcome, while an "o" indicates no effect.

SOURCES:

Beck EJ, Donegan C, Kenny C, Cohen CS, Moss V, Teny P, et al. An update on HIV testing at a London sexually transmitted diseases clinic: long-term impact of the AIDS media campaigns. Genitourin Med 1990;66:142-7.

Bortolotti F, Stivanello A, Noventa F, Forza G, Pavanello N, Bertolini A. Sustained AIDS education campaigns and behavioural changes in Italian drug abusers. Eur J Epidemiol 1992;8:264-7.

Bray F, Chapman S. Community knowledge, attitudes and media recall about AIDS. Sydney 1988 and 1989. Austr J Public Health 1991;15:107-13.

Bryce J, Pope RS. Ruff JA. The impact of the Michigan mass media campaign on hotline calls, knowledge levels, and requests for HIV counseling and testing. Sixth International Conference on AIDS, June 19-24, 1990, San Francisco [abstract no. F.D. 848].

Caron SL, Davis CM, Wynn RL, Roberts LW. "America Responds to AIDS," but did college students? Differences between March, 1987, and September, 1988. AIDS Educ Prev 1992;4:18-28.

Chileva A, Metodieff M. The mass media response to a national AIDS campaign. Tenth International Conference on AIDS, August 7-12, 1994, Yokohama [abstract no. PDO606].

Dubois-Arber F, Jeannin A, Zeugin P. Evaluation of AIDS prevention in Switzerland: behavioral change in the general population. Eighth International Conference on AIDS, July 19-24, 1992, Amsterdam [abstract no. PoD 5410].

Fox MP, Cortes E. The current relevance of mass media advertising in Brazilian AIDS prevention campaigns. Eighth International Conference on AIDS, July 19-24, 1992, Amsterdam [abstract no. PoD 5806].

Gentry EM, Jorgensen CM. Monitoring the exposure of "America Responds to AIDS" PSA campaign. Public Health Rep 1991;106:651-5.

Gerbert B, Maguire B. Public acceptance of the Surgeon General's brochure on AIDS. Public Health Rep 1989;104:130-3.

Hausser D, Lehmann P, Dubois-Arber F, Gutzwiller F. Evaluation of nationwide campaigns against AIDS in Switzerland. Fourth International Conference on AIDS, June 12-16, 1988, Stockholm [abstract no. 9553].

Helguera G, Acuna MI, Chavez-Peon F, Sepulveda J. Social mobilization in the prevention of AIDS. Sixth International Conference on AIDS, June 19-24, 1990, San Francisco [abstract no. F.C. 850].

Izazola JA, Vaidespino JL, Sepulveda J. Indicators of behavior modification due to the campaign for the prevention of AIDS in Mexico. Fourth International Conference on AIDS, June 12-16, 1988, Stockholm [abstract no. 9551].

Kaseka N, Jones D, Kalambay K, Walombua M, Doppagne A, Reyward W, et al. Contribution of a public mass-media and AIDS information campaign in AIDS knowledge, condom use and HIV seroincidence among employees of a large business in Kinshasa, Zaire. Eighth International Conference on AIDS, July 19-24, 1992, Amsterdam [abstract no. PoD 5546].

Keiser NH. Strategies of media marketing for "America Responds to AIDS" and applying lessons learned. Public Health Rep 1991;106:623-7.

Kyungu M, Eiger R, Kaombo K, Kambamba SA, Convisser J. The impact of an AIDS television campaign on an urban experience. Sixth International Conference on AIDS, June 19-24, 1990, San Francisco [abstract no. F.D. 846].

Lehmann P, Hausser D, Somaini B, Gutzwiller F. Campaign against AIDS in Switzerland: evaluation of a nationwide educational programme. Br Med J 1987;295:1118-20.

Maeda M, Inagaki T, Ishii A, Ashizawa M, Minamitani M. The effects of education campaign for AIDS/HIV through mass medias from 1992 to 1994. Tenth International Conference on AIDS, August 7-12, 1994, Yokohama [abstract no. 568D].

Margo G, MacDonald G, Schneider A, Dayrit M, Abad M, Consunjui B. The importance of social marketing techniques in creating effective media campaigns on AIDS. Seventh International Conference on AIDS, June 16-21, 1991, Florence [abstract no. W.D. 4273].

Mills S, Campbell MJ, Waters WE. Public knowledge of AIDS and the DHSS advertisement campaign. Br Med J 1986;293:1089-90.

Moatti JP, Dab W, Loundou H, Quenel P, Beltzer N, Anes A, et al. Impact on the general public of media campaigns against AIDS: a French evaluation. Health Policy 1992;21:233-47.

Rigby K, Brown M, Anagnostou P, Ross MW. Shock tactics to counter AIDS: the Australian experience. Psychol Health 1989;3:145-59.

Ross MW, Carson JA. Effectiveness of distribution of information on AIDS: a national study of six media in Australia. New York State J Med 1988;88:239-41.

Ross MW, Rigby K, Rosser BR, Anagnostou P, Brown M. The effect of a national campaign on attitudes toward AIDS. AIDS Care 1990;2:339-46.

Rukarangira NW, Ngirabakunzi K, Bihimi Y, Kitembo M. Evaluation of the AIDS information program, using mass media campaign, in Lumumbashi—Zaire. Sixth International Conference on AIDS, June 19–24, 1990, San Francisco [abstract no. F.D. 844].

Sekou D, Saihou C, Amie C, Theophilus G. A multidimensional approach to promote awareness of AIDS in the Gambia. Fifth International Conference on AIDS, June 4-9, 1989, Montreal [abstract no. W.E.P. 8].

Sepulveda J, Izazola JA, Valdespino JL, Mondragon M, Townsend J. Massive campaign for AIDS education, achievements and problems. Fifth International Conference on AIDS, June 4-9, 1989, Montreal [abstract no. T.G.O. 9].

Sherr L. An evaluation of the UK government health education campaign on AIDS. Psychol Health 1987;1:61-72.

Snyder LB. The impact of the Surgeon General's "Understanding AIDS" pamphlet in Connecticut. Health Commun 1991;3:37-57.

Stutz Steiger T, Wasserfallen F, Landert C, Dubois-Arber F, Obrist B, Somaini B. A media campaign in Switzerland targeted at the clients of prostitutes. Eighth International Conference on AIDS, July 19-24, 1992, Amsterdam [abstract no. PoD 5659].

Wasserfallen F, Stutz ST, Summermatter D, Hausermann M, Dubois-Arber F. Six years of promotion of condom use in the framework of the National Stop AIDS Campaign: experiences and results in Switzerland. Ninth International Conference on AIDS, June 6-11, 1993, Berlin [abstract no. WS-D27-3].

Weller IVD, Hindley DJ, Adler DW, Meldrum JT. Gonorrhea in homosexual men and media coverage of the acquired immune deficiency syndrome in London 1982-3. Br Med J Clin Res Educ 1984;289:1041.

Wober JM. Informing the British public about AIDS. Health Educ Res 1988;3:19-24.

Woods DR, Davis D, Westover BJ. "America Responds to AIDS": its content, development process, and outcome. Public Health Rep 1991;106:616-22.

REPRINTED FROM: Flora JA, Miabach EW, Holtgrave D. Communication campaigns for HIV prevention: using mass media in the next decade. In: IOM. Assessing the social and behavioral science base for HIV/AIDs prevention and intervention. Background papers. Washington, D.C.: National Academy Press, 1995:129-54.

APPENDIX

F

Recommended Interventions During the Periodic Health Examination for the Prevention of STDs, U.S. Preventive Services Task Force, 1996

RECOMMENDED INTERVENTIONS DURING THE PERIODIC HEALTH EXAMINATION FOR THE PREVENTION OF STDs, U.S. PREVENTIVE SERVICES TASK FORCE, 1996

Age Group (in years)	Interventions for General Population	Strength of Recommendation[a]	Interventions for Populations with High-Risk Sexual Behavior	Strength of Recommendation[a]
Birth–10	• Immunize for hepatitis B (birth, 1 month, 6 months; or 0–2 months, 1–2 months later, and 6–18 months; if not done in infancy, current visit and 1 and 6 months later). • Give ocular prophylaxis to prevent gonococcal ophthalmia neonatorum (for newborns).	A	• HIV testing (for infants of mothers at high risk for HIV)[b]	B
11–24	• Screen with Papanicolaou (Pap) test (for females who are sexually active at present or in the past, at least every 3 years. If sexual history is unreliable, begin Pap tests at age 18 years).	A	• RPR/VDRL (serological test for syphilis)[c]	A
	• Screen for chlamydia (for sexually active females < 20 years old).	B	• Screen for gonorrhea (for females)[d]	B
			• HIV[e]	A
			• Chlamydia (for females)[g]	B
			• Hepatitis A vaccine[h]	B

Age	Recommendation	Grade	Recommendation	Grade
	• Counsel for abstinence.*f*	B		
	• Counsel to avoid high-risk sexual behavior.*f*	B		
	• Counsel to use condoms/female barrier with spermicide.*f*	B		
	• Counsel to use contraception.	B		
	• Immunize for hepatitis B (if not previously immunized: current visits, 1 and 6 months later).	A		
25-64	• Screen with Papanicolaou (PAP) test (for women) who are or have been sexually active, at least every 3 years).	A	• RPR/VDRL*c*	A
			• Screen for gonorrhea (for females)*i*	B
	• Counsel to avoid high-risk sexual behavior*f*	B	• HIV*e*	A
	• Counsel to use condoms/female barrier with spermicide.*f*	B	• Chlamydia (for females)*j*	B
	• Counsel to use contraception.	B	• Hepatitis B vaccine*k*	A
			• Hepatitis A vaccine*l*	B

continued on next page

Age Group (in years)	Interventions for General Population	Strength of Recommendation[a]	Interventions for Populations with High-Risk Sexual Behavior	Strength of Recommendation[a]
>64	• Screen with Papanicolaou (Pap) test (for all women who are sexually active and who have a cervix. Consider discontinuation of testing after age 65 yrs. if previous regular screening showed consistently normal results).	A	• Hepatitis A vaccine[m]	B
			• HIV screen[e]	A
	• Counsel to avoid high-risk sexual behavior.[f]	B	• Hepatitis B vaccine[k]	A
	• Counsel to use condoms.[f]	B	• RPR/VDRL[c]	A
Pregnant women	During first visit:		• Screen for chlamydia (1st visit)[n]	B
	• Screen for hepatitis B surface antigen (HBsAg).	B	• Gonorrhea (1st visit)[o]	B
	• RPR/VDRL	A	• HIV (1st visit)[p] (see note)	A
	• Chlamydia (<25-year-olds)	B	• HbAg (3rd trimister)[q]	A
	• Offer to screen for HIV (universal screening is recommended for states, counties, or cities with an increased prevalence of HIV		• RPR/VDRL (3rd trimester)[r]	A

infection among pregnant women.
In low-prevalence areas, the choice
between universal and targeted
screening may depend on other
considerations).

- Counsel to avoid high-risk sexual   B
  behavior.[f]
- Counsel to use condoms.[f]   B

NOTE: The recommendations of the task force regarding the screening of pregnant women and newborns for HIV differ from those of the U.S. Public Health Service and some professional medical organizations. As examples, the U.S. Public Health Service recommends voluntary HIV testing for all pregnant women (Centers for Disease Control and Prevention, U.S. Public Health Service recommendations for human immunodeficiency virus counseling and voluntary testing for pregnant women, MMWR 1995;44(No. RR-7). The American Academy of Pediatrics recommends routine screening with consent of all pregnant women and HIV testing for infants whose mother's serostatus is unknown (American Academy of Pediatrics, Provisional Committee on Pediatric AIDS, Pediatr 1995;95:303-6). Determination of the appropriateness of these recommendations is beyond the charge of this committee. The following footnotes are direct quotations from the primary source.

[a]The letter "A" indicates that there is good evidence to support the recommendation that the condition be specifically considered in a period health examination. "B" indicates that there is fair evidence to support the recommendation that the condition be specifically considered in a period health examination.

[b]Infants born to high-risk mothers whose HIV status is unknown. Women at high risk include past or present injection drug users; persons who exchange sex for money or drugs and their sex partners; injection drug using, bisexual, or HIV-positive sex partners currently or in past; persons seeking treatment for STDs; blood transfusion during 1978–1985.

[c]Persons who exchange sex for money or drugs, and their sex partners; persons with other STDs (including HIV); and sexual contacts of persons with active syphilis. Clinicians should also consider local epidemiology.

continued on next page

[d]Females who have two or more sex partners in the last year; a sex partner with multiple sexual contacts; exchanged sex for money or drugs; or a history of repeated episodes of gonorrhea. Clinicians should also consider local epidemiology.

[e]Males who had sex with males after 1975; past or present injection drug use; persons who exchange sex for money or drugs and their sex partners; injection-drug using, bisexual, or HIV-positive sex partner currently or in the past; blood transfusion during 1978–1985; persons seeking treatment for STDs. Clinicians should also consider local epidemiology.

[f]The ability of clinician counseling to influence this behavior is unproven.

[g]Sexually active females with multiple risk factors including history of STD; new or multiple sex partners; age under 25; nonuse or inconsistent use of barrier contraceptives; cervical ectopy. Clinicians should also consider local epidemiology of the disease in identifying other high-risk groups.

[h]Persons living in, traveling to, or working in areas where the disease is endemic and where periodic outbreaks occur (e.g., countries with high or intermediate endemicity; certain Alaska Native, Pacific Island, Native American, and religious communities); men who have sex with men; injection or street drug users. Vaccine may be considered for institutionalized persons and workers in these institutions, military personnel, and day care, hospital, and laboratory workers. Clinicians should also consider local epidemiology.

[i]Women who exchange sex for money or drugs or who have had repeated episodes of gonorrhea. Clinicians should also consider local epidemiology.

[j]Sexually active women with multiple risk factors including history of STD; new or multiple sex partners; nonuse or inconsistent use of barrier contraceptives; cervical ectopy. Clinicians should also consider local epidemiology.

[k]Blood product recipients (including hemodialysis patients), persons with frequent occupational exposure to blood or blood products, men who have sex with men, injection drug users and their sex partners, persons with multiple recent sex partners, persons with other STDs (including HIV), travelers to countries with endemic hepatitis B.

[l]Persons living in, traveling to, or working in areas where the disease is endemic and where periodic outbreaks occur (e.g., countries with high or intermediate endemicity; certain Alaska Native, Pacific Island, Native American, and religious communities); men who have sex with men; injection or street drug users. Consider for institutionalized persons and workers in these institutions, military personnel, and day-care, hospital, and laboratory workers. Clinicians should also consider local epidemiology.

[m]Persons living in, traveling to, or working in areas where the disease is endemic and where periodic outbreaks occur (e.g., countries with high or intermediate endemicity; certain Alaska Native, Pacific Island, Native American, and religious communities); men who have sex with men; injection or street drug users. Consider for institutionalized persons and workers in these institutions, and day-care, hospital, and laboratory workers. Clinicians should also consider local epidemiology.

[n]Women with history of STD or new or multiple sex partners. Clinicians should also consider local epidemiology. Chlamydia screen should be repeated in 3rd trimester if at continued risk.

[o]Women under age 25 with two or more sex partners in the last year, or whose sex partner has multiple sexual contacts; women who exchange sex for money or drugs; and women with history of repeated episodes of gonorrhea. Clinicians should also consider local epidemiology. Gonorrhea screen should be repeated in the 3rd trimester if at continued risk.

[p]In areas where universal screening is not performed due to low prevalence of HIV infection, pregnant women with the following individual risk factors should be screened: past or present injection drug use; women who exchange sex for money or drugs; injection drug-using, bisexual, or HIV-positive sex partner currently or in the past; blood transfusions during 1978–1985; persons seeking treatment for STDs.

[q]Women who are initially HBsAg negative who are at high risk due to injection drug use, suspected exposure to hepatitis B during pregnancy, multiple sex partners.

[r]Women who exchange sex for money or drugs, women with other STDs (including HIV), and sexual contacts of persons with active syphilis. Clinicians should also consider local epidemiology.

SOURCE: U.S. Preventive Services Task Force. Guide to clinical preventive services. 2nd ed. Washington, D.C.: U.S. Department of Health and Human Services, 1996.

G
Summary of Workshop on the
Role of Managed Care Organizations in
STD Prevention

Thomas R. Eng[1]

INTRODUCTION

The IOM Committee on Prevention and Control of STDs invited a small number of representatives[2] from managed care organizations (Mcos); local, state, and federal health agencies; and an employer-purchasing coalition to a workshop on November 8, 1995, to advise the committee on the likely impact of managed care on STD-related services. The Los Angeles area was selected as the site of the workshop because of the substantial penetration of managed care and the high rates of STDs in California. The MCOs that participated in the workshop included a nonprofit group-model MCO (Kaiser Permanente Medical Group of Southern California), a for-profit primarily IPA (independent practice association) model MCO (CIGNA Healthcare of Southern California), and two publicly owned MCOs (Contra Costa Health Plan and Los Angeles County Community Health Plan). The workshop consisted of presentations by several participants followed by an open discussion of issues related to the role of managed care in STD prevention.

Major questions and issues addressed by workshop participants included:

- *STD-Related Activities of MCOs*: What types of curative and preventive

---

[1]Senior Program Officer, Institute of Medicine, Washington, D.C.
[2]Workshop participants included Bobbi Baron, Stanley Borg, Robert Bragonier, Jonathan Freedman, Carol Glaser, James Haughton, William Kassler, Paul Kimsey, Janet Kirkpartick, Gary Richwald, Tracy Rodriguez, Marilyn Keane Schuyler, Stanley Shapiro, and the IOM Committee on Prevention and Control of STDs.

services related to STD prevention are being provided by MCOs? How do MCOs handle confidentiality issues related to STDs, and who has access to this information? What are the experiences of MCOs that are serving populations at higher risk for STDs or participating in Medicaid managed care contracts?

• *Public/Private Partnerships*: What types of public/private partnerships related to STD prevention exist? What are the major barriers to successful public/private partnerships? How will MCOs that rely on publicly funded STD programs deliver STD-related services if public funding for these programs decreases or is eliminated?

• *Roles and Responsibilities:* What should be the roles and responsibilities of the public versus private sectors regarding STD prevention? How will decreased public funding and government oversight affect these various roles and responsibilities? How can MCOs coordinate their efforts with public agencies to improve the combined effectiveness of programs and to reduce duplication of efforts? What are the responsibilities of MCOs for the health of persons who are not plan beneficiaries? What incentives exist or need to be developed, and what barriers need to be addressed in order for MCOs to make STDs a priority?

• *Monitoring and Accountability*: How should MCOs, public health officials, purchasers, and accrediting organizations ensure quality and accountability and monitor performance of STD-related services? What is the role of purchasers in establishing STD prevention activities as priorities in MCOs?

WORKSHOP RESULTS

The following is a summary of the major issues that were discussed during the workshop. The perspectives reflected in this document do not necessarily represent the consensus of workshop participants or the committee.

Experiences of Two Privately Owned MCOs

CIGNA Healthcare of Southern California, a for-profit MCO that serves several southern California counties, is primarily comprised of a network of IPAs, medical groups, and individually contracted physicians (the staff-model component was sold in 1996). CIGNA serves a mostly commercial population of approximately 500,000 members but also has 108,000 Medi-Cal members. Anecdotally, rates of STDs among the commercial population have not increased in the last few years, but STD rates among Medi-Cal members have increased approximately two- to threefold. All STD-related services, including education, are triggered by and centered around patient visits to primary care providers. There is a system for automatic tracking and reporting of STDs, with nurses conducting patient follow-up for appointments. Although printed literature on STD-related topics is disseminated to providers, there has not been any STD-related provider training in the last few years. The MCO does not have specific guidelines to ensure confidentiality of STD-related care.

Kaiser Permanente of Southern California is a nonprofit, primarily group-model MCO serving several southern California counties. It is comprised of a medical group of 2,700 physicians and has an enrollment of approximately 2,200,000. Almost all beneficiaries are commercial members since Kaiser has only recently begun to accept Medi-Cal patients. Because of its centralized laboratory, Kaiser is able to closely monitor STD diagnoses and screening test results. To ensure that clinicians are aware of the latest trends in diagnoses and to further general information exchange, there are monthly teleconferences between physicians and laboratory personnel. Although Kaiser does not directly provide services to nonmembers, Kaiser has an unwritten policy to give prescriptions to nonmember partners of STD patients. In addition to sponsoring a clinic for teenagers, the MCO has an STD prevention program called "Secrets" (Appendix H) that is targeted towards adolescents. This program was largely initiated by pediatricians at Kaiser who had a strong interest in STD education for women and adolescents.

CIGNA and Kaiser represent two different types of MCO structures and missions. MCO structures range from relatively loosely organized networks of health care providers in IPAs to group- and staff-model organizations where the providers' practices are closely monitored. Missions of MCOs vary between the publicly operated, nonprofit organizations and the investor-owned, for-profit corporations. Many workshop participants believe that strong staff-model MCOs, such as Kaiser, may be more likely than IPAs to have the oversight structure and organization necessary to implement effective STD preventive services. Group- and staff-model MCOs also tend to have more centralized information systems that allow for better surveillance of health conditions and performance monitoring.

Experiences of Two Publicly Owned MCOs

The Los Angeles County Community Health Plan is one of only two publicly owned and operated MCOs in California. The MCO has an enrollment of approximately 115,000 persons, all of whom are medically or economically indigent. Because the MCO considers the enrolled population to be at high risk for STDs, the MCO conducts routine screening for gonorrhea and chlamydia as part of every pelvic exam and provides STD-related risk-reduction education with each health maintenance examination. One of the major problems that the MCO has encountered is the large turnover in eligibility for plan coverage, since eligibility is income-dependent. This problem hinders the establishment of longer-term relationships between providers and patients.

The Contra Costa Health Plan is the other county-sponsored and -operated staff-model MCO in California. It has an enrollment of approximately 24,000 persons, 65 percent of whom are Medicaid beneficiaries or other medically needy populations, including homeless persons. The Contra Costa Health Plan has a close collaborative relationship with the Contra Costa County Health Department. In a memorandum of understanding, the MCO and the county health department have outlined their specific roles and responsibilities for various health services, including STD-related care. The agreement covers STD-related education, reporting, contact investigation, and treatment. For example, when surveillance data indicate a specific problem within the catchment area of the MCO, the MCO will develop and implement a plan to provide STD-related risk-reduction information to all members in consultation with the county health department. One issue that the MCO has been dealing with is the conflict between the need for medical providers to know the treatment history of the individual and the patient's wish for confidentiality.

Because the Los Angeles County Community Health Plan and the Contra Costa Health Plan are both operated by local governments, they have built-in linkages with county health department activities and priorities. These linkages have allowed the MCOs and local health department programs to ensure that specific components of STD-related services are available. These MCOs, like other MCOs that serve large numbers of medically and economically needy persons, have found that the general package of managed care services developed for employer-sponsored or commercial populations may not be appropriate for indigent populations. There is a growing recognition that persons in publicly funded programs, such as Medicaid, have health care needs different from those of the commercial or general population.

Potential Strengths of MCOs in STD Prevention

Both opportunities and concerns were identified by workshop participants regarding the potential impact of managed care on STD prevention activities. The major potential strengths of MCOs in providing STD-related services include the following:

• *Coordination and integration of care.* STD-related services should be coordinated and integrated with primary care. Because MCOs provide all primary care for enrollees, they will be better able to coordinate and integrate STD-related care into primary care compared to specialized public STD clinics or fee-for-service providers.

• *Screening for STDs.* If MCOs adopt public health recommendations for screening of sexually transmitted infections as standard policy, the numbers of patients who will be screened will increase substantially compared to patients outside of the managed care environment, where screening decisions are up to individual health care providers and are not centralized.

• *STD-related data and information systems.* Given the potential of centralized automated information systems, there is a great potential for better information and data on STDs and STD-related services in managed care populations. The larger, more structured MCOs (such as group- and staff-model MCOs) are likely to have particularly useful patient population data. This assumption may not hold true for less-structured MCOs, such as some IPAs that lack centralized data systems. The information systems of publicly sponsored health insurance programs (e.g., Medicaid and Medicare) have been traditionally structured around the delivery of curative services on a fee-for-service basis and have not been particularly useful in evaluating public-health-related or preventive services.

• *Quality of STD-related care.* As a result of automated information systems, most MCOs have systems for monitoring quality of care and measuring performance. Standardized performance measures, such as the Health Plan Employer Data and Information Set (HEDIS) system coordinated by the National Committee on Quality Assurance, have the potential to greatly improve STD-related care in MCOs.

• *Accountability for services.* MCOs, by virtue of being organized systems of care, facilitate increased accountability of providers to purchasers and, ultimately, to beneficiaries. Purchasers are able to hold MCOs accountable by ensuring that specific services are available and delivered within the specifications of negotiated contracts and agreements. Through contract obligations, it may be possible to hold MCOs accountable for all aspects of STD-related care.

• *Preventive health.* Compared to traditional fee-for-service insurance companies, MCOs have emphasized preventive health services because many preventive health measures are cost-saving. Since MCOs are responsible for covering health conditions occurring within the enrollment period, they are more likely to emphasize health promotion and disease prevention and to encourage healthy behaviors among their enrolled populations compared to noncapitated providers.

• *Access to care.* Because the mission of MCOs and government regulations require that beneficiaries have convenient access to primary care services, MCOs are more likely to have greater access to care than dedicated public STD clinics. In addition, some communities that are currently at high risk for STDs do not have access to local public STD clinics.

• *Cultural barriers to care.* MCOs that serve populations at high risk for STDs are more likely to have providers of different cultural backgrounds and language capabilities than many public STD clinics or health plans that serve only commercial populations. These MCOs may be better able to provide culturally sensitive STD-related services to diverse populations than public STD clinics and health plans that do not serve high-risk populations.

Potential Limitations of MCOs in STD Prevention

The major potential limitations of MCOs in providing STD-related services include the following:

• *Confidentiality of services.* One of the major concerns regarding the ability of MCOs to deliver STD-related services is related to safeguarding the confidentiality of such services. Automated information systems and the team-oriented approach to care associated with most MCOs increase provider, employer, and potential public access to medically sensitive information. Ensuring confidentiality for STD-related services is especially critical for adolescents. It is important to allow adolescents to receive care without parental consent and to ensure that their parents are not notified of STD-related treatment through billing or other means.

• *Uninsured persons.* Inadequate access to health care for uninsured persons is a major barrier to STD prevention. Increasing competition resulting from the move towards managed care and reductions in publicly financed health care may reduce access. This may result from public hospitals and clinics shutting down or curtailing services and from decreasing eligibility thresholds for publicly financed programs such as Medicaid. Therefore, even if MCOs assume full responsibility for STD prevention and provide the same spectrum of services as public programs, public STD clinics may still be needed to provide services to persons who neither have private insurance nor qualify for Medicaid or other public assistance.

• *Quality of care.* Capitated payments for services encourage MCOs to limit costs. It is possible that MCOs, compared to providers who are reimbursed for their rendered services, may be less willing to conduct diagnostic and screening tests, thereby potentially compromising the quality of care. In addition, the short amount of time available for routine appointments may be a disincentive for MCO providers to become involved in patient education and prevention activities, since these activities require an investment of time.

• *Interest and mission.* STDs are not a priority for most MCOs, especially those that do not serve populations at high risk for STDs. It is logical to expect that MCOs serving high-risk populations, such as Medicaid participants, will be more interested in STD prevention than health plans serving lower-risk populations, such as employer-sponsored groups. An MCO's interest in STD prevention may also be dependent on its mission. The mission of the MCO is often closely aligned with the MCO's status as a nonprofit or for-profit organization. For example, nonprofit MCOs are more likely to reinvest their excess revenue in the organization, whereas for-profit MCOs are obligated to funnel a substantial portion of their profits to their stockholders or owners. The mission of for-profit MCOs, therefore, may be in conflict with providing services, such as preventive services, that are not cost-saving to the organization.

• *Variability of MCOs.* There is a wide spectrum of MCOs, and consequently there is a wide range of technical ability among MCOs in providing STD-related services. In general, MCOs that have greater service coordination and oversight (e.g., staff- and group-model MCOs) are likely to be more effective in STD prevention than MCOs with less infrastructure (e.g., IPAs). Given the limited experience of most MCOs in providing public health services, including STD-related services such as partner notification and outreach, even some of the best-organized MCOs may not have the technical expertise to take on full responsibility for STD prevention.

• *Training of providers.* Most health care providers, including those in MCOs, are not adequately trained to deliver the range of STD services offered by public STD clinics. This is particularly true for STD-related services that require specialized skills or experience, such as counseling for high-risk sexual behavior. For example, a survey conducted by the Pacific Business Group on Health showed that approximately 56 percent of enrollees in contracted staff-model MCOs reported that their physician or other health professional had not discussed STDs with them in the last three years (Pacific Business Group on Health, unpublished data, 1994). In addition, if we accept that STD-related care is specialty care that requires extensive training and experience, then it may not be cost-effective for MCOs to replicate the technical competency found in public STD clinics.

• *Disincentives for MCOs.* Cost-saving is a major incentive for MCOs to provide specific services to enrollees. Treating STDs is cost-saving because it averts more expensive treatment associated with treating complications of STDs. However, unless providing a specific benefit is shown to be cost-saving, MCOs may be reluctant to provide services that have not been rigorously evaluated, such as some behavioral change interventions. In addition, capitated payments for services may increase the risk of cost-shifting by MCOs. For example, MCOs may refer persons in need of STD-related services to public STD clinics to avoid assuming the costs of their care.

• *Patient preferences.* A recent multisite survey of STD clinic patients showed that most persons surveyed chose a public STD clinic over other providers because of the convenience of obtaining care without an appointment, lower costs, and other reasons (Celum et al., 1995). Irrespective of these issues, persons who currently receive episodic care at public STD clinics may not feel comfortable in receiving care through MCOs, where a longer-term relationship with a primary care provider would need to be established.

• *Services involving nonenrolled persons.* Many aspects of STD prevention, such as partner notification and referral, screening and case finding, and community education, may involve persons who are not members of the MCO. MCOs may not be able to provide services for nonmembers because of economic, legal, or other reasons.

• *Copayments.* The copayment required by most MCOs is usually assessed on a per-visit basis. These copayments, although nominal for most people, may be a substantial burden for some and a barrier to seeking appropriate STD-related care, especially for preventive services.

STDs as Priorities for MCOs

Most MCOs are currently not focused on STDs for various reasons. With some exceptions, there is generally insufficient awareness of STDs and their consequences among MCOs and other private sector health care providers. Some MCOs serving mainly commercial populations may not consider STDs to be a major problem because infection rates are perceived to be low. For MCOs to recognize STD prevention as a priority, workshop participants felt that an organized effort to educate MCOs regarding the broad consequences of STDs, such as infertility and cancer, and the potential cost savings associated with STD prevention is necessary. The most likely leaders in this effort are employer-purchaser groups, community-based organizations, and local health departments and other government agencies.

Role of Purchasers

The role and impact of purchasers of health services (e.g., employer groups and other coalitions) are likely to be significant in encouraging MCOs to provide STD-related services. Regardless of the type of MCO, all MCOs will be responsive to the needs of purchasers. MCOs seem willing to provide specific services as contract obligations if they consider the contract as desirable.

The Pacific Business Group on Health is a nonprofit employer-purchaser coalition of 29 large public and private employers in the San Francisco Bay Area. The organization represents more than three million employees, dependents, and retirees and negotiates terms and premiums for health plan contracts on behalf of approximately 15 member companies. The Pacific Business Group on Health has integrated the recommendations of the U.S. Preventive Services Task Force regarding clinical preventive services into their negotiated benefits packages and has implemented performance measures for many of these services. To ensure that MCOs are accountable for meeting performance goals, the Pacific Business Group on Health holds 2 percent of premium payments "at risk," pending a review of health plan performance.

Workshop participants suggested that the public health community encourage purchasers to consider STD prevention as a priority. Employers are interested in including preventive health services in their negotiated benefits packages, especially if the services are shown to be cost-saving for the company. However, some STD-related services may not be cost-saving, and these services will still need to be supported. Employers may be increasingly interested in the health of the general community, recognizing that employers within a region are essentially drawing from the same employee pool.

Initiatives of Local and State Health Departments

Many local and state health departments have been preparing themselves for the likely impact of managed care on the delivery of primary and public health services. The Los Angeles County Department of Health Services and the California Department of Health Services have both developed strategies to ensure that STD-related services will continue to be provided as more people are enrolled into managed care.

Los Angeles County had a 1995 budget of approximately $40 million for STD programs and operated a system of 10 public STD clinics. Funding for public STD clinics had been reduced as a result of county fiscal problems; 29 public clinics were in operation during the previous year. Historically, there was limited collaboration between the health department and MCOs in STD-related issues. In response to decreased funding for public health programs and increased enrollment of the Medicaid population into managed care, the health department recently clarified the specific roles and responsibilities of the local health department and participating MCOs in several major public health areas as part of the county's Medicaid (Medi-Cal) managed care contract. In this contract, health department and MCO responsibilities for specific aspects of STD prevention, such as treatment, disease reporting, and partner follow-up, are outlined. In addition, the contract requires that MCOs reimburse the county STD clinics for services provided to MCO members.

In January 1995, the California Department of Health Services required that all Medi-Cal managed care contractors in 12 counties have subcontracts with respective county or city health departments regarding responsibilities in nine public health areas, including STDs. The contracts would have to describe the general relationship between the local health department and the MCO, the responsibilities of the health department, the responsibilities of the MCO, and areas of shared responsibility.

The California Department of Health Services has also recently initiated the California Partnership for Adolescent Chlamydia Prevention. This is a statewide partnership bringing together government agencies, MCOs, academic health centers, and professional associations to address policy issues related to STDs among adolescents. This initiative also seeks to coordinate clinical preventive services for adolescents in managed care settings with community STD prevention activities and to coordinate all categorical state STD-related programs. Other components of this initiative include a media campaign targeted towards teenagers; development of screening, counseling, and education interventions; school-based programs; and training programs for health care providers.

Initiatives of Federal Agencies

The Centers for Disease Control and Prevention (CDC) established a Managed Care Working Group in January 1995 to foster partnerships between public health agencies and MCOs to improve public health. In a recent publication, the Working Group outlined its high priority areas for CDC's collaborative activities with MCOs and other health organizations, including prevention effectiveness and guidelines, Medicaid and managed care, research, and capacity development in public health agencies (CDC, 1995). The CDC recently initiated several collaborative activities with managed-care-related organizations. For example, a CDC epidemiologist is currently assigned on detail to the American Association of Health Plans (formerly Group Health Association of America) as a resource on public health issues. In addition, CDC staff have provided input regarding public health performance indicators, including STD-related indicators, to be used in the next version of HEDIS (3.0).

Funding for STD-Related Services

Given the recent and likely future reductions in public funding for public health services, many workshop participants believe that alternative funding streams for STD-related services, including public STD clinics, will need to be explored. Given that capitation encourages MCOs to keep costs down, there is a potential danger that MCOs may refer their patients with STDs to public STD clinics. In order to prevent this type of cost-shifting, local health departments will need to establish a mechanism for reimbursement of services.

CONCLUSIONS

The following are the major conclusions expressed by various workshop participants during the meeting. They do not necessarily represent a consensus of workshop participants or the conclusions of committee members.

• *Increase emphasis of STDs among MCOs.* Most MCOs are currently not focused on the problem of STDs. MCOs and other providers need to be encouraged to consider STD prevention as priorities. Changing "organizational norms" or the prioritization process of MCOs through methods similar to those used by employers and other purchasers should be considered. Additional incentives for MCOs to become more involved in STD prevention will have to be developed for many MCOs to offer comprehensive STD-related services.

• *Define roles and responsibilities.* The roles and responsibilities of MCOs, local public health departments, community-based organizations, and other stakeholders in STD prevention need to be clearly defined. In an era of limited resources for public health, it is important to identify what each potential provider of STD-related services does best and determine how each provider should function in an integrated system of STD-related services. Often, a formal mechanism for defining roles and responsibilities does not exist at the local level. A collaborative process for examining systems of STD-related services will need to be established. One possibility is for local health departments to organize a forum or other mechanism for the various stakeholders to come together and discuss their perspectives, with the goal of developing a strategy for coordinating STD-related services in the community. Strong leadership at the local level is necessary for this to be successful. Roles and responsibilities can also be defined through contract negotiations between purchasers and providers when appropriate, such as in the case of Los Angeles County's Medicaid managed care contracts. Mechanisms other than contract negotiations, however, should be available in communities that do not have opportunities to enter into formal contracts with MCOs.

• *Increase collaboration between public health agencies and employers and other purchasers.* Employers and other purchasers have an important role in ensuring that comprehensive STD-related services are available and that MCOs are accountable for their performance in delivering services. These purchasers need to be educated regarding the benefits of such services. Public health professionals should work with them to determine the preventive services that should be provided to beneficiaries. State and local governments that have Medicaid contracts with MCOs should ensure that responsibility for specific essential public health services, including STD prevention, is addressed through contracts or other agreements.

• *Increase collaboration between public and private sectors.* In light of decreasing public funds for public health, private/public partnerships should be developed to ensure availability of STD-related services. However, given the limited information and experience regarding both the effectiveness of public/private partnerships and the ability of some MCOs to provide such services, these partnerships should proceed cautiously. Publicly funded activities may need to be maintained until collaborative activities are evaluated and found to be effective. For example, the impact of reductions in federal funding for public STD clinics should be evaluated before clinic services are decreased.

• *Integrate services and increase effectiveness and efficiency of programs.* STD-related services, both preventive and curative, should be incorporated into primary care. As public funding for public health programs decreases, governments at all levels will need to maximize the effectiveness and efficiency of current programs. In collaboration with private sector health organizations, governments will need to objectively evaluate the effectiveness of various STD-related programs and integrate and coordinate services.

• *Maintain public STD-related services.* Even if MCOs assume increasing responsibility for STD prevention, persons who do not have private insurance, or do not qualify for Medicaid or other public assistance, will need to rely on public STD-related services. This may be particularly important if the numbers of the uninsured increase. Therefore, services provided by public STD clinics should be maintained and delivered by public STD clinics or by other publicly funded programs in high-incidence areas. However, in communities where STD incidence is low, it may be appropriate for STD-related services to be delivered by alternate providers.

• *Protect confidentiality of STD-related services.* MCOs and other providers of STD-related services should safeguard the confidentiality of STD-related services, especially for adolescents. States that do not have laws ensuring complete confidentiality of STD-related services for adolescents should consider them.

• *Train providers.* Health care providers, including those in MCOs, are not adequately trained in the spectrum of STD-related services. MCOs should provide training to their staff in both curative and noncurative preventive health, especially management of high-risk behaviors.

• *Tailor MCO services for high-risk groups.* The general managed care packages of services developed for commercial populations may not be appropriate for indigent populations. MCOs and other providers should develop the capacity to address the unique needs of the high-risk populations that they serve. MCOs that serve indigent populations and others at high risk for STDs will need to tailor the traditional package of health services for commercial populations to the health care needs of high-risk populations.

• *Educate policymakers.* Local, state, and federal policymakers in private and public health agencies and organizations should be educated regarding the issues associated with managed care in STD prevention. Local health departments, in particular, should develop expertise on issues related to managed care and public health. In addition, legislators at all levels should have a good understanding of these issues.

• *Conduct further research.* Many policy and funding decisions regarding STD-related programs are being made in the absence of good data on program effectiveness. Additional research regarding the effectiveness of various interventions in STD prevention needs to be conducted to support data-based decision-making. A mechanism for sharing information and experiences regarding effective or innovative STD prevention programs should be developed. Information on "best practices" should be available to all stakeholders in STD prevention. Evaluation or research components should be built into public/private partnerships.

• *Explore new sources of funding.* New sources of funding for STD-related services should be considered. One potential source of funding for public health programs is payments assessed against publicly funded nonprofit hospitals and health plans that convert to for-profit status. Another potential source is a "tax" levied on MCOs and health insurance companies to pay for public health activities that benefit their enrolled populations.

REFERENCES

CDC (Centers for Disease Control and Prevention). Prevention and managed care: opportunities for managed care organizations, purchasers of health care, and public health agencies. MMWR 1995;44(No. RR-14).

Celum CL, Hook EW, Bolan GA, Spauding CD, Leone P, Henry KW, et al. Where would clients seek care for STD services under health care reform? Results of a STD client survey from five clinics. Eleventh Meeting of the International Society for STD Research, August 27-30, 1995, New Orleans, LA [abstract no. 101].

H
STD-Related Services Among Managed Care Organizations Serving High-Risk Populations

Kimberly H. Greene,[1] Thomas R. Eng,[2] Patrick H. Mattingly,[3] and Paul D. Cleary[3]

INTRODUCTION

Managed care organizations (MCOs) are increasingly enrolling persons from groups potentially at high risk for STDs, particularly Medicaid beneficiaries. There is limited information, however, regarding the scope of services for STDs among MCOs. A previous study of reproductive health services in MCOs collected limited information on STD-related services and activities (Kaiser/Group Health Association of America, 1994), and data on reproductive health and managed care (Bernstein et al., 1995; Delbanco and Smith, 1995) have recently been published. These data suggest that, although there is variability in the extent of coverage of reproductive health services, most MCOs are providing comprehensive reproductive health services. In order to obtain preliminary data regarding STD-related services among MCOs, we surveyed a limited number of MCOs that were considered likely to serve persons at high risk for STDs. The survey collected information regarding their STD-related services and potential prevention activities.

METHODS

A convenience sample of 45 MCOs was surveyed. Thirty-nine MCOs were

[1]Candidate, Masters in Public Health Program, George Washington University, Washington, D.C.
[2]Senior Program Officer, Institute of Medicine, Washington, D.C.
[3]Member, IOM Committee on Prevention and Control of STDs, Washington, D.C.

selected on the basis of their likelihood of serving populations at high risk for STDs, such as having a high proportion of Medicaid enrollees and being located in an inner-city area. The remaining six MCOs were referred to us by MCOs who heard about the survey. Data were collected regarding MCO characteristics; STD-related data collection and analysis; STD-related preventive and curative clinical services; confidentiality policy; and community activities. Surveys were mailed and followed up with telephone calls from December 1995 through February 1996. Respondents who indicated that the MCO had significant activities in STD prevention or services were contacted to obtain details. The small sample size precluded analysis of correlations between variables. A median and range are reported for enrollment and demographic figures.

RESULTS

The survey response rate was 60 percent (27/45). Of those responding to the survey, 6 MCOs (22 percent) described their structure as a sole staff/group model; 11 MCOs (40 percent) described a mixed model that included a staff/group model component; and 10 (37 percent) described their organizations as a combination of IPA, indemnity and/or PPO models. The plans had a median enrollment of 85,000 persons (range: 6,500–2,500,000). Twenty-five MCOs served Medicaid populations, representing, on average, 16 percent of their enrollment (range: 0–100 percent). For MCOs reporting demographic data (24), the median proportion of the enrolled population that was African American or Hispanic was 50 percent (range: 4–95 percent); the median proportion of adolescents age 15–24 was 15 percent (range: 10–70 percent); and the median proportion of women age 14–44 years was 27 percent (range: 10–60 percent). Forty-eight percent of the respondents were nonprofit organizations and 30 percent were among the 50 largest MCOs in the United States. Respondents were located in the Pacific (41 percent), mid-Atlantic (37 percent), New England (7 percent), East-North Central (7 percent), Mountain (4 percent), and Southern (4 percent) regions of the country.

Selected responses are summarized in Table H-1. Standardized patient history forms were used by 15 organizations (65 percent) to collect information about previous STD diagnoses and by 16 organizations (73 percent) to document a history of sexual activity. This type of information was used by 14 MCOs (52 percent) to define groups at high risk of STDs. Eight MCOs (30 percent) reported using data analysis to implement changes in STD-related activities, and four organizations (16 percent) had established performance criteria for STD-related outcomes or process measures for STD-related care.

Seven MCOs (26 percent) reported that they did not use any published STD treatment guidelines, and six (22 percent) used more than one published protocol. The Sexually Transmitted Diseases Treatment Guidelines published by the Centers for Disease Control and Prevention were used by 18 organizations (67 per-

TABLE H-1   STD-Related Activities of Managed Care Organizations
(MCOs), 1996

Characteristic	Percentage of Affirmative Responses[a]
MCO includes questions regarding previous diagnoses of STDs on standardized patient history forms.	73 (16/22)
MCO includes questions regarding sexual activity on standardized patient history forms.	65 (15/23)
MCO has performance criteria for STD-related outcomes or process measures for STD-related care.	16 (4/25)
MCO has used data analysis to implement changes in STD-related activities.	30 (8/27)
MCO requires parental permission for adolescents/children (under age 18) to receive treatment for an STD or other STD-related services.	8 (2/26)
MCO notifies parents of STD-related care provided to their children through billing or other means.	0 (0/24)
MCO has a specific policy for ensuring adolescent and adult confidentiality regarding STD-related care.	52 (13/25)
MCO has a policy requiring or encouraging health care providers to discuss sexual activity and related issues during routine adolescent health care visits.	78 (21/27)
MCO has STD-related activities specifically targeted towards adolescents.	46 (12/26)
MCO offers routine screening for chlamydia automatically to all women of childbearing age.	39 (10/26)
MCO has a specific or categorical STD prevention program.	0 (0/26)
MCO provides STD-related services to the general community, including people not enrolled in the MCO.	22 (6/27)
Case-finding	7 (2/27)
Community screening for STDs or related conditions	4 (1/27)
Partner identification/notification	15 (4/27)
Other	11 (3/27)
MCO has a formal training program in STD-related topics for its health care staff.	33 (9/27)

[a]Number responding yes/total number responding to question.

cent), and four MCOs (15 percent) followed internally produced guidelines. Twenty MCOs (74 percent) guaranteed acute care for all conditions within 48 hours; however, these policies did not usually specify STDs or any other specific clinical condition. Within the MCO staff, primary care providers most frequently provided STD-related care (100 percent), followed by obstetricians/gynecologists (96 percent). Other providers of STD-related care included specialists (48 percent), publicly sponsored STD clinics (41 percent), and non-MCO health facilities (19 percent). Four health plans (15 percent) required patients to obtain referrals to other physicians or providers to obtain STD-related care.

Most MCOs (92 percent) permitted adolescents to obtain STD-related care without obtaining parental permission, and none notified parents of this care. Thirteen plans (52 percent) adhered to a specific policy that guaranteed adolescent and adult confidentiality, but most of these were general nondisclosure policies that did not specifically refer to STDs or STD-related care. However, preventive medicine guidelines were more specific: 21 MCOs (78 percent) required or encouraged health care providers to discuss sexual activity during routine adolescent health care visits; 12 (46 percent) had an STD-related activity specifically targeted towards adolescents; and 10 (39 percent) automatically offered chlamydia screening to all women of childbearing age (15–44 years). None of these health plans had a specific or categorical STD prevention program at the time the survey was conducted.

Five MCOs (19 percent) provided STD-related services to nonenrolled populations in their communities by participating in case-finding, screening for STDs or related conditions, and partner identification/notification. Three organizations (11 percent) routinely referred patients with STDs to public facilities for treatment and/or preventive services; and seven (26 percent) referred their patients for such public health activities as contact-tracing and partner notification. Contractual agreements that specified STD-related care were rare: one MCO had a contract with a purchasing group that specified STD-related services to be provided, and six MCOs (22 percent) had contracts or agreements with government agencies that specifically addressed STD-related services. However, these contracts and agreements almost always referred specifically to HIV-related services.

Five MCOs (19 percent) conducted STD-related clinical or epidemiological research. Most frequently, this research addressed HIV-related issues. Nine MCOs (33 percent) reported a formal training program in STD-related topics for health care staff, usually in the form of continuing medical education; and 13 (48 percent) had plans for future STD-related programs or activities.

CONCLUSIONS

There are several limitations to these survey data. Because of the small sample size and sample selection, these data should be considered preliminary and may not be representative of MCOs serving high-risk populations. In addition, although the survey specifically requested that all questions be answered for STDs other than HIV, some respondents may not have consistently adhered to this request. Thus, there is a possibility of asymmetric data collection. Nevertheless, this survey does provide a modicum of insight into the STD-related activities of some MCOs serving high-risk populations.

Most MCOs reported providing a basic level of services. However, because a significant proportion of the survey respondents served populations at high risk for STDs, it is likely that typical MCOs in the United States would have substantially lower levels of involvement in STD prevention activities than those reported in this survey. In general, surveyed MCOs screened for prior STD diagnosis and sexual activity; made STD-related care accessible through primary care providers; used treatment guidelines; and guaranteed availability of acute care within 48 hours. However, few MCOs provided services beyond the expected scope of clinical practice. For example, only 22 percent of MCOs reported providing services to the general community or to sexual partners who were not plan enrollees. No MCO had a specific or dedicated STD prevention program.

Only a third of MCOs had STD-related topics in a formal training program. Further interviews with MCOs suggested that three main factors prompted the planning of STD-specific continuing medical education programs and departmental meetings: desire to improve the quality of care; physician requests for further education; and recognition of organizational weaknesses by MCO-affiliated/employed health care providers. A few MCOs have relied upon printed materials for educational outreach. For example, FHP in San Diego, CA, developed preventive health guidelines for adolescents that are distributed to all primary care providers; Humana Health Care Chicago has developed a teen care manual; and Kaiser Permanente provided, in its quarterly newsletter, information for its physicians on confidentiality and consent/disclosure requirements for minors.

When MCOs with special activities in STD prevention were interviewed, they frequently discussed and highlighted various programs or activities for adolescents. For example, The Community Health Plan of Los Angeles has created a teen clinic that focuses on preventive care, particularly the psychosocial component of health issues, such as family planning, HIV testing, depression, and sexual activity. Several other organizations sponsored teen clinics that were in various stages of development and received varying levels of support.

Particularly interesting STD-related programs or activities are briefly described in the following pages. The effectiveness of many of these programs has not been formally evaluated. However, these programs and activities may serve as models for other MCOs that wish to develop activities in STD prevention.

Educational Theater Programs
Kaiser Foundation Health Plan, Inc.
Pasadena, CA
Kaiser Permanente Medical Care Corporation
Oakland, CA[4]

Kaiser Permanente's educational theater programs use live theater in an innovative approach to community health promotion for children and adolescents. Kaiser Permanente supports five programs promoting communication and healthy decision-making: "Secrets," "Nightmare on Puberty Street," "Intersections," "R.A.V.E.S.," and "Professor Bodywise's Traveling Menagerie." Respectively, these address sexual health and HIV/STD issues; peer pressure, emotions, and sexuality; communication and conflict resolution; "real alternatives to violence for every student"; and health, hygiene, and resistance to peer pressure.

These prevention programs are intended mainly for young audiences. They are shown to high school students ("Secrets" and "Intersections"), middle school students ("Nightmare on Puberty Street," "Intersections," and "Secrets") and elementary school students ("Professor Bodywise" and "R.A.V.E.S."). All of the programs are available for adult and community audiences. In order to encourage participation in the process of health promotion, Kaiser Permanente distributes educational and other materials to parents. In addition, children receive supplemental materials in school, and supportive classroom resources are provided to educators.

All five productions are funded as a nonprofit community service of Kaiser Permanente. The plays were created with the assistance of an advisory committee of health care practitioners, community leaders, school officials, teachers, parents, students, and a team of theater professionals. When a play is launched, both Kaiser enrollees and the general community are sent promotional information and are invited to free screenings. Subsequently, HMO and community members are welcome to attend program showings, but specific invitations are not tendered. Each Kaiser Permanente region selects those productions it wishes to support; hence, not every production is shown in every region.

"Secrets," "Nightmare on Puberty Street," and "Intersections" all touch on issues related to STDs, but "Secrets" is particularly relevant. It addresses the issues of self-control, self-esteem, and prevention as they pertain to sexuality and sexual health, and it advocates both abstinence and safer sex. The program focuses on HIV/STD transmission, symptoms, and treatment, and it emphasizes adolescent susceptibility to infection. Each performance is followed by a ques-

---

[4]Other Kaiser Permanente regions may also produce some or all of these educational theater programs. The support materials that accompany performances are designed to meet each community's needs and may vary from region to region.

tion-and-answer session during which the actors, who are also trained HIV/AIDS educators, respond to audience queries.

"Secrets" is performed daily at area schools and is often incorporated into the standard sex education curriculum. Two weeks prior to a showing, a team member from Kaiser Permanente visits the school to distribute resource manuals, provide teacher and parent guides, and supply a copy of the Kaiser Permanente video entitled "It Won't Happen to Me." This award-winning video is a recording of an interview with an HIV-infected woman who gave birth to an HIV-infected child. There has been no formal evaluation of "Secrets," but anecdotal evidence and focus groups reflect a positive response in the community.

Teenage Health Center
Kaiser Permanente of Southern California
Panorama City, CA

Kaiser Permanente of Southern California responded to the special needs of patients age 13 to 20 by forming the Teenage Health Center. The center's goal is to provide a full range of health care services to teens and to help them maintain and improve their physical and emotional health. The clinic seeks to increase access to appropriate care for adolescents and deliver health services in a proactive and preventive manner. For example, no referrals are required to use the center, and patients can call a hotline number for medical advice. In order to achieve its goals, the center employs two physicians, two nurses, a social worker, and two health educators. Many of the staff members have been specifically trained to work with adolescents. The center's varied health services include routine gynecological care and treatment of sexually transmitted diseases. Social and psychological services are available, and the center sponsors a number of health education opportunities, addressing such issues as reproductive health, birth control, HIV testing and counseling, and STDs.

A critical and unique element of treatment at the Teenage Health Center is the psychosocial assessment administered to all incoming patients. This questionnaire seeks information on sexuality, contraception, history of STDs and childbearing, and other health-related topics. The intention of the questionnaire is to identify potential or existing problems such as depression, suicide, or pregnancy in order to provide truly comprehensive health services. A survey tool was recently used to evaluate the effectiveness of the Teenage Health Center as compared to traditional primary care. Data indicate that those teens seeking care at the Teenage Health Center were significantly more satisfied with the care they received than adolescents seeking health services through traditional routes. Greater satisfaction was linked with increased likelihood that the adolescent patient would discuss sensitive issues with his/her health care provider. This is of critical importance in STD-related care.

Safer Sex Campaign
Group Health Cooperative of Puget Sound
Seattle, WA

In 1992, a prime-time television documentary entitled "Sexual Survival" aired on KING 5 TV in Seattle. This program specifically targeted adolescents and explicitly described the acquisition, symptoms, identification, and treatment of a number of STDs. It was a component of the "Safer Sex Campaign," which was cosponsored by the Group Health Cooperative (GHC), Planned Parenthood, and KING 5 TV; the program was developed with the assistance of an advisory board composed of representatives from local community-based organizations. "Sexual Survival" was supplemented by two workshops called "Parent Talk: Teaching Your Child About Sexuality," and "Safer Choices: Sex in the 90's." In addition, GHC, KING 5 TV, and Planned Parenthood developed three educational pamphlets and two videos for distribution.

Community response to the program was evaluated by quantifying program viewers and workshop participants. "Sexual Survival" had a market share of 39 percent, with an estimated 500,000–750,000 viewers. There were four favorable responses for every unfavorable one among the 350 calls received in the hour-and-a-half following the broadcast (10–11:30 PM). The ratio jumped in the following week, when favorable calls outnumbered the unfavorable by 10 to 1. Workshop participation was high: "Parent Talk" was conducted 66 times and served 1,000 people; "Safer Choices" had 235 participants in 23 workshops. In addition to these measures of participation, the campaign was featured on "NBC Nightly News," and GHC received hundreds of letters of support.

GHC continues to distribute the pamphlets created as a part of the Safer Sex Campaign in its clinics. One of the pamphlets ("What is an STD?") defines the term "sexually transmitted diseases"; supplies summaries of the six most common STDs, including HIV; provides a risk assessment quiz; furnishes descriptions of common STD-related symptoms, high-risk behaviors, and STD prevention measures; and lists area clinics and resources. The second pamphlet ("Parent Talk: Teaching Your Child About Sexuality") makes both general and specific suggestions to help parents serve as their children's primary sexuality educators. Age- and developmentally appropriate information and approaches are recommended and selected community resources are cited. The third pamplet ("Safer Choices: Sex in the 90's") defines safer sex, furnishes a list of high-risk behaviors, and discusses attitudes and communication techniques as they relate to effective safer sex negotiations.

Despite the relative success of the program, GHC does not plan to replicate it and is now shifting its STD prevention focus from the community to the individual patient. Currently, GHC's intention is to encourage providers to make prevention education a regular part of the patient-provider interaction. GHC has recently received funding to study the best ways to incorporate HIV/STD risk assessment and prevention counseling into primary care visits. The study will use a systems approach, focusing on the entire health care team. Training, materials, and other practice supports will be developed to help primary care providers play a more consistent role in HIV/STD prevention efforts.

MY Health: Minority Youth Health Project
Group Health Cooperative of Puget Sound
Seattle, WA

The Minority Youth Health Project (MY Health), a Group Health Cooperative (GHC) community program, is one of seven such interventions funded by the National Institutes of Health (NIH). Its purpose is to "prevent violence, pregnancy, sexually transmitted diseases, and substance abuse in 10–14 year old youths in Seattle." Seattle's diverse racial and ethnic groups include Vietnamese, Latino, and African American populations, making this project's target audience especially unique. In order to appropriately target this audience and to encourage innovative approaches to changing youth health behaviors, GHC has worked with the University of Washington, the city of Seattle, a local minority health coalition, and target population focus groups.

MY Health takes three main approaches to encourage behavior modification: parenting, youth intervention, and community coalition mobilization efforts. Attention has primarily been focused upon the promising youth intervention and community coalition mobilization efforts. These efforts approach behavior change in very different ways. In the youth intervention program, a small group of students is exposed to health education messages. With the assistance of group leaders, they create an innovative health promotion product. Through their work, they learn entrepreneurial skills and enhance their knowledge of health.

The community coalition mobilization effort convened community focus groups to assess significant youth health problems in their communities, providing each group with $8,000 per year to implement creative interventions to these issues. The African American community focus group, one of those selecting STDs as a priority issue, designed and executed a particularly creative project. Approximately two dozen adolescents, chosen from Garfield High School, worked closely with experts in music and video production to produce unique music videos focusing on health promotion and disease prevention. This approach employs the peer education approach that has become popular and that appears, anecdotally, to be moderately successful. A second round of this program is just beginning.

Current and past efforts to support and enhance the MY Health Project derive from GHC's commitment to both health promotion/disease prevention and community service in its tightly knit health care community. The project's goals fit in with GHC's general program objectives. In addition, both the director of the municipal hospital and the local minority health coalition identified minority youth health as a priority issue and encouraged GHC to pursue the Minority Youth Health Project.

Developing Long-Term Substance Abuse Prevention and Career Development Programs for African American Youth
Healthcare Management Alternatives, Inc.
Philadelphia, PA

In 1990, Healthcare Management Alternatives, Inc. (HMA) developed and piloted a general prevention program for "at-risk" students (identified by faculty and administrators) at Audenried High School in Philadelphia. Although HMA continues to sponsor the intervention, it is no longer involved in daily administration activities. Currently, 30 students are enrolled in the program. During the school year, they attend weekly classes led by an HMA-trained counselor where they discuss and learn about STDs and HIV/AIDS, pregnancy prevention, violence, decision-making, self-esteem, substance abuse, goal-setting, conflict resolution, and career development.

One of the program's goals is to improve health knowledge and attitudes about risky behaviors, including those related to adolescent sexuality, STDs, and HIV/AIDS. In order to measure the effect of the classroom activities on attitudes and behaviors, enrolled students are asked to fill out a pre- and postprogram behavior assessment questionnaire (adapted from the national Youth Risk Behavior Survey) at the beginning and end of each school year.

In 1993, data collected using the pre- and postprogram questionnaires were used to assess the program's impact. The evaluation found a small decrease in the number of sexually active students; a moderate increase in the proportion of students utilizing condoms, birth control pills, or both; and a significant decline in the percentage of students with multiple sex partners and in the number of students engaging in unprotected sex. Overall, the 1993 evaluators concluded that the program had a positive impact on the students. The current ninth-grade participants will be followed through high school in order to perform a similar evaluation. A long-term assessment of the 1993 participants who have graduated from high school is planned.

Watts/Jordan School-Based Health Clinic
Watts Health Foundation
Los Angeles, CA

Watts Health Foundation (WHF), in conjunction with the Los Angeles Board of Education, established a health care clinic at Jordan High School in 1987. It is one of three such clinics that, with parental consent, supplies free and comprehensive medical care, psychological services, and health education to students. During 1993 and 1994, the three clinics handled 10,400 patient visits. Patients sought assistance in three major areas during these visits: medical services (57 percent of visits); mental health services (27 percent); and health education (7 percent). Other (unspecified) concerns prompted the remaining 9 percent of visits. Patients sought reproductive health care, including contraceptives and pregnancy tests, in 22 percent of these visits.

The Watts/Jordan School-Based Health Clinic serves a low-income population in South Central Los Angeles that is 70 percent Latino and 30 percent African American. The 11 pregnant and 18 parenting girls currently seen by the clinic represent the relevance of teen pregnancy, parenting, and sexuality to these adolescents. Therefore, the clinic conducts HIV/STD education as a part of its health education program. These prearranged sessions are run by either a health educator or peer educator, and require advance registration by interested students. Sessions consist of a group discussion on STDs (e.g., chlamydial infection, syphilis, gonorrhea, vaginitis, and HIV/AIDS), which is supplemented by educational activities.

A good portion of the clinic's publicity and success derives from the work of its teen advocates. Each year, four students undergo a six-week summer training program in reproductive health. They speak to classes, conduct outreach, run the above-mentioned educational groups, and are responsible for bringing into the clinic teens who are not "consented" (i.e., those whose parents have not yet consented to allow them to access care through the school-based clinic). The teen advocates provide an invaluable service because they are able to reach students who would not willingly speak with adults and who are not aware that the clinic exists.

The Watts/Jordan School-Based Health Clinic, like the other two clinics, does not bill students for services. Medi-Cal is billed to help cover the uninsured but does not fully cover medical services.

REFERENCES

Bernstein A, Dial T, Smith M. Women's reproductive health services in health maintenance organizations. West J Med 1995;163[Suppl]:15-18.

Delbanco S, Smith M, eds. Reproductive health and managed care: a supplement to the Western Journal of Medicine. West J Med 1995;163[Suppl].

Kaiser/Group Health Association of America. Survey on HIV/AIDS and reproductive health care. Menlo Park, CA: The Henry J. Kaiser Family Foundation, 1994.

Examples of Community-Based Programs for Providing Clinical Services for STDs

The following are brief descriptions of innovative programs for providing STD-related clinical services that were visited by the committee during its site visits to the Chicago and Atlanta areas in June 1995. Because most of these programs have not been systematically evaluated for effectiveness, the committee does not necessarily endorse these specific programs but rather encourages agencies and organizations to consider these examples as a basis for developing collaborations to improve STD-related services.

West End Medical Centers, Inc.
Atlanta, GA

The West End Medical Centers, Inc., has been providing comprehensive primary health care services to residents in low-income communities since the early 1970s. The health center was established in 1972 by Atlanta University Center to serve its students as well as employer groups, the medically indigent, and Medicare and Medicaid beneficiaries. In 1976, reincorporated as the independent West End Medical Centers, Inc., the health center refocused its services on the nearly 49,000 residents in the West End and Nash/Washington communities. In addition to its main health center, West End Medical Centers operates health centers in several public housing projects and communities, including an AIDS clinic in an inner-city high-rise apartment building, and serves approximately 28,000 residents. The centers also operates a school-based clinic at a local high school, which provides a full range of episodic care for teenagers.

The centers provides primary care pediatrics, internal medicine and obstetrics/gynecology services, dental care, nutritional counseling, health education, social services, radiology, and laboratory services. Of 55,000 patient visits annually, approximately 45 percent are for pediatric care, 28 percent are for obstetrics/gynecology services, 10 percent are for dental care, and the remaining 17 percent are for adult medicine, including geriatrics. All 12 physicians at the centers have admitting privileges at two or more hospitals and provide 24-hour coverage for health center patients. The centers emphasizes preventive care, including nutrition counseling, management of chronic health problems to improve quality of life, and participation in community health fairs and screening programs. The centers provides WIC vouchers and, under an arrangement staffed by the county, conducts WIC certification at the centers.

The centers have a well-developed and comprehensive STD program. STD-related services are provided through regular primary health care services rather than through a separate STD clinic. All persons seeking family planning and obstetrics services are offered STD testing. Individuals who suspect they may have an STD make an appointment with their regular provider, who conducts an examination and orders all necessary lab tests. At the time of the diagnosis the client receives counseling. Follow-up is conducted by the staff social worker, and a staff member conducts partner notification and contact-tracing in cooperation with the Fulton County STD program. The West End Medical Centers, Inc., appears to represent a model community-based program, with strong community ties and a high-quality medical and public health program.

Planned Parenthood/Chicago Area
Chicago, IL

Planned Parenthood of the Chicago Area (PP/CA) operates six health centers that provide reproductive health care services to approximately 16,000 women annually. These services include birth control education and contraceptives, pregnancy testing, screening and treatment for STDs, and HIV counseling and testing. Three of the health centers are operated on a standard fee basis, and the others are operated on fees based on a sliding scale of income. PP/CA offers comprehensive medical services for women and adolescents, linking the adolescents to communities through their school-based programs. Funded by Title X funds, state funds, private donations, and grants from a local foundation, the aim of PP/CA is to provide the highest quality services in a comfortable and attractive environment, regardless of a client's ability to pay. The program offers a wide range of preventive screening including chlamydia, gonorrhea, syphilis, HIV counseling and testing, and Pap smears, in addition to contraception counseling and services. The program seeks to provide a "medical home" for adolescents, and many teenagers have become accustomed to receiving services at the Planned Parenthood Clinics.

PP/CA operates a community outreach program in several high schools called the "Linked Services Project." This program provides sexuality education to ninth-grade students using a seven-week curriculum. Topics include anatomy, basic sexuality, responsible health, HIV and other STD prevention, and birth control. The project employs educators who are from the same communities as the students, thus creating a level of trust between the teenagers and the educators. One of the goals of the program is to help link students to medical services at either a Planned Parenthood clinic or other community health center. The Linked Services project attempts to link all aspects of the teens' lives through their school, home, and community. The Linked Services Project evolved out of a request received in 1987 from the Chicago Vocational High School to assist them in developing an innovative teenage pregnancy prevention program. The pilot program took three years to develop and serves as a model for similar projects in other local schools. PP/CA is expanding the program, initially to the schools in communities that already have Planned Parenthood clinics. This program appears to be successful and has a high level of community involvement and support from school administrators.

West Town Neighborhood Health Center: Young Adult Clinic
(Chicago Department of Public Health)
Chicago, IL

The Young Adult Clinic is an STD clinic for teenagers, located in the West Town Neighborhood Health Center, a Chicago public health clinic. The Young Adult Clinic is staffed by a bilingual, bicultural nurse clinician and is operated by the Chicago Department of Public Health. The Young Adult Clinic was established to reduce the risk of HIV infection and other STDs among Hispanic youth, specifically Puerto Rican youth. The clinic provides comprehensive health services, including STD screening, HIV counseling and testing, pregnancy testing, condom distribution, and family planning services. Located across the street from Roberto Clemente High School, the Young Adult Clinic has established close ties with the students and school administration. The clinic is open on weekdays and two evenings per week. Sex partners of STD patients are also evaluated in the clinic. As a publicly sponsored facility, the clinic utilizes the state public heath laboratory, and disease reporting is automated. The clinic also works closely with Vida/SIDA's peer educators (see below).

Vida/SIDA
Chicago, IL

Vida/SIDA, established in 1988 by the Puerto Rican Cultural Center, is an innovative community-based program dedicated to teaching youth about HIV and STD prevention. Vida/SIDA is an outreach program, largely designed and staffed by teens, that trains teens to become peer educators in HIV and STD prevention. These teens serve as peer outreach workers in schools and the community and serve as "peer experts" not only for HIV and other STDs, but for other reproductive health and general health issues as well. The program has established a close working relationship with the Young Adult Clinic and encourages teens to use the clinic for HIV and other STD testing and treatment or general health care. Part of the teens' outreach work includes conducting presentations in various high schools in a five-part series that includes topics such as HIV, STD, and pregnancy prevention, substance abuse, and violence. The program has also extended its outreach presentations to middle schools. These activities are supported by the local school council.

To coordinate an effective prevention strategy in the West Town community of Chicago, Vida/SIDA brought together community health and educational organizations in West Town to form the West Town STD/HIV Prevention Network. The network brings together many community agencies that work together to develop new, interrelated prevention programs. Working with the Young Adult Clinic, Vida/SIDA is able to refer youths to the clinic for STD-related or other services. While the program appears to be running well, peer educators report that there is a common perception in the adolescent community that STDs are "no big deal." Although the program has strong support from the community and school board, it has not been formally evaluated. Vida/SIDA is currently working in collaboration with the CDC to establish a formal evaluation process.

West Central Health District
Columbus, GA

The West Central Health District (District 7) is composed of 16 counties with a total population of approximately 450,000, with 22 percent of residents living below the federal poverty level. The largest health clinic in the district is located in Columbus and is staffed by "expanded role" nurses who work under the standing protocols and supervision of physicians. These nurses have been specifically trained in STD-related care at the regional STD training center and also receive periodic training updates at the center. Other counties in the district have health department clinics of varying sizes that provide STD screening and treatment. In two counties that do not have physicians available to treat STDs, patients frequently have to cross county lines for STD treatment.

Contact-tracing is conducted for syphilis only, but West Central Health District staff are skeptical of the effectiveness of this service. Staff have proposed that efforts should be focused in high morbidity areas within the district. STD screening and treatment and HIV testing and counseling are also integrated into family planning services provided by the health department. The Columbus Health Department operates separate clinics for teenagers that provide comprehensive health services such as prenatal care, STD screening, and pre- and post-HIV counseling and testing. In general, the private physicians in the community have not been interested in providing STD-related services and prefer to refer patients to the health department. Public health officials from Columbus are currently conducting outreach to physicians in private practice to involve them more fully in the diagnosis and reporting of STDs.

The West Central Health District programs collect fees from the Medicaid program for services. The staff is very concerned about changes that will occur with the implementation of Medicaid managed care and is looking for a niche in a managed care environment. The staff also expressed concern about the impact of block grants for HIV, STD, and TB and agreed that STDs are not a high priority in rural areas. They are in the process of working with private providers to arrange a public/private partnership and have begun discussions with a local hospital. The director of the program has personally approached all the private sector providers in the area to arrange a public/private partnership.

The Emory/Grady Teen Services Program
Atlanta, GA

The Emory/Grady Teen Services Program, a collaboration between Emory University and Grady Memorial Hospital, is a nationally acclaimed program that seeks to provide continuity of care for adolescents at risk for unintended pregnancy. The program has a school-based education component and a clinical component. The Teen Services Program has a formal agreement with the Atlanta Public Schools to provide 10 classroom periods of reproductive health education to all eighth-grade students, most of whom are from low-income families. The program educates 4,500 students each year through this agreement. "Postponing Sexual Involvement" is a component of the 10-hour outreach program in the Atlanta schools designed to help teens avoid early sexual involvement. Five sessions of the "Postponing Sexual Involvement" educational series are taught by Grade 11 and 12 students under the supervision of the hospital staff. The teen-led sessions are designed to help younger teens develop skills and resist social and peer pressures to begin sexual intercourse before they are able to take full responsibility for the consequences of their actions. The older youth also serve as role models, showing that they can be successful teenagers without being sexually involved. One session of the educational series is devoted exclusively to HIV infection and other STDs. The program emphasizes prevention of high-risk behaviors and STDs rather than providing detailed information on each STD.

Two special after-school family planning clinics (supported by Title X funds) are held at Grady Hospital each week. Nearly 1,200 sexually active female adolescents age 16 and younger are seen in these clinics annually. Once enrolled, adolescents continue to receive their care in these clinics until age 18 or graduation from high school. At Grady Hospital, each counselor sees patients from assigned schools who come for family planning services at least three or four times a year. Teen Services' nurses and counselors are assigned responsibility for a "case load" of individual schools and thus are able to have consistent interactions with teachers and students at those schools. Male adolescents also come to the clinic for counseling and condoms, but other reproductive health services for them are handled through referrals. In addition, STD education, screening, and treatment are available in the family planning clinic. While STD prevention is not the focus of the Teen Services Program, it has been integrated into education and clinical services.

Results of evaluations of the school education component of the program indicate that teens who have participated in the program are five times more likely to postpone sexual activity in the eighth grade, and the rate of initiation of sexual intercourse is reduced by a third through the ninth grade (Howard and McCabe, 1990). In the service/clinical program, 80 percent of young mothers remain pregnancy-free during their teenage years. The program has recently begun a comprehensive message, "Free to Be," which means drug-free, HIV-free, and pregnancy-free. The program is based on the notion that the same skills are needed to avoid drugs, drinking while driving, sexual involvement, and unprotected sexual intercourse.

REFERENCE

Howard M, McCabe JB. Helping teenagers postpone sexual involvement. Fam Plann Perspect 1990;22:21-6.

Committee and Staff Biographies

COMMITTEE

NANCY E. ADLER, Ph.D., is vice chair of the Department of Psychiatry and director of the Health Psychology Program, both at the University of California, San Francisco (UCSF). In addition, she is professor of medical psychology in the Departments of Psychiatry and Pediatrics at UCSF. She received her B.A. in psychology from Wellesley College and her Ph.D. in social psychology from Harvard University. Between 1972 and 1977, Dr. Adler was assistant professor and associate professor of psychology at the University of California, Santa Cruz. Among her many honors, Dr. Adler has been elected a fellow of four divisions of the American Psychological Association, and she is a member of the Academy of Behavioral Medicine Research. She was elected to the IOM in 1994. Dr. Adler conducts research in the area of health psychology. She has published extensively on the psychosocial aspects of abortion, including the emotional responses of women following therapeutic abortion, on unintended pregnancy in adolescent and adult women, and on reproductive and contraceptive decision-making among adolescents. Her recent work is examining the influence of socioeconomic status on health.

E. RICHARD BROWN, Ph.D., is founder and director of the UCLA Center for Health Policy Research, and he is professor of public health in the UCLA School of Public Health. He is also president of the American Public Health Association. Dr. Brown received his Ph.D. in sociology of education from the University of California, Berkeley. Dr. Brown has written extensively about a broad range of health policies, programs, and institutions, with emphasis on issues that affect the access of low-income people to health care. His most recent research has focused on health insurance coverage and the effects of lack of coverage and other factors on access to health services. He served as a senior consultant to the President's Task Force on National Health Care Reform, for which he worked full time for several months in early 1993. Dr. Brown has developed bills in the California legislature and in the U.S. Senate, where he has served as health policy advisor to two senators. He has presented invited testimony to numerous committees in both houses of the U.S. Congress and in the California legislature and has provided consultation to private, local, state, federal, and international agencies.

WILLIAM T. BUTLER, M.D., is chancellor of Baylor College of Medicine in Houston, Texas, having served previously as president from 1979 to 1996. He is a professor of internal medicine and of microbiology and immunology. Dr. Butler received his B.A. from Oberlin College and his M.D. from Western Reserve University in Cleveland. After residency training in internal medicine at the Massachusetts General Hospital in Boston, he completed a research fellowship in bacteriology and immunology at Harvard Medical School. Before joining the Baylor faculty in 1966, Dr. Butler served as chief clinical associate in the Laboratory of Clinical Investigation at the National Institute of Allergy and Infectious Diseases (NIAID). In 1991, he served as chairman of the Association of American Medical Colleges. He was elected to the IOM in 1990 and is also a member of many professional organizations, including the American Association of Immunologists, the American Society for Clinical Investigation, and the Infectious Diseases Society of America. He has authored more than 140 scientific publications in the fields of immunology and infectious diseases.

VIRGINIA A. CAINE, M.D., is director of the Marion County Health Department in Indianapolis, Indiana. She is also associate professor of medicine in the Division of Infectious Diseases at the Indiana University School of Medicine. Dr. Caine received her M.D. from the State University of New York, Upstate Medical School, in Syracuse. She completed her residency in internal medicine at the University of Cincinnati Medical School and a fellowship in infectious diseases at the University of Washington Medical School in Seattle. Between 1981 and 1984, Dr. Caine was assistant professor of medicine in the Divisions of Infectious Diseases and Obstetrics and Gynecology at the Johns Hopkins University School of Medicine. During that time, she also served as associate medical director in the Clinic for Sexually Transmitted Diseases of the Baltimore City Health Department. Dr. Caine has served as a member and expert panelist on many national, state, and regional committees, including the Centers for Disease Control and Prevention (CDC) expert panel on Sexually Transmitted Diseases Guidelines and the CDC's Healthy People 2000 Progress Review for Sexually Transmitted Diseases. Dr. Caine is a member of numerous professional societies, including the

National Medical Association, where she is chair of the Infectious Disease and AIDS Sections.

DAVID D. CELENTANO, Sc.D., M.H.S., is professor of social and behavioral sciences in the Department of Health Policy and Management at the Johns Hopkins University School of Hygiene and Public Health. He is also professor of epidemiology and international health. Dr. Celentano is a behavioral scientist with extensive experience in leading investigations of social and behavioral epidemiology in the fields of HIV/AIDS, STDs, substance abuse, and cancer. He has been active in HIV/AIDS research since 1984, when he assisted in the development of the assessment strategy for the Multi-Center AIDS Cohort Study (MACS) of the natural history of HIV infection in gay and bisexual men. He is an active contributor in the ALIVE study, the largest longitudinal study of HIV infection in injection drug users. Since 1990, he has been conducting investigations on HIV infection in Thailand. Dr. Celentano received his B.A. in psychology, his M.H.S. in mental hygiene, and his Sc.D. in behavioral sciences from Johns Hopkins University. Dr. Celentano is a member of the International AIDS Society, the American Sexually Transmitted Disease Association, and the Society for Epidemiological Research.

PAUL D. CLEARY, Ph.D., is a professor in the Departments of Health Care Policy and Social Medicine at Harvard Medical School. He also holds appointments as lecturer and associate professor in the Department of Behavioral Sciences at the Harvard School of Public Health and as visiting associate professor in the Department of Sociomedical Sciences at the Columbia University School of Public Health. Dr. Cleary received both his B.S. in physics and his Ph.D. in sociology from the University of Wisconsin. Dr. Cleary is editor of *The Milbank Quarterly* and a consulting editor of the *Journal of Culture, Medicine and Psychiatry*. His research interests focus on health behavior, screening and risk assessment, assessment of health outcomes, and health policy. Between 1989 and 1992, Dr. Cleary was a member of the local advisory committee for the Eighth International Conference on AIDS. He is currently a member of the Data Monitoring Board for the Department of Veterans Affairs and a member of the Committee on Higher Degrees in Health Policy. Dr. Cleary is a member of many professional societies, including the American Association for the Advancement of Science and the American Association of Health Services Research, and he was elected to the IOM in 1994.

MARGARET A. HAMBURG, M.D., is commissioner of health for New York City. She received her M.D. from Harvard Medical School and completed her residency in internal medicine at the New York Hospital-Cornell Medical Center. Dr. Hamburg began her service in the NYC Department of Health in June 1990 as deputy commissioner for Family Health Services. In that position she was responsible for child health, school and adolescent health, day care, dental health services, lead poisoning control, families with special needs, maternity services and family planning, and substance abuse. Between 1986 and 1988, she worked for the federal assistant secretary for health in the areas of disease prevention and health promotion. From 1988 to 1990, Dr. Hamburg was a senior member of the National Institute of Allergy and Infectious Diseases (NIAID), first as special assistant to the director and then as assistant director of the Institute. While at NIAID, she was instrumental in shaping AIDS research strategies and policies. Dr. Hamburg has extensive research experience in the areas of biology of addictions, behavioral sciences, and child development. She serves on many health-related committees and organizations and is the author of numerous scientific articles. Dr. Hamburg was elected to the IOM in 1994.

KING K. HOLMES, M.D., Ph.D., is director of the Center for AIDS and STD, professor of medicine, and adjunct professor of microbiology and epidemiology at the University of Washington in Seattle. Dr. Holmes received his A.B. from Harvard, his M.D. from Cornell University Medical College, and his Ph.D. in microbiology from the University of Hawaii. He completed a residency in internal medicine at the University of Washington. Dr. Holmes has written and conducted extensive research in the areas of STDs, AIDS, etiology and natural history of cervical neoplasia, and surveillance of gonorrhea. He is a member of the editorial boards of many scientific journals, including *Sexually Transmitted Diseases* and *Genitourinary Medicine*. Dr. Holmes is a member of numerous national and international committees, including the NIH Office of AIDS Research, the WHO Expert Advisory Panel on Venereal Infections, and the Board of Scientific Counselors at the CDC Center for Infectious Diseases. Dr. Holmes has received numerous honors and awards, including the City of Medicine Award and the Bristol-Myers Squibb Infectious Diseases Research Award. He is a fellow of the American Association for the Advancement of Science and the American Academy of Microbiology and was elected to the IOM in 1987.

EDWARD W. HOOK III, M.D., is professor of medicine and epidemiology at the University of Alabama at Birmingham (UAB) Schools of Medicine and Public Health and is a senior scientist at the UAB AIDS Center. He also serves as the medical director of the STD Control Program of the Jefferson County Health Department in Birmingham. Dr. Hook received his M.D. from Cornell University Medical College and completed his internship and residency in internal medicine at the University of Washington Affiliated Hospitals in Seattle. Between 1985 and 1992, Dr. Hook was a member of the faculty of the Johns Hopkins University School of Medicine and School of Hygiene and Public Health. During that time, he also served as chief of the Sexually Transmitted Diseases Clinical Services at the Baltimore City Health Department. Dr. Hook is past president of the American Venereal Disease Association, serves on the editorial board of the journal

404

THE HIDDEN EPIDEMIC

Clinical Updates in Infectious Diseases, and is a member of the advisory board of the Alabama State Department of Public Health. He has published extensively in the field of STDs on such topics as the diagnosis and treatment of gonorrhea and syphilis and the interrelationship between HIV and STDs.

LORETTA SWEET JEMMOTT, Ph.D., R.N., F.A.A.N., is associate professor of nursing and the director of the Office of HIV Prevention Research at the University of Pennsylvania School of Nursing. She is also an associate at the Center for Population Studies at the University of Pennsylvania and an associate at the HIV Center for Clinical and Behavioral Studies of Columbia University. Dr. Jemmott received her B.S.N. from Hampton Institute. She received her M.S.N. in child, adolescent, and family psychiatric mental health nursing and her Ph.D. in education, specializing in human sexuality education, from the University of Pennsylvania. Over the past 10 years, Dr. Jemmott has been involved in a line of research designed to elucidate the psychosocial factors that underlie HIV risk behaviors among African American adolescents and women. She has designed and tested theory-based, culturally appropriate interventions to reduce those risks. Dr. Jemmott has published extensively in the areas of HIV/AIDS prevention, adolescent sexual behavior, and condom use among African American adolescents. She has received many honors, including the Congressional Merit Recognition Award, the Outstanding Research Award from the Northern New Jersey Black Nurses Association, and the Governor of New Jersey's Nurse Merit Award in Advanced Nursing Practice. She is a fellow in the American Academy of Nursing and a member of the National Institute of Nursing Research's Advisory Council.

DOROTHY MANN is executive director of the Family Planning Council for Southeastern Pennsylvania, Inc., where she has served in this position since 1977. The Council provides family planning services to low-income women and sponsors programs in cancer and genetic screening, maternity services, and STD/HIV research and training. Ms. Mann received her B.A. in anthropology and history from Bennington College, and completed all the requirements for her M.A. in anthropology at Columbia University. She has conducted extensive research in the areas of family planning, sexuality education, and abortion and contraceptive services for teenagers. Ms. Mann is a member of numerous professional and national organizations, including the National Family Planning Association, the Philadelphia AIDS Coalition, and the AIDS Advocacy Coalition.

PATRICK H. MATTINGLY, M.D., is senior vice president of planning and development at Harvard Pilgrim Health Care in Brookline, Massachusetts, and previously served as president and medical director of the Harvard Community Health Plan of New England in Providence, Rhode Island. Dr. Mattingly received his M.D. from Harvard Medical School. He trained in internal medicine at Harvard and completed a residency in pediatrics at the University of Washington in Seattle. Between 1981 and 1990, Dr. Mattingly served as president and chief executive officer of the Wyman Park Health System, an integrated health care system, which he merged into the Johns Hopkins Health System. During 1989 and 1990, Dr. Mattingly served as an IOM scholar in residence with the Council on Health Care Technology. He is a member of many professional organizations, including the Group Health Association of America, the American College of Physician Executives, and the Rhode Island Anti-Drug Coalition. Dr. Mattingly is a member of the Rhode Island Health Services Council and is president of The HMO Group Insurance Company Ltd.

KATHLEEN E. TOOMEY, M.D., M.P.H., is state epidemiologist and director of the Epidemiology and Prevention Branch of the Division of Public Health in Georgia. She is an adjunct professor in the Divisions of Epidemiology and International Health at Emory School of Public Health in Atlanta. She received her A.B. in biology from Smith College and her M.D. and M.P.H. from Harvard University. After completing her residency in family medicine at the University of Washington in Seattle in 1982, she served for three years as the clinical director of the Kotzebue Service Unit with the Indian Health Service in Alaska. In 1985, Dr. Toomey was selected as a Pew Health Policy Research Fellow at the University of California, San Francisco, Institute for Health Policy Studies. From 1987 to 1993, she held a number of positions within the Division of STD/HIV Prevention at the CDC, including Epidemic Intelligence Service Officer and associate director. In 1991, Dr. Toomey served on the health staff of U.S. Senator John Chafee, drafting health care legislation. She has received many honors and awards, including the CDC Award for Contributions to the Advancement of Women and the Public Health Service Plaque for Outstanding Leadership. Her research interests include health services research, women's health and reproductive health policy, and the epidemiology and prevention of STDs and HIV/AIDS. She is a member of many professional and national organizations, including the Board of Directors of the Alan Guttmacher Institute and the APHA Program Development Board.

A. EUGENE WASHINGTON, M.D., M.P.H., M.Sc., is professor and chair of the Department of Obstetrics, Gynecology, and Reproductive Sciences at the University of California, San Francisco. He is also director of the Medical Effectiveness Research Center for Diverse Populations at UCSF. Dr. Washington received his B.S. from Howard University, his M.D. from the University of California, San Francisco, his M.P.H. from the University of California, Berkeley, and his M.Sc. from Harvard University. He completed residencies in preventive medicine at Harvard University and in gynecology and obstetrics at Stanford University. Dr. Washington has published extensively on topics in his major areas of research, which include effectiveness of health services, prevention of diseases in women, STD prevention and management policy, and patient preference in health care decision-making. He is a member of the Editorial Boards of *Family Planning Perspectives* and *Infectious Diseases in Obstetrics and Gynecology*. Dr. Washington has served as a member of many national and international committees, including the U.S. Preventive Services Task Force and the Board of the International Society for STD Research. He is currently a member of the Advisory Committee for the National Breast and Cervical Cancer Early Detection and Control Program, DHHS, and a member of the National Advisory Committee for the Arthur Ashe Fellowships in AIDS Care, Harvard AIDS Institute.

CATHERINE M. WILFERT, M.D., is professor of pediatrics and microbiology at Duke University. Dr. Wilfert graduated from Harvard Medical School and completed an internship and residency in pediatrics at Boston City Hospital and the Children's Hospital Medical Center in Boston. After a fellowship in pediatrics in the Division of Infectious Diseases at Children's Hospital Medical Center, she joined the faculty at Duke University. Dr. Wilfert's clinical investigations have included vaccine trials in children and, more recently, therapeutic trials for pediatric HIV infection. She is the principal investigator of the pediatric AIDS Clinical Trials Unit (ACTU) at Duke, which has been operating since 1987. Her other responsibilities have included serving as chair of the Advisory Committee on Immunization Practices for the CDC, a member of the Microbiology and Infectious Diseases Advisory Committee to NIAID, and a member of the Advisory Committee to the Center for Biologics Evaluation and Research at FDA. Dr. Wilfert was the first chair of the Pediatric Committee of the pediatric ACTU, and she continues to be involved in the national organization of multicenter trials.

JONATHAN M. ZENILMAN, M.D., is associate professor in the Division of Infectious Diseases at Johns Hopkins University School of Medicine. He also holds joint appointments in the Department of Obstetrics and Gynecology and in the Department of Immunology and Infectious Diseases at the Johns Hopkins University Schools of Medicine and Public Health. Dr. Zenilman received his B.A. in chemistry from Cornell University and his M.D. from the State University of New York at the Downstate Medical Center in Brooklyn. He completed a residency in internal medicine and was a fellow of infectious diseases at the Kings County Hospital Center in Brooklyn. Between 1985 and 1989, Dr. Zenilman served as an Epidemic Intelligence Service Officer and as clinical research investigator at the CDC. At that time, he coordinated the publication of the *1989 Sexually Transmitted Disease Treatment Guidelines* and developed the National Gonococcal Isolate Surveillance Project. Dr. Zenilman is on the editorial board of the journals *Sexually Transmitted Diseases* and *Genitourinary Medicine*, serves as a consultant to the journal *AMA Drug Evaluations*, and as a reviewer for *The Journal of the American Medical Association*. Dr. Zenilman has received many honors and awards, including the American Foundation for AIDS Research (AmFAR) Scholar Award and a U.S. Public Health Service Unit Citation. He is a member of many professional organizations, including the American Association for the Advancement of Science and the Infectious Disease Society of America. Dr. Zenilman served on the Committee on Prevention and Control of STDs from January 1995 through September 1995.

IOM STAFF

THOMAS R. ENG, V.M.D., M.P.H., is a senior program officer at the IOM for the Committee on Prevention and Control of STDs. He was most recently an American Association for the Advancement of Science (AAAS) Congressional Fellow in the U.S. Senate, where he served as a health policy advisor to Senator Paul Simon on issues including health care financing and reform, public health, maternal and child health, and food and drug regulation. During his fellowship, Dr. Eng developed and wrote legislation to provide universal health care coverage for children and pregnant women. He was recently on detail from the CDC to the Peace Corps, where he served as the latter agency's epidemiologist and worked in numerous developing countries. In addition, he has worked in two state health departments and was a preventive medicine resident and Epidemic Intelligence Service Officer with the CDC. Dr. Eng received his degree in veterinary medicine from the University of Pennsylvania and in public health from Harvard University. He has received several awards from the U.S. Public Health Service and the International Society for Travel Medicine, and he is a member of various professional organizations, including the American Public Health Association.

LESLIE M. HARDY, M.H.S., is currently a senior policy analyst in the office of the Assistant Secretary for Planning and Evaluation (ASPE). Prior to her position at ASPE she was senior program officer at the IOM, where she was study director for the Committee on Prevention and Control of STDs. She has been with the IOM since 1986 and most recently directed the IOM's Roundtable for the Development of Drugs and Vaccines Against AIDS, a group composed of leaders from government, the pharmaceutical industry, academia, and patient advocacy groups. The Roundtable convened workshops and conferences to identify and help resolve impediments to the rapid availability of safe, effective drugs and vaccines for HIV infection and AIDS. During her tenure with the Roundtable, Ms. Hardy wrote and edited several workshop reports on topics including the development of effective therapies for AIDS-related infections, gene therapy for HIV infection, government and industry collaboration in HIV/AIDS drug development, and enhancing heterogeneity in HIV/AIDS clinical studies. Prior to the Roundtable, Ms. Hardy served as study director for the IOM committee that produced the 1991 report *HIV Screening of Pregnant Women and Newborns*. She also formerly served as staff officer for the IOM/NAS AIDS Activities Oversight Committee, which produced the study report *Confronting AIDS: Update 1988*.

During her work with the AIDS Oversight Committee, she focused on issues pertaining to the delivery and financing of health care for people with HIV infection, stress among HIV/AIDS care providers, and the care of neuropsychologically impaired people with AIDS. Ms. Hardy received her bachelor of arts degree in zoology and botany from Duke University and her master of health science degree in maternal and child health from the Johns Hopkins University School of Hygiene and Public Health. Ms. Hardy served as the senior program officer on this project through July 1995.

JENNIFER K. HOLLIDAY is a project assistant at the IOM for the Committee on Prevention and Control of STDs. Ms. Holliday has been with the IOM for four years. She previously worked as a project assistant with the Roundtable for the Development of Drugs and Vaccines Against AIDS. Prior to joining the IOM, Ms. Holliday worked as registrar for the Art in Embassies Program at the U.S. Department of State, where she managed the return of art collections from American embassies to lending institutions, private collectors, and individuals. Ms. Holliday received her B.A. in Southwest Studies from Colorado College.

MARISSA WEINBERGER FULLER, M.H.S., is a research associate at the IOM for the Committee on Prevention and Control of STDs. Prior to joining the IOM, she was a policy analyst at the National Governors' Association (NGA) in the Health Policy Studies Division. Her primary area of research involved maternal and child health. She published several issues of the *MCH Update*, a publication highlighting state initiatives to improve maternal and child health. She also authored the report *Improving Coordination Between Medicaid and Title II of the Ryan White CARE Act*, prepared for the Health Care Financing Administration. Prior to joining NGA, Ms. Fuller was the outreach coordinator at a community health center in New York City. She received her A.B. in political science from Barnard College and her M.H.S. degree in health policy from the Johns Hopkins University School of Hygiene and Public Health.

MICHAEL A. STOTO, Ph.D., is director of the Division of Health Promotion and Disease Prevention of the IOM. He received an A.B. in statistics from Princeton University and a Ph.D. in statistics and demography from Harvard University and was formerly an associate professor of public policy at Harvard's John F. Kennedy School of Government. A member of the professional staff since 1987, Dr. Stoto directed the IOM's effort in support of the Public Health Service's Healthy People 2000 project and has worked on IOM projects addressing a number of issues in public health, health statistics, health promotion and disease prevention, vaccine safety and policy, and AIDS. Most recently, Dr. Stoto served as study director for the IOM committee that produced *Veterans and Agent Orange: Health Effects of Herbicides Used in Vietnam*. Dr. Stoto is coauthor of *Data for Decision: Information Strategies for Policy Makers* and numerous articles in statistics, demography, health policy, and other fields. He is a member of the American Public Health Association, the American Statistical Association, the International Union for the Scientific Study of Population, the Population Association for America, and other organizations.

Index

3 5282 00411 5062